MOBILIZING CIVIL SOCIETY'S RESPONSE TO STIGMA AND DISCRIMINATION IN CENTRAL ASIA

MOBILIZING CIVIL SOCIETY'S RESPONSE TO STIGMA AND DISCRIMINATION IN CENTRAL ASIA

Anna Alexandrova, editor

international debate education association
New York – Amsterdam – Brussels

Published by
The International Debate Education Association
400 West 59th Street
New York, NY 10019

Library of Congress Cataloging-in-Publication Data
Mobilizing civil society response to stigma and discrimination in central Asia / Anna Alexandrova, editor.
    p. ; cm. — (Sourcebook on contemporary controversies)
  ISBN-13: 978-1-932716-34-4

1. AIDS (Disease)—Patients—Civil rights—Asia, Central. 2. HIV-positive persons—Civil rights—Asia, Central. 3. AIDS (Disease)—Social aspects—Asia, Central. 4. AIDS (Disease)—Asia, Central—Psychological aspects. 5. Stigma (Social psychology)—Asia, Central. 6. Discrimination—Asia, Central. I. Alexandrova, Anna, 1976-
II. International Debate Education Association. III. Series.
  [DNLM: 1. Acquired Immunodeficiency Syndrome—psychology—Central Asia. 2. Acquired Immunodeficiency Syndrome—psychology—China. 3. Acquired Immunodeficiency Syndrome—psychology—Russia. 4. HIV Infections—psychology—Central Asia. 5. HIV Infections—psychology—China. 6. HIV Infections—psychology—Russia. 7. Health Policy—Central Asia. 8. Health Policy—China. 9. Health Policy—Russia. 10. Human Rights—Central Asia. 11. Human Rights—China. 12. Human Rights—Russia. 13. Prejudice—Central Asia. 14. Prejudice—China. 15. Prejudice—Russia. 16. Sexual Behavior—psychology—Central Asia. 17. SexualBehavior—psychology—China. 18. Sexual Behavior—psychology—Russia.
WC 503.7 M687 2007]
  RA643.86.A783M63 2007
  362.196'979200958—dc22
                                    2007019693

Designed by Herman Bonomo
Printed in the USA

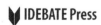 **IDEBATE Press**

IDEA SOURCEBOOKS
ON CONTEMPORARY CONTROVERSIES

The International Debate Education Association (IDEA) has dedicated itself to building open and democratic societies through teaching students how to debate. The IDEA Sourcebooks on Contemporary Controversies series is a natural outgrowth of that mission. By providing students with books that show opposing sides of hot button issues of the day as well as detailed background and source materials, the IDEA Sourcebooks on Contemporary Controversies give students the opportunity to research issues that concern our society and encourage them to debate these issues with others. IDEA is an independent membership organization of national debate programs and associations and other organizations and individuals that support debate. IDEA provides assistance to national debate associations and organizes an annual international summer camp.

Contents

Introduction

STIGMA, DISCRIMINATION, SOCIAL EXCLUSION AND HIV/AIDS

Used in Ancient Greece for the mark burned or cut into the body to distinguish slaves from citizens, the word *stigma* is now defined as a "mark of shame or discredit"[1] that reduces an individual "from a whole person to a tainted, discounted one."[2]

Social stigma has profound effects across a wide range of outcomes, including one's well-being, self-esteem, and self-perception. Experts agree that stigma is rooted in three conditions:

- Assumed deviant or immoral behavior (e.g., the mentally ill, people who abuse alcohol and/or drugs, people who engage in sexual relationships with members of the same sex, etc.).

- Physical disfigurement (e.g., the overweight, people with leprosy, etc.)

- Membership—actual or perceived—in marginalized groups (religious, ethnic, racial populations or communities, etc.).[3]

Discrimination and exclusion are essential aspects of stigmatization. Exclusion is often based on social consensus in the culture; it is rooted in a social, not a personal identity, and is often considered justified or legitimate.[4]

Stigma is often divided into felt stigma and enacted stigma.[5] While felt stigma defines perceived or actual threats or dangers should the particularities of stigma be known (i.e., being gay), enacted stigma refers to the real experiences of discrimination and exclusion.

In 1987, Jonathan Mann, then the director of the World Health Organization, recognized the significance of stigma and discrimination related to HIV and AIDS. This stigma is a complex social phenomenon explained, in part, by the special nature of HIV and its deep associations with many sensitive social topics—the fear of epidemics and death; the significance of sex in love, passion, and reproduction; and the euphoria and devastation of illicit drugs.

In many instances, the communities most vulnerable to HIV are also those that are the most stigmatized, either for their "deviant" behavior or for their membership in marginalized groups. The association of these communities with HIV and AIDS further deepens the existing stigma and often adds a new layer of symbolic AIDS stigma,[6] used to express prejudices and dislike of the traditionally marginalized populations.

Twenty-five years into the epidemic, dealing with HIV- and AIDS-related stigma and discrimination remains a problem for those trying to prevent and address the disease. Although the problem is global, this work focuses on AIDS-related stigma in Central Asia.

THE HIV AND AIDS EPIDEMIC IN CENTRAL ASIA

Over the past few years, Central Asia has witnessed a dramatic increase in the rate of HIV and AIDS infections. Officially reported cases jumped from approximately 500 in 2000 to over 12,000 in 2004. According to official statistics, in April 2006, 6,081 people in Kazakhstan were living with HIV and AIDS. Uzbekistan has recently seen a surge of new infections: in 1999, 28 people were diagnosed with the virus; in 2005, 2,016 new infections were reported, bringing the official total to 7,800.[7] The number of unreported cases is thought to be much higher; the U.S. Centers for Disease Control and Prevention estimates that some 90,000 people in Central Asia are living with HIV and AIDS.[8] The epidemic, which is concentrated among young people, is driven by injecting drug use.

Although the numbers are alarming, international experts believe that should effective HIV prevention, treatment, care, and support measures be introduced immediately, the region can avert a major public health crisis that would have serious detrimental effects on security and stability. The international community has responded by providing financial support and technical assistance to the decaying public health systems in the region. The United Nations, foreign assistance agencies of numerous governments, and international and national foundations have supported HIV prevention efforts in the region since the mid-1990s. In 2005, the World Bank launched an ambitious five-year US$27 million project designed to strengthen regional coordination and policy development, increase local skills and resources, and fund initiatives to prevent HIV and sexually transmitted infections (STIs). Yet, efforts to contain the epidemic have been hindered by deep-rooted stigma and discrimination against people living with HIV and AIDS as well as many of the populations at risk for the disease.[9]

STIGMA AND HIV/AIDS IN CENTRAL ASIA

HIV- and AIDS-related stigma in Central Asia takes many forms. People living with HIV and AIDS (PLHA) experience discrimination in access to health services, employment, and housing, and especially in their communities.

> Stigma also concerns people with diseases other then HIV, for example, those with TB also often get stigmatized. But there is a big difference between TB and HIV in as much as TB can be treated, and HIV is lethal. The imminent death from HIV is one of the reasons why people living with HIV in Kazakhstan face heightened stigma and discrimination. In practice, I saw a lot of cases of stigmatization, especially coming from their status being disclosed by public health workers. Pursuant to the confidentiality breach and resulting disclosure of their HIV status, I saw people being ostracized in their families and communities.

> For example, when talking to a man who was diagnosed with HIV when he was 46 years old when being treated for TB, I found out that his status was disclosed to his neighbors by the TB clinic's staff. Following this, his neighbors, who were people he had been close to for a number of years, cut all communications with him, and would turn away when passing him on the street! Unfortunately, this is not the only example of HIV discrimination in Kazakhstan, and as a result of widespread stigma and discrimination, people are afraid to go through HIV test; they are not motivated to disclose their status, live an active life, and HIV-activists find it difficult to openly work inside the community and fight for their rights.

> *Testimony of Z. from Almaty, Kazakhstan.*
> *Z. is a person living with HIV, and an activist*
> *in HIV/AIDS movement in Kazakhstan.*
> *Due to the high level of stigma and discrimination,*
> *Z. requested that the name is withheld.[10]*

Certain populations—drug users, sex workers, and men who have sex with men (MSM)—continue to bear the heavy burden of official mistrust and bias. This, in turn, limits their access to health care and other social services, and increases their vulnerable to rights abuses, thus increasing their risk of acquiring HIV.

In Central Asia, those most at risk of HIV and AIDS belong to populations that are often already stigmatized and face discrimination: injection drug users, sex workers, and MSM. All countries in Central Asia are experiencing an epidemic of injection drug use. With cheap heroin smuggled from war-torn Afghanistan and fields of opium poppies naturally found throughout the region, injection drug use has grown and is now the most prevalent cause of HIV transmission in the region. The criminalization of drug use and drug users has severely limited access to effective addiction treatment. For example, although harm reduction services that include needle exchange, condom distribution, and voluntary HIV and STI testing and counseling are available throughout Kazakhstan, they reach only a sliver of the population in need of these services. Stigma and prejudice against injection drug users is widespread and deep-rooted, and although several steps have been taken to eradicate this prejudice and subsequent stigma, these measures are just the first on a long series needed to achieve this goal.

Sex workers face deep-rooted stigma, especially in conservative and religious parts of Central Asia. Girls working the streets and highways in Central Asia are especially at risk of violence and acquiring HIV, but further suffer from police corruption and discrimination. Often without the proper residential registration documents, they are also unable to access free public health services. This further increases their vulnerability to HIV and sexually transmitted infections. Close proximity to drug trafficking routes and relatively inexpensive, accessible drugs, in part, pre-disposes many sex workers to injection drug use, thus adding another layer of stigma to this already highly stigmatized population. Legal vagueness about the status of their work provides sex workers with no opportunities for redress and allows for widespread discrimination from communities and police authorities.

MSM is another traditionally stigmatized group at increasing risk for HIV and AIDS unless society addresses existing stigma. According to the 2003 Human Rights Watch report, in Kazakhstan, gay men experience such severe stigma and discrimination that they were effectively excluded from harm reduction and other HIV prevention efforts underway in the country. In Kyrgyzstan, sodomy laws were repealed in 1998, but as late as 2005, most of Bishkek's gay men still choose to keep their sexual orientation a secret for fear of public censure and isolation from family and friends.[11] Turkmenistan and Uzbekistan both have sodomy laws that punish gay relationships with prison sentences. Not surprisingly, therefore, the 2006 UNAIDS Report on the Global AIDS Epidemic found that Eastern Europe and Central Asia lags significantly in reaching out to gay men with any kind of prevention programming. According to the report, in 2005 HIV prevention efforts covered only 4% of this population group in Eastern Europe and Central Asia.[12]

Respect for and adequate protection of human rights and freedoms can help combat stigma and provide victims of discrimination with tools for recourse. Yet, in countries and regions such as Central Asia, with long histories of poor human rights records, marginalized populations often face widespread discrimination, including blatant acts by local authorities. The situation has improved somewhat in the past few years. For example, Kazakhstan has ratified the International Covenant on Economic, Social and Cultural Rights (ICESR), committing governments to secure the right of all citizens to health care, and the International Covenant on Civil and Political Rights.[13] The latter covenant is important for combating HIV and AIDS because it obliges the signatories to secure "the right of everyone to the highest attainable standard of physical and mental health" (article 12). The ratification of the ICESR is also significant because it requires nations to submit reports on the implementation of the rights enshrined in the treaty to an independent body of experts—the Committee on Economic, Social and Cultural Rights. However, despite the recent positive changes in some countries of Central Asia, the region remains known for its low standards of human rights protection. This lack of protection mechanisms worsens the existing stigma and exacerbates discrimination of vulnerable populations and marginalized communities.

Some experts on HIV prevention believe that access to antiretroviral treatment for PLHA is associated with the overall reduction of the stigma of the disease.[14] The general limited access to antiretroviral treatment for PLHA in many Central Asian countries also means that traditionally marginalized groups have even less access to treatment.

Ineffective laws and policies exacerbate stigma for sex workers. For example, laws mandating incarceration of those involved in prostitution communicate the norm that sex work is socially unacceptable. This social unacceptability, reflected in myths, public attitudes, and discrimination, drives sex workers further underground. Fear of discrimination by healthcare workers stops sex workers from seeking treatment, while fear of incarceration and abuse prevents them from reporting violent "johns" to the police. Overall, this fear of authorities inhibits sex workers from adopting healthier choices, thus facilitating the spread of HIV in this population. Self-lacerating shame and self-discrimination further lower their quality of life and render it even more difficult to make long-term decisions, such as using condoms for protection from disease.

> Say, I work the highway. A police truck approaches. You are grabbed and forced inside. Of course, they [police] curse you all the way. You spend some time in that truck, they drive you all over the city looking for others. Then they [police] bring you to ROVD (District Department for Interior Affairs, police station), right in the hands of the superior at the anti-drugs and prostitution department. It's important to behave yourself, as otherwise you will probably be beaten. Police make you write why you were on the highway "prostituting yourself." They maintain you should admit in writing that you are a prostitute. Sometimes this is when you can try and bribe the officer with an offer of free sex. This works maybe once in every 10 times that you try. After you have admitted in writing they can either let you go, but keep your passport, or bring you to the STI clinic for compulsory tests. In the STI clinic, if you test positive for something or other, you can end up staying there for up to 30 days, and you pay for your own treatment. Of course, you are tested for HIV. If you are "clean"—then police pick you up from the STI clinic, and back to ROVD again you go, where you have to write yet another paper, where you say that you will pay the administrative fine and will not work as a prostitute any longer. The Court decides whether or not to fine you. After this—you are a free bird. The police will not touch you for at least three days on the highway, because the STI clinic will not take you again in such a short period of time.

> *Testimony from Dushanbe, Uzbekistan.*[15]

ATTACKING THE PROBLEM OF STIGMA—GENERAL APPROACHES

Approaches for combating HIV- and AIDS-related stigma and discrimination have included: encouraging self-disclosure of HIV status; staging aggressive media campaigns that stressed the importance of taking control over one's behavior; and encouraging famous people with HIV to publicly disclose their serostatus.[16] Yet the effectiveness of these approaches is questionable, and evidence suggests that policy and decision makers need to exercise caution when adopting them. For example, public disclosure of one's serostatus can lead to violence, as some suggest that "living in areas where stigma and seroprevalence are both high may create pressures to publicly prove one's own seronegativity by rejecting or attacking others who are known to be HIV-positive."[17]

Researchers still need to conduct rigorous longitudinal investigations into the causes of stigma in Central Asia and the effectiveness of different approaches in combating it, yet a number of studies have shown that efforts to combat stigma and discrimination have succeeded when the following actions were at play:[18]

- building political will and commitment to sufficient funding;

- actively involving people and communities living with or affected by HIV and AIDS in prevention and advocacy efforts;

- addressing related fears and behavioral myths about HIV combined with active non-government organization (NGO) involvement in information campaigns, and

- addressing human rights violations of traditionally marginalized populations and PLHA.

During his keynote address at the 2006 XVI International AIDS Conference in Toronto, Dr. Peter Piot, UNAIDS executive director, called on the governments and donors to:

- make the reduction of stigma, discrimination, and gender inequalities explicit programmatic priorities;

- devote political and programmatic efforts and resources to emphasize the reduction of stigma, discrimination, and gender inequality; and

- rapidly conduct operational research on stigma and discrimination and feed the findings of such research without delay into national programs.[19]

He further called on governments, NGOs, and activists to closely monitor stigma and discrimination and to unite efforts, both at the national and community levels, against stigma and harmful gender norms. By initiating public debate on the issues of stigma and discrimination, and addressing the most harmful myths surrounding traditionally marginalized populations—MSM, intravenous drug users, and commercial sex workers—civil society organizations can turn commitments into action and help reverse the tide of HIV and AIDS by addressing another epidemic, that of stigma and discrimination.

Experts agree that to deliver the commitments found in the international human rights instruments, national commitment is key to success.[20] Sustained action at the country level should include the commitment to reduce stigma and discrimination and to improve the human rights situation of the most vulnerable populations. Measures should include: reforming policies and repealing laws that impede access to prevention and care; educating the community and policy makers; actively involving PLHA in developing policy, and investing in social mobilization to address HIV and AIDS.

Civil society actors, including NGOs and community groups, have an important role to play in holding governments responsible for their commitments. Historically, the first AIDS-service NGOs that emerged in the Newly Independent States (NIS) of the Soviet Union in response to the HIV epidemic among injecting drug users included many former staff from local AIDS centers—government institutions that were responsible for prevention, treatment, and support. As the epidemic evolved, new NGOs and associations emerged, and many of them now include community activists and PLHA. As providers of needle and syringe exchange services, counseling, referral, and outreach, civil society organizations that include representatives of the vulnerable populations and PLHA know best what works in their communities and often have the best opportunities for advocacy.

Central Asia Addresses HIV– and AIDS–Related Stigma

In 2006, most Central Asian governments adopted a regional policy on HIV and AIDS prevention designed, in part, to address the problem of stigma. This policy was rooted in three documents: the Millennium Development Goals, specifically MDG 6, which called for a halt to and reversal of the spread of HIV and AIDS by 2010; the 2001 United Nations Declaration of Commitment on HIV/AIDS, pledging to combat HIV- and AIDS-related stigma and discrimination; and, the United Nations General Assembly Political Declaration on HIV/AIDS, which "recognized that addressing stigma and discrimination is ... a critical element in combating HIV/AIDS epidemic."[21]

This commitment to HIV and AIDS prevention efforts was further reinforced at the 2006 UN General Assembly meeting on HIV and AIDS, when Kyrgyzstan's Acting Deputy Prime Minister, Ishengul Boldjurova, emphasized the importance of her nation humanizing drug policy and revising current laws and policies to ensure they are in accordance with the country's international commitments. Her statement represented an important step toward fighting the deep-rooted stigma and discrimination surrounding drug use in Kyrgyzstan. Hopefully, lessening the stigma will allow for successful HIV prevention efforts among drug users.

Presenting at the same event, Anatoly Belonog, the vice-minister of healthcare of Kazakhstan, especially noted the importance of fighting HIV- and AIDS-related stigma and discrimination, saying that "fighting stigma and discrimination, [attaining] respect for human rights, providing medical care, including treatment of AIDS-related diseases, and insuring social protection to people living with HIV/AIDS and their full participation in social and productive life" were among the political priorities of his government.[22] Both speakers reiterated their governments' commitments to attaining the objectives set out in the UN declarations of commitment. The public commitments of these governments, together with the key international documents, human rights treaties (the Convention on the Elimination of All Forms of Discrimination against Women, the Convention on the Rights of the Child, and the International Covenant on Economical, Cultural and Social Rights), and national laws, form the policy framework used to develop national HIV and AIDS prevention strategies.

CIVIL SOCIETY TAKING ACTION

Since the late 1990s, Central Asia, and particularly Kazakhstan and Kyrgyzstan, has seen a dramatic increase in the activities of community groups and civil society organizations. These organizations were especially important in effective project implementation, delivering much needed support to populations at risk and initiating long-needed prevention services, such as needle and syringe exchange and information dissemination. In many cases, special associations or networks were formed to facilitate lobbying and advocacy efforts (for example, the Kazakh Association of Organization Working on the Issues of HIV/AIDS and Drug Use, http://www.hivngokz.org).

MOBILIZING CIVIL SOCIETY RESPONSE

Mobilizing Civil Society Response to Stigma and Discrimination in Central Asia has been developed in collaboration with activists and professionals from

Kazakhstan to ignite public debate around the issues of HIV- and ADS-related stigma and discrimination, and to draw the attention of the governments of Central Asia, and Kazakhstan in particular, to the international commitments and the existing policy framework that need to be considered when identifying programmatic priorities for national HIV and AIDS prevention strategies.

The anthology offers readers general theoretical background on stigmatization and exclusion; studies of groups experiencing stigma; articles on stigma, law, and human rights; and discussions of the importance of involving civil society organizations in advocacy efforts. With limited research on stigma and discrimination in Central Asia, the articles draw on the experiences of populations from China, the United States, and where available, other countries of the NIS, as well as personal testimonies from activists and professionals from the region. Some of the key findings from research efforts in this guide can be extrapolated to the AIDS-related stigma in the Central Asia and will help governments and organizations increase their understanding of stigma and discrimination and deepen their anti-stigma advocacy efforts in this region. Debaters may also find it useful in understanding stigma and discrimination in their own cultures.

NOTES

1. *Merriam-Webster Online Dictionary*, s.v. "stigma," http://www.m-w.com/dictionary/stigma (accessed August 31, 2006).

2. E. Goffman, *Stigma: Notes on the Management of Spoiled Identity* (Englewood Cliffs, NJ: Prentice Hall, 1963), 3.

3. E. Goffman referred to the above-mentioned stigmatizing conditions as "blemishes of individual character," "abominations of the body," and "tribal stigmas." See E. Goffman, *Stigma: Notes on the Management of Spoiled Identity.*

4. B. Major and C. Eccleston, "Stigma and Social Exclusion," in *The Social Psychology of Inclusion and Exclusion*, eds. D. Abrams, M. Hogg, and J. Marques (Psychology Press: New York, 2005), 66.

5. A. Malcolm, P. Aggleton, et al., "HIV Related Stigmatization and Discrimination: Its Forms and Contexts," *Critical Public Health* 8, no. 4 (1988): 347–370.

6. G. Herek, "Thinking about AIDS and Stigma: A Psychologist's Perspective," *The Journal of Law, Medicine and Ethics* 30, no. 4 (Winter 2002): 594–607 at 598.

7. As reported by Interfax Kazakhstan in "HIV/AIDS is Growing Fast in the Republic of Kazakhstan," June 15, 2006.

8. USAID, Central Asian Republics Regional Program, "Health Profile: Central Asia HIV/AIDS" (background document, November 2004), http://www.usaid.gov/our_work/global_health/aids/Countries/eande/caregion.html

9. Activists and experts agree that the region can improve the situation surrounding HIV- and AIDS-related stigma and discrimination. However, although trends have been encouraging, consistent efforts are needed to fully address these deep-rooted problems.

10. The interview was conducted by Assel Janaeva, OSI-Kazakhstan, specifically for this publication.

11. Antoine Blua, "Central Asia: Gays Say Tolerance Improving, but Still a Long Way to Go," Radio Free Europe, January 20, 2005, http://www.sodomylaws.org/world/kazakhstan/kznews001.htm (accessed August 30, 2006).

12. UNAIDS, 2006 Report on the Global AIDS Epidemic: A UNAIDS 10th Anniversary Edition (May 2006, Geneva), p.57.

13. Kazakhstan ratified the International Covenant on Economic, Social and Cultural Rights and the International Covenant on Civil and Political Rights on January 24, 2006.

14. "Access to Treatment Associated with Declining HIV Stigma in Botswama," aidsmap, http://www.aidsmap.com/en/news/4112593B-475C-4C48-AF5C-757009D96741.asp (accessed April 14, 2007).

15. This testimony is taken from *Sex Work, HIV/AIDS and Human Rights in Central and Eastern Europe and Central Asia*, eds. A. Sarang and J. Hoover (Central and Eastern European Harm Reduction Network, July 2005), p. 42.

16. G. Herek, "Thinking about AIDS and Stigma: A Psychologist's Perspective," *The Journal of Law, Medicine and Ethics* 30, no. 4 (Winter 2002): 594–607.

17. Ibid., 602.

18. L. Brown, K. Macintyre, and L. Trujillo, "Interventions to Reduce HIV/AIDS Stigma: What Have We Learned," *AIDS Education and Prevention* 15, no. 1 (2003): 49–69.

19. Dr. Peter Piot, "How to Reduce the Stigma of AIDS," (keynote address, Symposium at the XVI International AIDS Conference, Toronto August 12, 2006, http:// data.unaids.org/pub/Speech/2006/200608012_SP_Piot_Stigma%20speech_en.pdf. (accessed June 4, 2007).

20. See panel outcomes "Stigma and Discrimination: the Undoing of Universal Access?" at the XVI International AIDS Conference, http://www.kaisernetwork.org/health_cast/hcast_index.cfm?display=detail&hc=1837 (accessed December 27, 2006).

21. Political Declaration on HIV/AIDS, A/RES/60/262 (adopted June 16, 2006), http://www.un.org/ga/aidsmeeting2006/declaration.htm (accessed August 31, 2006).

22. 2006 High-Level Meeting on AIDS, Webcast, http://www.un.org/webcast/ga/aids/2006/parallelsegmentB-02june06.html (accessed August 31, 2006).

PART 1:
Defining Stigma and Discrimination

To better understand the intrinsic links between HIV- and AIDS-related stigma and health, human rights, laws, and policies, we need to define stigmatization in terms of its psychological and social factors. Social and psychological factors, such as fears of death, lack of knowledge, and misunderstandings related to the transmission of HIV, often are central to the persistent enactment and experience of stigma. Better understanding of these factors will allow for a more effective response to stigmatization.

Challenging individual attitudes and conduct so that society accepts HIV as a virus, not a moral judgment, and tackling the persistent negative opinions of traditionally marginalized populations remain the primary objectives for AIDS activists, along with influencing laws and policies to support changes in understandings and behaviors.

The anthology opens up with Gregory M. Herek's "Thinking About AIDS and Stigma: A Psychologist's Perspective," which provides key definitions of stigma, prejudice, and discrimination. It describes the impact of stigma in a variety of social interactions and explores the effectiveness of common responses to stigma.

Thinking About AIDS and Stigma: A Psychologist's Perspective

*by Gregory M. Herek**

It is now clear that vulnerability to becoming infected with HIV derives directly from stigma and discrimination (and, more broadly, violations of human rights and dignity) occurring within each society. Thus, we have learned that to uproot the HIV/AIDS epidemic, as well as to protect and promote health more generally, human rights and dignity must be protected and advanced. When the history of AIDS and our time is written, the inextricable links between health and societal stigma, discrimination, human rights, and dignity may be recognized as our most important contribution.[1]

Jonathan Mann

As Jonathan Mann observed, the problem of AIDS-related stigma is inextricably bound to issues of health, human rights, and the law. Such stigma translates into feelings of fear and hostility directed at people with HIV.[2] It finds expression in avoidance and ostracism of people with HIV, discrimination and violence against them, and public support for punitive policies and laws that restrict civil liberties while hindering AIDS prevention efforts. Being the target of stigma inflicts pain, isolation, and hardship on many people with HIV, while the desire to avoid it deters some from being tested for HIV, seeking treatment, or practicing risk-reduction.[3]

AIDS-related stigma and its attendant prejudice and discrimination are significantly shaped by misunderstanding and fear of HIV disease, coupled with social attitudes toward the people who contract it and the conditions under which it is transmitted. Thus, social psychological factors play a central role in the maintenance, enactment, and experience of stigma, and a better understanding of them will permit a more effective response to stigma. In the present article, I provide a brief introduction to social psychological theory and research concerning AIDS-related stigma.

I begin by considering what stigma is and I distinguish it from two related constructs, prejudice and discrimination. Next, I briefly describe the contours of contemporary AIDS-related stigma in the United States, using findings from my own empirical research to illustrate key patterns. Then I explore some reasons HIV is stigmatized and how this stigma is enacted in social encounters. I also discuss the distinction between stigma based mainly on fear of HIV transmission (instrumental stigma) and that based mainly on preexisting attitudes toward the groups disproportionately affected by HIV (symbolic stigma). In the final section, I reflect on various strategies for reducing AIDS stigma.[4]

DEFINING STIGMA

English usage of "stigma" dates back at least to the 1300s.[5] The term derives from the same Greek roots as the verb "to stick," that is, to pierce or tattoo. The earliest recorded English usage of stigma referred to the cluster of wounds manifested by Catholic saints, which corresponded to the wounds of the crucified Jesus. These stigmata were said to appear regularly, sometimes bleeding, in conjunction with important religious feast days.

Religious stigmata signified holiness, but stigma more commonly has had a thoroughly negative connotation. Taken literally, it refers to a visible marking on the body, usually made by a branding iron or pointed instrument. But the "mark" could also be a nonphysical condition or attribute. A 1907 textbook of psychiatry described a form of psychopathology known as a Stigmata of Degeneration, for example,[6] and the Oxford English Dictionary notes a reference in 1859 to the "stigmata of old maidenhood."[7]

Historically, then, the meaning of stigma has had two components. First, it refers to an enduring condition or attribute. It is a mark borne by an individual. Second, that mark is negatively valued by the larger group or society. Whether it was physical or figurative, the mark was commonly understood to signify that the individual carrying it was criminal, villainous, or otherwise deserving of social ostracism, infamy, shame, and condemnation. Thus, not only are stigmatized individuals marked, but the larger group or society in which they live is characterized by a shared knowledge about the negative evaluation associated with the mark. People might vary in their personal responses, but everyone knows how society regards those who possess a particular stigma. As Erving Goffman pointed out in what is generally considered the classic sociological text on stigma, the stigmatized and the "normal" (his term for the nonstigmatized) are social roles, and all parties to any given interaction regardless of their own status—know the expectations associated with each role.[8]

The two roles are not simply complementary or symmetrical. Rather, they are characterized by a clear power differential. Sometimes the power difference itself is a basis for stigma, as when the poor and members of minority ethnic groups are stigmatized. Alternatively, members of society's ingroups may lose their advantaged status as a result of developing a stigmatized condition (e.g., schizophrenia or AIDS) or identity (e.g., as a homosexual or criminal). In either case, stigmatized individuals have less power and access to resources than do "normals."

Based on these considerations, we can define stigma as an enduring condition, status, or attribute that is negatively valued by a society and whose possession consequently discredits and disadvantages an individual. This definition allows us to distinguish stigma from two other relevant constructs: prejudice and discrimination. These words have somewhat different meanings for lawyers and social scientists. I use them here in their social psychological sense.

Prejudice is a negative attitude—that is, an evaluation or judgment—toward members of a social group.[9] As an attitude, it involves emotions such as fear, disgust, anger, and contempt. Whereas stigma resides in the structure and relations of society, prejudice resides in the minds of individuals. One can be prejudiced against any individual or group regardless of how they are evaluated by the rest of society. But personal prejudice is a manifestation of stigma only when it reflects society's negative judgment of the target. A member of a stigmatized minority can harbor prejudice against members of the dominant majority, for example, but it is still the minority individual who is stigmatized, not those in the majority.

Discrimination is behavior. It refers to differential treatment of individuals according to their membership in a particular group.[10] Discrimination, the act, is distinct from prejudice, the attitude. Attitudes often find expression in an individual's ongoing pattern of behavior, but many intervening variables can affect that relationship.[11] Establishing a causal link between a person's general attitudes and her or his behavior in a particular situation is especially difficult. Thus, the relationship between attitudes and overt behavior is complex, hard to predict, and often indirect.[12] Prejudice is only one element that potentially contributes to discriminatory conduct. Whether or not an individual discriminates in any specific instance depends on her or his having the motivation and ability to enact the behavior, and on the environment facilitating or hindering action.[13] Like prejudice, individual acts of discrimination are distinct from stigma. One can discriminate against members of any group, but such behavior is a manifestation of stigma only when society as a whole condones or encourages it.

Discrimination and overt expressions of prejudice are not necessary for stigma to affect its targets. Many stigmatized individuals regulate their own behavior to avoid others' hostility and abuse. Recognizing this fact, British sociologist Graham Scambler distinguished between enacted stigma (overt acts of discrimination) and felt stigma (a stigmatized person's internal sense of shame and fear of persecution).[14] Felt stigma motivates individuals with a stigmatized condition to attempt to pass as members of the nonstigmatized majority. Successful passing reduces their likelihood of actually being the target of enacted stigma, but also significantly disrupts their lives and is likely to increase their psychological distress. A valuable insight provided by Scambler's model is that actual discrimination need not occur for stigmatized people to suffer as a result of their status. They may restrict their own behavior and limit their own opportunities out of a sense of vulnerability resulting from felt stigma. This feeling of vulnerability is likely to persist in the absence of overt stigma. Even a few dramatic enactments of stigma (e.g., violence, discrimination, or ostracism directed at one individual) can heighten the sense of felt stigma among all members of the target group.

AIDS AND STIGMA

Having AIDS or being HIV-positive meets the criteria described above for a stigmatized condition: HIV infection is an enduring characteristic that relegates an infected individual to a socially recognized, negatively evaluated category. AIDS-related stigma is manifested in prejudice, discounting, discrediting, and discrimination directed at people perceived to have AIDS or HIV and at the individuals, groups, and communities with which they are associated.[15]

AIDS stigma is a worldwide phenomenon. People with HIV in different nations are subjected to varying degrees of personal rejection, social ostracism, discrimination, violence, and, in many countries, laws and policies that deprive them of basic human rights.[16] In the United States, press accounts and personal testimony since the first cases were detected in 1981 have told stories of people with AIDS—as well as those merely suspected of having the disease—being evicted from their homes, fired from their jobs, and shunned by family and friends.[17] Although the prevalence of enacted AIDS stigma over the years has not been precisely determined, these anecdotal reports have been corroborated by experimental research and questionnaire and interview studies with people with HIV[18] as well as reviews of litigation.[19] In addition, public opinion surveys conducted in the early years of the epidemic revealed widespread fear of AIDS, lack of accurate information about its transmission, and willingness to support draconian public policies that would restrict civil liberties in the name of fighting the disease.[20]

After more than two decades of AIDS, we might expect stigma to have diminished to undetectable levels. Unfortunately, this is not the case. For example, my own national surveys throughout the 1990s showed that although support for quarantine and public identification of people with AIDS—the most punitive aspects of AIDS stigma—had diminished considerably by the end of the decade, one-fifth of those surveyed in 1999 still feared people with AIDS and one-sixth expressed disgust toward them or supported their public labeling. In addition, the surveys revealed that more covert forms of stigma persisted. Even as recently as 1999, roughly one-fourth of respondents felt uncomfortable having contact with a person with AIDS. Nearly one-third of respondents said they would avoid shopping at a neighborhood grocery store whose owner had AIDS.[21]

The surveys also revealed troubling signs that the sorts of beliefs and opinions that provide a foundation for AIDS stigma continue to be widespread. The proportion of adults believing that a person infected with HIV through sex or drug use deserves to have AIDS increased over the decade, peaking in 1997 at 28 percent. In response to a question phrased in less harsh language, approximately one-half of respondents said that people with AIDS are responsible for their illness.[22] As elaborated below, when people are perceived to be personally responsible for having an undesirable condition, they generally are subjected to greater stigma than if their situation is perceived to be beyond their control.[23]

Of further concern is the fact that although members of the public understand how HIV is transmitted, they are much less knowledgeable about how it is not transmitted. In my surveys, the proportions of respondents overestimating the risks posed by some forms of casual social contact were actually higher at the end of the decade than in 1991, with between 42 percent and 51 percent believing in 1999 that HIV can be spread through sharing a drinking glass, being sneezed on, or using a public toilet.[24] Similar results have been reported by other researchers.[25] Those who believe that HIV can be spread through casual social contact are probably more likely to fear contact with those who have HIV and may be more willing in the future to support punitive policies that violate their human rights under the guise of protecting public health. Such fears may partly account for the widespread support that my surveys recorded for mandatory testing of various groups, including pregnant women, immigrants, and people judged to be at risk for getting AIDS. Although such support declined somewhat between 1997 and 1999, mandatory testing continued to he favored by most respondents.[26]

The Social Psychology of AIDS Stigma
Why AIDS Is Stigmatized

In the field of social psychology, we have generally focused more on how stigma affects face-to-face interactions than on why a particular mark is stigmatized.[27] Nevertheless, past theory and research highlight three characteristics that seem particularly relevant to understanding AIDS stigma.[28]

First, as noted earlier, the stigma attached to an undesirable condition tends to be more intense when that condition is understood to be the bearer's responsibility. An illness is likely to be stigmatized if it is perceived as having been contracted through voluntary and avoidable behaviors, especially behaviors that evoke social disapproval. Such an illness tends to evoke responses of anger and moralism rather than pity or empathy.[29] Because the common routes of HIV in the United States include male-male sex and behaviors associated with injecting drug use, it is not surprising that people with HIV are regarded by a significant portion of the public as responsible for their condition and consequently are stigmatized.[30] Indeed, research in the United States consistently reveals hierarchies of stigma associated with HIV according to who gets infected and how. Gay and bisexual men with AIDS are more stigmatized than heterosexual women with the disease. People who contracted AIDS through sex with multiple partners or sharing needles receive the most hostile reactions, with the least negative evaluations going to those who were infected through receiving contaminated blood products.[31]

Second, greater stigma is associated with conditions that are lethal and incurable. AIDS has been widely perceived to be a fatal condition since the earliest days of the epidemic.[32] Although new drug regimens now offer realistic hope that HIV disease may be transformed from a fatal malady to a chronic illness, these regimens are not effective for everyone who takes them and many with HIV cannot tolerate them or do not have access to them. For the foreseeable future, therefore, most of the U.S. public will probably continue to perceive AIDS as invariably fatal.

Third, greater stigma is associated with a condition when it is perceived to pose a risk to others. More negative attitudes are directed at a stigmatized person to the extent that others believe they can be physically, socially, or morally tainted by interacting with him or her.[33] Perceptions of danger and fears of contagion have surrounded AIDS since the beginning of the epidemic,[34] and are evident in Americans' continuing overestimation of the transmission risks posed by casual social contact.[35]

Stigma and Social Interactions

What happens when a person possessing a stigmatized condition interacts with others? When addressing this question, it is important first to specify the type of individual with whom the stigmatized person interacts. When both parties possess the stigmatized characteristic (for simplicity, let us consider the case of a dyad), it may have little effect on the interaction. Minority status may be stigmatized in most of society, but typically not in gatherings of individuals from the minority group itself. Shared stigma can create a bond between individuals when they perceive themselves to be members of a group that is set apart from the rest of society. A consensus may even emerge whereby members of the majority group are disparaged. It is important to recognize, however, that such micro-climates of stigma—in which the stigmatized turn the tables on "normals"—cover extremely small areas of the social map.

When only one party to an interaction possesses the stigmatizing characteristic, her or his "normal" counterpart may not know about it. For example, being gay or asymptomatically infected with HIV is usually concealable, which permits the stigmatized individual to pass as a "normal." When the stigmatized member of a dyad successfully passes, the "normal" party believes that the interaction is occurring between two "normals." However, the individual who is passing knows that her or his stigmatized condition might be exposed at any time with an ensuing change in status. In Goffman's terms, she or he is "discreditable."[36] The stigmatized person's central concern in such interactions, according to Goffman and others, is the management of information, that is, preventing the "normal" from learning about the mark.[37]

Like other stigmatized people, those with HIV who are passing as uninfected may divide the world into two camps: a large group to whom they disclose nothing about their serostatus and a small group of individuals who know about their diagnosis and are relied upon for help in keeping the secret. Sometimes these intimates put themselves in the role of protecting the person with HIV from prejudice or rejection by others and, in the course of filling this role, become acutely sensitive to the diagnosis and its attendant problems. People with HIV may also find themselves having to rely for help in protecting their secret upon others who, although they are not known personally, are able to detect their condition. These might include others with HIV as well as individuals whom Goffman labeled "the wise,"[38] e.g., healthcare professionals and lay individuals active in the AIDS community. The wise are "persons who are normal but whose special situation has made them intimately privy to the secret life of the stigmatized individual and sympathetic with it, and who find themselves accorded a measure of acceptance, a measure of courtesy membership in the clan."[39]

Once the "normal" knows that the other party is marked, the latter individual is "discredited" (again using Goffman's terminology).[40] The discredited no longer need to worry about passing, but they face different problems, the most obvious of which are overt expressions of stigma in the form of rejection, discrimination, or violence. Even if such enactments of stigma do not occur, however, they must manage the "normal's" impression of them. They may feel uncertain as to what others are really thinking of them and may perceive that they are under closer scrutiny than nonstigmatized individuals in comparable interactions. Their minor accomplishments may be considered too remarkable, whereas minor failings may be interpreted as a direct expression of their illness. Others might stare at them, especially if they manifest lesions, lipodystrophy, or other physical signs of illness. Strangers may feel free to strike up personal conversations about AIDS or offer unwanted help.

Of course, most people with HIV move through multiple social worlds in the course of a single day. Their stigma may be known in some of those worlds while they pass as uninfected in others. Hence, at various times they are likely to find themselves in both the discredited and discreditable roles. Even when the stigmatized person's status is known, the stigma's effect on the social interaction may vary according to how much the stigmatized condition actually disrupts the interaction or is perceived by others as repellent, ugly, or upsetting. For example, it is relatively easy to overlook the condition of an HIV-infected person who is asymptomatic, whereas the physical manifestations of advanced AIDS are readily evident in social interactions and often evoke distress from observers.[41]

The partners, family members, and close friends of those with HIV, as well as the professionals and volunteers who work with them or provide AIDS services or advocacy, often experience what Goffman called a "courtesy stigma."[42] They are stigmatized through their close association with AIDS, those with HIV, and the many outgroups associated with HIV, including gay people and drug users. This secondary form of stigma creates challenges for those who are subjected to it. The loved ones of people with HIV, for example, may find that they are isolated from others. Caregivers and advocates may find that their work is more difficult and stressful as a result of stigma, or they may be deterred from working with those with HIV.[43]

Instrumental and Symbolic Stigmas

Given that AIDS is generally regarded as a degenerative and fatal disease, that HIV is transmissible, and that HIV infection is widely perceived to be the infected person's responsibility, AIDS probably would have evoked stigma regardless of which social groups it first affected. In the United States and many other countries, however, AIDS-related stigma has another layer of meaning because of the widely perceived association between HIV and disliked sectors of the population, especially gay and bisexual men and injecting drug users (IDUs). Recognizing this fact, many social scientists have found it useful to differentiate between two types of reactions to people with HIV.

The first type, labeled "instrumental AIDS stigma," derives mainly from fear of AIDS as a communicable and lethal illness along with a desire to protect oneself from it. Instrumental stigma reflects the apprehension likely to be associated with any transmissible and deadly illness. The second type of reaction, referred to as "symbolic AIDS stigma," results from the use of AIDS as a vehicle for expressing hostility toward other groups that were already stigmatized before the epidemic began.[44] It is based on the metaphorical social meanings attached to AIDS, the people who get it, and the ways in which it is transmitted. As Susan Sontag observed, illnesses such as cancer and AIDS have often been interpreted not as amoral biological phenomena, but rather in terms of good and evil, virtue and vice, punishment and innocence.[45] Symbolic AIDS stigma derives its force from the association of HIV with disliked groups. The specific groups linked to AIDS in symbolic stigma vary somewhat across cultures, depending on the local epidemiology of HIV and preexisting prejudices.[46] In the United States, symbolic AIDS stigma has focused principally on male homosexuality and, to a lesser extent, IDUs.

Even though gay and bisexual men constitute a shrinking portion of U.S. AIDS cases, much of the American public continues to equate AIDS with homosexuality.[47] Moreover, individuals who closely associate AIDS with homosexuality harbor more negative attitudes toward gay men than those who do not.[48] At the same time, some segments of society have had different experiences with the epidemic and, consequently, make different symbolic associations to AIDS. In the African-American community, for example, AIDS has affected not only gay and bisexual men, but also a substantial number of injecting drug users, with the consequence that symbolic AIDS stigma is linked to attitudes toward both groups.[49]

RESPONDING TO AIDS STIGMA

How can we best respond to HIV-related stigma? In the remainder of this article, I briefly offer a social psychological perspective on this question. Unfortunately, the empirical research literature on the effectiveness of various strategies for challenging AIDS stigma and its consequences is sparse. Relatively few antistigma interventions have been attempted, fewer still have been reported at professional conferences or in print, and adequate assessments of outcomes have been rare.[50] My discussion, therefore, is necessarily speculative, although it draws upon social psychological theory and, when possible, empirical research.

As a starting point, Table 1 summarizes the results of follow-up analyses that I conducted with data from a 1999 national telephone survey of 1,335 English-speaking adults.[51] The statistics presented in the table describe how strongly respondents' scores on a measure of AIDS-related stigma[52] were associated with various social, psychological, and demographic characteristics.[53]

The first column of data in Table 1 reports correlation coefficients, which characterize the strength of association between each individual variable and the measure of AIDS stigma.[54] As shown in the table, respondents' stigma scores tended to be higher to the extent that they expressed negative attitudes toward gay men and did not understand that HIV is not transmitted through casual social contact (e.g., sharing a drinking glass, using a public toilet). In addition, respondents who expressed beliefs consistent with the psychological construct of authoritarianism—which is associated with a generalized tendency toward prejudice[55]—tended to have higher scores for stigma, as did older respondents and those who did not personally know anyone with HIV Stigma

TABLE 1. STRENGTH OF ASSOCIATIONS BETWEEN AIDS STIGMA AND OTHER VARIABLES				
Variable	Correlation	Regression Coefficients		T
	(r)	Standardized (β)	Unstandardized (b)	
Inaccurate beliefs about casual contact	0.39	0.278	0.178	10.71
Negative attitudes toward gay men	0.39	0.266	0.197	9.81
Authoritarianism	0.26	0.100	0.185	3.78
Age	0.21	0.125	0.016	4.97
Number of people with AIDS known	−0.18	−0.091	−0.146	−3.63
Considers sex acceptable only in marriage	0.24			
Educational level	−0.19			
Political ideology (high = liberal)	−0.17			
Believes sex is mainly for procreation	0.15			
Importance of religion	0.13			
Frequency of religious attendance	0.12			
Income	−0.11			
Employment status (employed = 1)	−0.11			
Rural/small town residence	0.11			
Sex (male = 1)	0.10			

All correlation coefficients and T-values are significant at $p < 0.001$.
R^2 (adjusted) = .277, $F (5, 1179)$ = 91.61, $p < 0.001$.

also tended to be higher among respondents who held traditional opinions about sex—i.e., those who believed that it is mainly for purposes of procreation or is acceptable only between married people—and among respondents who had less formal education, described themselves as politically conservative, accorded religion a high level of importance in their life, attended religious services frequently, had a lower income, were unemployed, resided in a small town or rural area, or were male.

This pattern of correlations paints a preliminary picture of the groups of people in U.S. society who are most likely to harbor stigmatizing attitudes toward people with AIDS. While informative and thought-provoking, however, the correlations are of limited value in guiding the construction of stigma-reduction interventions. Many of them are extremely small.[56] In addition, some of the variables are correlated with each other as well as with AIDS stigma. Compared with the less educated, for example, people with more years of schooling generally tend to be less prejudiced toward minority groups and also are more likely to be knowledgeable about topics such as HIV transmission. Consequently, the strong correlation between AIDS stigma and knowledge about casual contact might actually result from the fact that both are correlated with educational level. A statistical technique called multiple regression is useful here because it permits assessment of the relationship between AIDS stigma and each of the other variables while statistically controlling for all of these interrelationships.

The remaining columns in Table 1 report the end result of a series of regression analyses. Ultimately, five variables from the correlation analysis emerged as the most important predictors of AIDS stigma: beliefs about casual contact, attitudes toward gay men, authoritarianism, age, and personal contact with people with AIDS. When the variables' relationships to AIDS stigma were all analyzed simultaneously, these five proved to be the major factors underlying stigma scores for this particular sample. The standardized regression coefficients (beta, reported in the second data column) give an indication of the relative importance of each variable in explaining variation in AIDS stigma scores.[57] I use these findings as the starting point for my discussion of interventions to combat AIDS-related stigma.

Information Campaigns

Early in the epidemic, it became clear that simply providing information about HIV and how it is transmitted would not be adequate to stop the spread of AIDS. At the same time, knowledge about HIV transmission clearly is a necessary, albeit not sufficient, prerequisite for risk reduction. What about for stigma? Table 1 shows that one of the best predictors of stigmatizing attitudes is the belief that casual contact can transmit HIV. Can information campaigns make a dent in HIV-related stigma?

I believe they can. Social reactions to a disease evolve as new information about the illness becomes available and is widely disseminated. Historically, the stigma associated with some diseases declined dramatically when the disease etiology was understood and cures or effective treatments were developed. This is illustrated in Charles Rosenberg's account of three nineteenth century cholera epidemics in the United States.[58] Between the 1832 and 1866 epidemics, Americans progressed from regarding cholera as a moral punishment for sinners to understanding its connections with poor sanitation and public health practices.

When the 1832 epidemic struck, neither physicians nor members of the general public understood that cholera is transmitted through bacterial infection. Physicians believed that it was caused by the introduction of poisons into the atmosphere, e.g., from decaying matter. People were thought to be predisposed to succumb to these poisons as a result of certain conditions, including excessive sexual activity, intemperance, and idleness. Consequently, prostitutes and their customers, the poor, blacks, and immigrants all were regarded as "risk groups" for cholera. Because no effective treatment was available, public attention centered on prevention efforts, which often took a highly moralistic tone (e.g., closing saloons). Most Americans viewed cholera as a direct punishment from God or a consequence of failing to observe Nature's laws. Although physicians proclaimed (incorrectly) that cholera was not contagious, many members of the public avoided the sick. Hospitals for cholera patients provoked community protest ranging from petitions to arson.[59]

In the subsequent 1849 and 1866 cholera epidemics, scientific understanding of the disease increased and public attitudes changed. Once it was known that the cholera bacillus spread primarily through the vomitus and excrement of infected individuals, massive public health campaigns were mounted to destroy contaminated bedding and clothing, improve sewage disposal, purify public water supplies, and clean up cities. Outmoded moralistic conceptualizations yielded to a new respect for public health and medicine as Americans became familiar with the germ theory of disease and realized that purely material practices could prevent the spread of cholera. As Rosenberg pointed out, this shift in the paradigm for cholera did not reflect the culture's decrease in piety; rather, it was based on advances in scientific understanding that made the moralistic approach to cholera increasingly irrelevant.[60]

The story of cholera offers some hope for combating HIV-related stigma. We do not yet have a cure for AIDS but we understand how HIV is transmitted, and this understanding should help to reduce stigma. Unfortunately, there are at least three reasons why our advanced knowledge about HIV does not have a greater impact on stigma. First, the public remains surprisingly ill-informed about the disease. Whereas scientific understanding of HIV and AIDS has increased dramatically since the epidemic began, the public's knowledge has not followed suit. As noted earlier, my own surveys show that the proportion of American adults who incorrectly believe that HIV can be transmitted through casual social contact or donating blood actually increased over the decade of the 1990s.[61]

The fact that much of the public has never completely understood the viral transmission of AIDS is apparent in responses to survey questions about the

HIV risks associated with male homosexual behavior. In four national telephone surveys conducted between 1991 and 1999, I consistently found that a disturbingly large minority of U.S. adults equated any male homosexual behavior—even sex between two uninfected men—with HIV transmission.[62] In a 1997 survey, for example, nearly one-fourth of the respondents believed that an uninfected man could get AIDS from one sexual encounter with another uninfected man, even if they used condoms. Without condoms, more than four respondents in ten believed that a man could get AIDS through sex with an uninfected man.[63] In that survey, respondents who incorrectly believed that all male-male sex spreads AIDS also expressed significantly more negative attitudes toward gay men, which suggests that the association between AIDS stigma and antigay attitudes was buttressed by a belief system equating AIDS with sex between men.

These data point to the importance of reinvigorating public education efforts about HIV transmission and going beyond simple slogans like, "You can't get AIDS from shaking hands." The American public needs to understand why they can't get AIDS from shaking hands, other forms of casual contact, donating blood, or having sex (even unprotected sex) with an uninfected partner.

A second reason knowledge about HIV has not reduced stigma as much as it might is that some sectors of the public simply do not believe the scientific data about HIV Mistrust of experts is especially high among African-Americans, many of whom have long believed that HIV represents a genocidal government conspiracy targeting blacks.[64] In a 1991 national survey, for example, 20 percent of blacks believed that AIDS is being used as a form of genocide against minority groups, compared to 5 percent of whites. Individuals who distrusted government and scientific sources of AIDS information also were more likely to stigmatize people with AIDS, mainly by avoiding social contact with them and supporting draconian policies that would isolate them.[65]

A third reason knowledge about HIV does not inevitably reduce stigma is that a considerable portion of AIDS-related stigma is symbolic and, consequently, unlikely to be affected by information campaigns. (The importance of confronting symbolic stigma is discussed below.) However, instrumental stigma also plays an important role in shaping reactions to AIDS. As shown in Table 1, misinformation about casual contact is a substantial predictor of AIDS stigma, even when attitudes toward gay men and other relevant variables, such as education, are statistically controlled. It is this component of stigma that is most likely to be affected by AIDS educational campaigns.

In mounting campaigns to provide accurate and credible information about AIDS, it is important that we do not further reinforce existing stigma. I noted earlier, for example, that the proportion of adults in the United States who perceive people with AIDS as responsible for their condition and therefore, to many, blameworthy—increased over the decade of the 1990s. This trend maybe an unintended consequence of public education efforts that have portrayed HIV prevention entirely in terms of individual decision-making. The flipside of messages stressing the importance of taking control of one's personal behavior to prevent HIV is that those who do not exercise such control may deserve whatever bad consequences follow. If so, health educators face the challenge of communicating the importance of protecting oneself from AIDS without promoting increased blame for individuals who become infected.

Mindful of these limitations, I believe we will have at least a limited impact on HIV-related stigma if we reenergize our public education efforts and address the specific problems I have outlined here. In contrast to cholera in the nineteenth century, we should not expect increased knowledge about HIV transmission to largely eradicate stigma. But without such knowledge, we cannot expect much progress at all.

Self-Disclosure of Serostatus

Another approach to stigma reduction has been to encourage people with HIV to disclose their serostatus to others. The hope is that uninfected individuals will be less likely to stigmatize people with HIV if they personally know someone who is infected. HIV infection is concealable, which makes it possible for many with HIV to "pass" as uninfected in routine social interactions. Controlling who knows that they are infected not only helps them to avoid the stigma associated with AIDS and related statuses (e.g., being gay or an IDU), but also allows them to preserve their privacy and maintain a sense of normalcy in their own lives. Passing, however, is often stressful. Keeping important information about oneself a secret can have negative consequences for one's mental and physical health.[66] The demands of passing can disrupt relationships, requiring those with HIV to create distance from others in order to avoid disclosing their diagnosis. This may prevent them from receiving much needed social support. Moreover, hiding their diagnosis may reinforce a sense of shame about being infected, or may cause them to feel inauthentic—that they are living a lie.

On the other hand, people with HIV have legitimate concerns about personal rejection, discrimination, and even violence if others know their serostatus. It is understandable, then, if the admonition to people with HIV to disclose to others—not only sexual partners, but also family, friends, co-workers, and even strangers—meets with resistance. It is appropriate that they should want to know that "coming out of the closet"—i.e., disclosing their serostatus—will have a positive effect or, at the least, will not cause them harm.

My use of the phrase "coming out" to describe self-disclosure of HIV status intentionally invokes the metaphor used by gay men and lesbians to describe the process whereby they reveal their sexual orientation to others. The expectation that coming out as an HIV-positive person will help to reduce AIDS-related stigma is based to a significant extent on the experiences of gay and lesbian people in the United States and other Western nations. Indeed, the U.S. public's attitudes toward homosexuality have moderated during the past few decades and one likely reason is that increasing numbers of heterosexual Americans now know that they have a gay or lesbian friend or close relative.

This effect has been explained with reference to what social psychologists call the contact hypothesis. As originally described by Gordon Allport, it holds that many forms of prejudice can be reduced by equal-status contact between majority and minority groups in the pursuit of common goals.[67] Empirical data generally support the contact hypothesis, albeit with qualifications.[68] Research also suggests that its tenets are applicable to heterosexuals' attitudes toward lesbians and gay men. Heterosexuals who personally know someone who is gay are likely to hold more favorable attitudes toward gay people generally.[69]

Because HIV in the United States was first reported among gay men, and because the epidemic here has disproportionately affected the gay community, it is not surprising that the process of disclosing one's HIV status has often been conceptualized in a manner that parallels how we think about disclosing one's sexual orientation. Indeed, many gay men with AIDS have characterized HIV disclosure as a second coming out. Moreover, consistent with the finding that heterosexuals who know a gay person have lower levels of sexual prejudice than others, empirical research has shown that uninfected Americans who personally know someone with HIV express less prejudice against people with AIDS than do uninfected individuals who lack personal contact.[70] This association is demonstrated in Table 1, which shows that personally knowing someone with AIDS was an important predictor of lower levels of AIDS stigma in the 1999 survey.

It remains to be seen whether or not a similar correlation will be found in other cultures. Coming out as a person with HIV seems intuitively like a vastly different experience in the United States compared to countries with extremely high rates of HIV infection, as is the case in many African nations. In the latter societies, individuals who do not personally know someone living with AIDS or HIV are probably in the minority. Yet, anecdotal reports suggest that AIDS stigma is widespread in many of these countries. In addition, the coming out model of HIV self-disclosure may have important limitations in such societies for several reasons. Living in an area where stigma and seroprevalence are both high may create pressures to publicly prove one's own seronegativity by rejecting or attacking others who are known to be HIV-positive. In addition, to the extent that those with HIV are perceived to be similar to oneself, it becomes difficult to take refuge in the belief that "it can't happen to me." Consequently, the fact that heterosexual behavior is the predominant transmission mode for HIV in those countries may mean that members of the majority ingroup (i.e., heterosexuals) experience a greater sense of personal threat from HIV-infected individuals than is the case in societies where most people with HIV are (or are perceived to be) members of outgroups (e.g., homosexuals, injecting drug users). Yet another difference is that vast numbers of people with HIV in those societies are women, a group already lacking in power.

Thus, whether and to what extent self-disclosure of HIV status is an effective antidote to stigma in developing countries remains an empirical question. At the least, it seems likely that the social psychological processes underlying self-disclosure (for both the HIV-infected discloser and the uninfected recipient of that disclosure) will be different from those commonly observed in the United States.

Vicarious Contact with People with AIDS

A related strategy that is often advocated for reducing AIDS stigma is to encourage famous people who are HIV-infected to publicly disclose their serostatus. The underlying assumption is that members of the public will be affected by such an announcement in much the same way that they would be affected by learning that a close friend is infected. The difference between the two situations, of course, is that people have direct contact with friends but most have only vicarious contact with celebrities.

Expectations about the beneficial effects of vicarious contact with a famous person with HIV were discussed extensively in the United States when basketball star Earvin "Magic" Johnson revealed his HIV infection in 1991. The president of one AIDS organization commented on the effect of Johnson's announcement: "The main thing that raises awareness of HIV or AIDS is to know someone who has it. Now everybody in America knows someone with HIV."[71] In similar fashion, a *Sports Illustrated* writer compared Johnson's disclosure to the shock of learning that a member of one's own family has AIDS.[72] Social scientists also speculated that the effect of Johnson's announcement on those without AIDS would be similar to that of having personal contact with someone who did have the disease.[73]

Magic Johnson's announcement provided an unusual opportunity to study the effects of celebrity disclosure on AIDS stigma. As it happened, my colleagues and I had completed a national telephone survey on HIV-related stigma one year earlier and were preparing to field a follow-up version of that survey when Johnson made his serostatus public.

When we reinterviewed respondents, we asked them whether Johnson's announcement had affected their opinions. We also compared their follow-up attitudes and beliefs to their initial survey responses from one year earlier.

Johnson's disclosure did not result in dramatic reversals of attitudes, but it appeared to reduce stigma in those who had expressed the most extreme negative attitudes in the initial survey. Their AIDS-related attitudes moderated somewhat in the follow-up survey, but still remained generally more negative than those of the rest of the sample. The effect of vicarious contact was considerably weaker than that of direct contact: Survey respondents who personally knew someone with AIDS or HIV manifested substantially less AIDS stigma than those who lacked such contact.

These findings derive from what is effectively a single case study. Public disclosure by other celebrities with HIV may well have a different impact. However, given Magic Johnson's prominence, the public's high regard for him, and the way in which he disclosed (e.g., the fact that he revealed his serostatus while still in apparent good health), public reactions to his disclosure may well be as positive as we are likely to see in response to any celebrity disclosure. If this is true, the potential for reducing stigma through vicarious contact with people with HIV is probably limited.

Confronting Symbolic Stigma

As explained earlier, AIDS-related attitudes often serve as a vehicle for expressing hostility toward disliked groups that have been linked with the epidemic. Because its roots lie in these other prejudices, symbolic AIDS stigma is unlikely to be affected by factual information about HIV Instead, such information tends to be interpreted in a manner that reinforces stigma. Consider, for example, information about transmission. Increased knowledge about how cholera was spread helped to reduce stigma in the nineteenth century. In the AIDS epidemic, however, knowledge about the routes of HIV transmission has often been used to promote antigay stigma, as when then-Representative William Dannemeyer (R-CA) cited the epidemic as a reason for reinstating sodomy laws in the 1980s.[74] Indeed, since the early years of AIDS, antigay activists have promoted symbolic stigma by blaming the gay community for starting the epidemic and portraying homosexuals as ongoing dangers to themselves. They also have admonished heterosexuals to avoid homosexuals, arguing that HIV and various AIDS-related diseases could be spread through casual contact, while they actively campaigned to prevent AIDS education programs from providing explicit information to gay and bisexual men about how to protect themselves sexually from HIV.[75]

The continuing potency of symbolic AIDS stigma is evident in the regression analysis reported in Table 1: Attitudes toward gay men were a prime predictor of AIDS stigma in the 1999 national survey; authoritarianism—an indicator of generalized prejudice—was a secondary predictor. The strong associations between Americans' AIDS-related attitudes and their attitudes toward gay people suggest that AIDS stigma will not be eliminated unless stigma, prejudice, and discrimination based on sexual orientation are also confronted. Unfortunately, the research literature on reducing sexual prejudice is of limited scope (though not as limited as the research on reducing AIDS stigma). Most studies in this area have focused on one of two routes by which sexual prejudice might be counteracted: through exposure to information or through personal contact with lesbians or gay men.[76]

In one type of study, experimental designs have been used to compare the attitudes of heterosexuals (typically college students) before and after they are exposed to information about homosexuality or the gay community (e.g., through a film, a speaker, or an entire course on gender or sexuality).[77] Most of these investigations have documented reductions in research participants' prejudice after the educational program. Unfortunately, they have not identified the reasons why attitudes change. We do not know whether prejudice decreases because educational programs provide factual information and refute stereotypes about gay people, because they create an opportunity for developing positive feelings toward a specific gay person (e.g., a speaker), or because they promote general social norms of tolerance. It is also possible that such programs simply cue participants to subsequently give unprejudiced questionnaire responses regardless of their own true attitudes. The conclusions from this type of study have been further limited by self-selection bias: Participants who choose to be exposed to an educational program (e.g., by enrolling in a sexuality course) are probably different in important ways from other heterosexuals. For example, they may be more receptive to new information about sexual minorities in the first place.

In the second category of studies are the previously mentioned reports showing that personally knowing a gay man or lesbian is associated with lower levels of sexual prejudice among heterosexuals.[78] The link is especially strong when heterosexuals know several gay people, when they report having close friends who are gay (rather than mere acquaintances), and when their relationship has included open discussion of the other person's homosexuality.[79] An important limitation is that studies of this type have been mainly descriptive. The question of causality—whether contact reduces prejudice or whether heterosexuals low in prejudice are more likely to have contact with openly gay people has not been resolved. Most likely, contact and attitudes each exert some effect on the other. Consistent with social psychological theory and with empirical research on other types of prejudice,[80] it is reasonable to assume that contact reduces prejudice.

Both types of studies—experimental assessments of educational programs and surveys of interpersonal contact—have focused on attitudes rather than behavior. We have virtually no empirical data directly assessing how to reduce enactments of antigay stigma, such as discrimination or violence. Nor have systematic studies been conducted to determine that reducing an individual's antigay prejudice will result in diminished AIDS-related stigma. Heterosexuals with more positive attitudes toward lesbians and gay men would be unlikely to use AIDS as a vehicle for expressing sexual prejudice, but they might be susceptible to other forms of symbolic stigma (e.g., expressions of hostility toward IDUs).[81] As with interventions for reducing AIDS stigma, this remains an area where empirical research is urgently needed.

Other Responses to Stigma

Consistent with my psychological perspective in this article, I have highlighted strategies for fighting stigma that focus on individuals. I do not wish to imply, however, that such strategies are sufficient by themselves. We also need structural antistigma interventions, including legal and policy initiatives and political mobilization. Although an extended discussion of macro-social strategies is beyond the scope of this article (and my own expertise), I offer a few reflections relevant to such strategies.

In the United States, laws have been enacted to mitigate the effects of AIDS stigma, ranging from local ordinances prohibiting discrimination on the basis of HIV status to the federal Americans with Disabilities Act. In addition to their direct benefits to people with HIV, such laws are likely to lessen AIDS stigma for several reasons. They communicate the norm that AIDS-related discrimination is socially unacceptable. They motivate organizations to develop implementation plans that typically include methods for avoiding discrimination, such as guidelines for accommodating the needs of HIV-infected persons in the workplace. And, by making it safer for those with HIV to be open about their serostatus, antidiscrimination laws can increase the number of opportunities that uninfected people have to interact with those who are infected, which, in turn, may reduce prejudice.

Yet, as Scott Burris has pointed out, the benefits of legislation are limited.[82] For one thing, people with HIV often remain unaware that laws protecting them even exist. For another, whereas laws may reduce enacted stigma, actual discrimination need not occur for people with HIV to suffer from the effects of AIDS-related stigma. As noted earlier, felt stigma motivates many people with HIV to constrict their own behavioral options to avoid ostracism, discrimination, and violence. Laws may have a negligible impact on felt stigma, especially in the short term.

Another limitation of relying on the law is that it can also be used as a vehicle for the expression of stigma. Throughout the epidemic, legislators and activists have repeatedly attempted to enact statutes and implement policies that are hostile toward people with HIV. As Burris observed:

Our law does as much to stigmatize people with HIV, gay people, poor people, and drug users as it does to protect them. From the succession of Helms Amendments restricting HIV education to recent legislation requiring the discharge of the HIV infected from military service, there is a prostigma plank for every antistigma one in the government's AIDS platform.[83]

Many—perhaps most—of those prostigma planks can be understood as expressions of symbolic stigma. They translate moral condemnation of stigmatized outgroups and behavior into public policy. In doing so, they not only reinforce stigma, but have probably made the epidemic worse. For example, a considerable body of social science research on HIV prevention demonstrates the importance of creating culturally sensitive HIV-prevention programs that are tailored to their target audience, imparting information that is clear and explicit, providing instruction on safe sex behavior, and enlisting social and community support for individuals who are trying to reduce their risk.[84]

However, federally funded AIDS prevention programs have been effectively prevented from meeting these criteria in their outreach to gay and bisexual men because they have been barred from portraying homosexuality in a positive light, promoting sexual activity, or distributing materials that federal officials judge to be obscene.[85] In a similar vein, the abstinence-only curriculum legally mandated for federally funded sex education programs in the public schools ensures that male adolescents who engage in same-sex behavior (regardless of whether they will eventually identify as gay, bisexual, or heterosexual) will not receive information about how to protect themselves from HIV. And whereas syringe exchange programs have been shown to be effective in reducing HIV transmission among IDUs, the federal government has opposed their implementation, largely on the premise that such programs condone injecting drug use.[86]

These are examples of how, as Jonathan Mann observed in the epigraph to this article, stigmatized status is linked to risk for HIV Because gay and bisexual men and IDUs belong to social outgroups, reducing their risk for HIV infection is a lower government priority than promoting moral condemnation of their behavior. These laws and policies increase felt stigma, not only among people with HIV but also among uninfected gay and bisexual people (women as well as men) and IDUs. Any effort to reduce AIDS-related stigma inevitably must confront these laws and policies.

This observation points to the necessity of locating efforts to eradicate HIV-related discrimination within the larger context of cultural power relations. As noted earlier, stigma is premised on power differentials. A group's relative powerlessness, however, does not mean that it must resign itself to being stigmatized. Indeed, recent history provides many examples of outgroups that have successfully challenged society's negative evaluation of a particular attribute or condition, such as homosexuality, mental illness, and racial and ethnic minority status. Such challenges were based on political mobilization among members of the stigmatized group as well as their "normal" allies. In like fashion, political organizing clearly has played a central role in shaping how society has responded to the AIDS epidemic.[87] It will continue to be important for creating responses to AIDS stigma that challenge the structural bases of disempowerment that are so closely linked to such stigma.[88]

CONCLUSION

As Jonathan Mann observed, stigma and discrimination are the enemies of public health not only because they inflict suffering on people with HIV and undermine efforts to prevent the further spread of HIV, but also because they heighten vulnerability to HIV infection among individuals and groups. "For this reason," he wrote, "preventing discrimination toward HIV-infected people and people with AIDS has been made an essential part—for the first time in history—of the public health strategy to prevent and control the global epidemic."[89]

In this antistigma project, lawyers, health professionals, human rights advocates, and social scientists will all benefit from each other's insights and expertise. We need to change the law and public policy so that they censure AIDS stigma rather than sanction it. At the same time, we must change individual attitudes and behaviors so that people understand that HIV is a virus, not a moral judgment, and that those who contract it are human beings, not symbols. Thus, institutional and individual change must be central objectives in an antistigma project. Part of the challenge we face is to keep both goals in sight.

ACKNOWLEDGMENTS

An earlier version of this paper was presented at the conference Health, Law and Human Rights: Exploring the Connections, co-sponsored by the American Society of Law, Medicine & Ethics and the Temple University Beasley School of Law, in Philadelphia on September 30, 2001. I gratefully acknowledge the support I received while writing this paper from the University of California, Davis, and from the National Institute of Mental Health through an Independent Scientist Award (K02 MH01455). I thank Scott Burris for his insightful comments on a preliminary draft.

NOTES

1. J. Mann, "Preface," *The Impact of Homophobia and Other Social Biases on AIDS* (San Francisco: Public Media Center, 1996): at 3, available at <http://www.publicmediacenter.org/pdfs/stigma.html>.

2. The category of "people with HIV" includes people diagnosed with AIDS as well as those who are asymptomatic. In the present article, I generally frame the discussion in terms of people with HIV. The exception is in my discussion of some public opinion data and some specific incidents that refer specifically to people with AIDS.

3. G.M. Herek, "Illness, Stigma, and AIDS," in P.T. Costa, Jr., and G.R. VandenBos, eds., *Psychological Aspects of Serious Illness: Chronic Conditions, Fatal Diseases, and Clinical Care* (Washington, D.C.: American Psychological Association, 1990): 107–50; G.M. Herek and E.K. Glunt, "An Epidemic of Stigma: Public Reactions to AIDS," *American Psychologist*, 43 (1988): 886–91; M.A. Chesney and A.W Smith, "Critical Delays in HIV Testing and Care: The Potential Role of Stigma," *American Behavioral Scientist*, 42 (1999): 1162–74.

4. My discussion provides only a brief and somewhat idiosyncratic introduction to social psycholog-ical thinking about stigma and HIV Readers who desire additional information about stigma in general will find the following sources helpful: E. Goffman, *Stigma: Notes on the Management of Spoiled Identity* (Englewood Cliffs, New Jersey: Prentice-Hall, 1963); J. Crocker, B. Major, and C. Steele, "Social Stigma," in D.T. Gilbert, S.T. Fiske, and G. Lindzey, eds., *The Handbook of Social Psychology*, vol. 2, 4th ed. (Boston: McGraw-Hill, 1998): 504–53; E.E. Jones et al., *Social Stigma: The Psychology of Marked Relationships* (New York: W.H. Freeman, 1984); B.G. Link and J.C. Phelan, "Conceptualizing Stigma," *Annual Review of Sociology*, 27 (2001): 363–85. For more detailed discussions of HIV-related stigma, see the papers in G.M. Herek, ed., "AIDS and Stigma," a thematic issue of *American Behavioral Scientist*, 42, no. 7 (1999).

5. The source for my comments about the etymology of stigma is the *Oxford English Dictionary* (1971 edition).

6. *Oxford English Dictionary* (1971): at 954.

7. *Id.*

8. Goffman, *supra* note 4.

9. J.H. Duckitt, *The Social Psychology of Prejudice* (New York: Praeger, 1992): at 7–24.

10. *Id.* at 9.

11. I. Ajzen and M. Fishbein, *Understanding Attitudes and Predicting Social Behavior* (Englewood Cliffs, New Jersey: Prentice Hall, 1980); A.H. Eagly and S. Chaiken, eds., *The Psychology of Attitudes* (Fort Worth, Texas: Harcourt Brace Jovanovich, 1993); I. Ajzen, "Nature and Operation of Attitudes," *Annual Review of Psychology*, 52 (2001): 27–58; M. Fishbein and I. Ajzen, *Belief, Attitude, Intention, and Behavior* (Reading, Massachusetts: Addison-Wesley, 1975).

12. Eagly and Chaiken, *supra* note 11; Ajzen and Fishbein, *supra* note 11.

13. Ajzen and Fishbein, *supra* note 11; F. Heider, *The Psychology of Interpersonal Relations* (New York: John Wiley & Sons, 1958).

14. G. Scambler, *Epilepsy* (London: Routledge, 1989): at 56–57. I am grateful to Scott Burris for making me aware of Scambler's work.

15. G.M. Herek et al., "AIDS and Stigma: A Conceptual Framework and Research Agenda," *AIDS and Public Policy Journal*, 13, no. 1 (1998): 36–47.

16. J.M. Mann, D.J.M. Tarantola, and T.W. Netter, eds., *AIDS in the World* (Cambridge: Harvard University Press, 1992); Panos Institute, *The 3rd Epidemic: Repercussions of the Fear of AIDS* (Budapest: Panos Institute, 1990); P. Aggleton, *HIV and AIDS Related Stigmatization, Discrimination and Denial: Research Studies From Uganda and India* (Geneva: UNAIDS, 2000); C.S. Goldin, "Stigmatization and AIDS: Critical Issues in Public Health," *Social Science and Medicine*, 39 (1994): 1359—66; A. Malcolm et al., "HIV-Related Stigmatization and Discrimination: Its Forms and Contexts," *Critical Public Health*, 8 (1998): 347–70.

17. For more extensive discussion of how AIDS-related stigma has been enacted, see Herek, *supra* note 3; Herek and Glunt, *supra* note 3; National Association of People with AIDS [NAPWA], *HIV in America: A Profile of the Challenges Facing Americans Living with HIV* (Washington, D.C.: NAPWA, 1992).

18. A.C. Gielen et al., "Women's Disclosure of HIV Status: Experiences of Mistreatment and Violence in an Urban Setting," *Women and Health*, 25, no. 3 (1997): 19–31; R. Klitzman, *Being Positive: The Lives of Men and Women with HIV* (Chicago: Ivan R. Dee, 1997); S. Zierler et al., "Violence Victimization After HIV Infection in a U.S. Probability Sample of Adult Patients in Primary Care," *American Journal of Public Health*, 90 (2000): 208–15; NAPWA, *supra* note 17; S. Page, "Accommodating Persons with AIDS: Acceptance and Rejection in Rental Situations," *Journal of Applied Social Psychology*, 29 (1999): 261–70; B.L. Fife and E.R. Wright, "The Dimensionality of Stigma: A Comparison of Its Impact on the Self of Persons with HIV/AIDS and Cancer," *Journal of Health and Social Behavior*, 41 (2000): 50–67.

19. L.O. Gostin, "The AIDS Litigation Project: A National Review of Court and Human Rights Commission Decisions, Part I: The Social Impact of AIDS," *JAMA*, 263 (1990): 1961–70; L.O. Gostin, "The AIDS Litigation Project: A National Review of Court and Human Rights Commission Decisions, Part II: Discrimination," *JAMA*, 263 (1990): 2086–93; L.O. Gostin and D.W Webber, "The AIDS Litigation Project: HIV/AIDS in the Courts in the 1990s, Part 1," *AIDS and Public Policy Journal*, 12 (1997): 105–21; L.O. Gostin and D. Webber, "The AIDS Litigation Project: HIV/AIDS in the Courts in the 1990s, Part 2," *AIDS and Public Policy Journal*, 13 (1998): 3–19.

20. S.M. Blake and E.B. Arkin, *AIDS Information Monitor: A Summary of National Public Opinion Surveys on AIDS: 1983 Through 1986* (Burlingame, California: Down There Press, 1988); E. Singer and T.F. Rogers, "Public Opinion and AIDS," *AIDS and Public Policy Journal*, 1 (1986): 1–13; T.F. Rogers, E. Singer, and J. Imperio, "AIDS: An Update," *Public Opinion Quarterly*, 57

(1993): 92–114; G.M. Herek and E.K. Glunt, "AIDS-Related Attitudes in the United States: A Preliminary Conceptualization," *The Journal of Sex Research*, 28 (1991): 99–123; Herek, *supra* note 3.

21. G.M. Herek, J.T. Capitanio, and K.F. Widaman, "HIV Related Stigma and Knowledge in the United States: Prevalence and Trends, 1991–1999," *American Journal of Public Health*, 92 (2002): 371–77, at 372–75.

22. *Id.* at 372.

23. B. Weiner, "AIDS from an Attributional Perspective," in J.B. Pryor and G.D. Reeder, eds., *The Social Psychology of HIV Infection* (Hillsdale, New Jersey: Lawrence Erlbaum, 1993): 287–302.

24. Herek, Capitanio, and Widaman, *supra* note 21, at 373.

25. D.A. Lentine et al., "HIV-Related Knowledge and Stigma—United States, 2000," *Morbidity and Mortality Weekly Report*, 49 (2000): 1062–64.

26. For more findings from the survey, see Herek, Capitanio, and Widaman, *supra* note 21. See also J.P Capitanio and G.M. Herek, "AIDS-Related Stigma and Attitudes Toward Injecting Drug Users Among Black and White Americans," *American Behavioral Scientist*, 42 (1999): 1148–61; G.M. Herek and J.P Capitanio, "AIDS Stigma and Sexual Prejudice," *American Behavioral Scientist*, 42 (1999): 1130–47.

27. In his classic analysis of stigma, for example, Goffman paid relatively little notice to how a particular characteristic or condition comes to be stigmatized in the first place, taking this to be largely a given, a part of the social structure. Instead, he focused mainly on how stigma affects face-to-face encounters.

28. E.g., Goffman, *supra* note 4; Jones et al., *supra* note 4.

29. Weiner, *supra* note 23.

30. E.g., Capitanio and Herek, *supra* note 26; Herek and Capitanio, *supra* note 26.

31. E.g., Herek and Capitanio, *supra* note 26.

32. Blake and Arkin, *supra* note 20.

33. Goffman, *supra* note 4; Jones et al., *supra* note 4.

34. Herek, *supra* note 3.

35. Herek, Capitanio, and Widaman, *supra* note 21. For analyses of how beliefs about casual contact interact with prejudice against people with HIV, see G.M. Herek, "The Social Construction of Attitudes: Functional Consensus and Divergence in the U.S. Public's Reactions to AIDS," in G.R. Maio and J.M. Olson, eds., *Why We Evaluate: Functions of Attitudes* (Mahwah, New Jersey: Lawrence Erlbaum, 2000): 325–64; G.M. Herek and J.P Capitanio, "Symbolic Prejudice or Fear of Infection? A Functional Analysis of AIDS-Related Stigma Among Heterosexual Adults," *Basic and Applied Social Psychology*, 20 (1998): 230–241; Herek and Capitanio, *supra* note 26.

36. Goffman, *supra* note 4, at 4.

37. *Id.*; Jones et al., *supra* note 4.

38. Goffman, *supra* note 4, at 28.

39. *Id.*

40. *Id.* at 4.

41. Klitzman, *supra* note 18.

42. Goffman, *supra* note 4, at 28–31.

43. C.C. Poindexter and N.L. Linsk, "HIV-Related Stigma in a Sample of HIV-Affected Older Female African American Caregivers," *Social Work*, 44 (1999): 46–61; A. van der Straten et al., "Managing HIV Among Serodiscordant Heterosexual Couples: Serostatus, Stigma and Sex," *AIDS Care*, 10 (1998): 533–48; M. Snyder, A.M. Omoto, and A.L. Crain, "Punished for Their Good Deeds: Stigmatization of AIDS Volunteers," *American Behavioral Scientist*, 42 (1999): 1175–92.

44. Herek, *supra* note 35; Herek and Capitanio, *supra* note 35; J.B. Pryor, G.D. Reeder, and S. Landau, "A Social-Psychological Analysis of HIV-Related Stigma: A Two-Factor Theory," *American Behavioral Scientist*, 42 (1999): 1193–211.

45. See generally S. Sontag, *Illness as Metaphor* (New York: Farrar, Straus and Giroux, 1978); S. Sontag, *AIDS and Its Metaphors* (New York: Farrar, Straus and Giroux, 1989).

46. Goldin, *supra* note 16; Malcolm et al., *supra* note 16; Mann, Tarantola, and Netter, *supra* note 16. Panos Institute, *supra* note 16; R. Sabatier, *Blaming Others: Prejudice, Race and Worldwide AIDS* (Philadelphia: New Society, 1988).

47. Herek, *supra* note 35; Herek and Capitanio, *supra* note 26.

48. Herek and Capitanio, *supra* note 26.

49. Capitanio and Herek, *supra* note 26; M.T. Fullilove and R.E.I. Fullilove, "Stigma as an Obstacle to AIDS Action," *American Behavioral Scientist*, 42 (1999): 1117–29.

50. For a review, see L. Brown, L. Trujillo, and K. Macintyre, *Interventions to Reduce HIV/AIDS Stigma: What Have We Learned?* (New York: Population Council, 2001).

51. The total 1999 sample included 666 respondents who were recontacted after participating in a similar 1997 survey as well as 669 new respondents. Some data from the 1999 interviews with the recontacted participants have been reported elsewhere (Herek, Capitanio, and Widaman, *supra* note 21). Respondents were included in the present analyses only if they identified themselves as heterosexual in a screening question. Because of missing data for some variables, the sample size for the correlation coefficients shown in Table 1 ranged from 1,197 to 1,258. For the regression analysis, the sample size was 1,185. Details about the sampling methods, response rates, interview procedures, and other aspects of the methodology, including the

wording of individual items, are reported in Herek, Capitanio, and Widaman, *supra* note 21; G.M. Herek, "Gender Gaps in Public Opinion About Lesbians and Gay Men," *Public Opinion Quarterly*, 66 (2002): 40–66; G.M. Herek, "Heterosexuals' Attitudes Toward Bisexual Men and Women in the United States," *Journal of Sex Research*, 39 (2002): in press.

52. This index was computed by counting the number of stigmatizing responses each person gave to nine different items designed to measure various aspects of AIDS-related stigma. The items assessed the extent to which respondents felt angry, disgusted, and afraid of people with AIDS; would avoid interacting with a person with AIDS in an office; would have their child avoid an HIV-infected schoolmate; would refrain from shopping at a neighborhood grocery store whose owner had AIDS; supported quarantining people with AIDS; believed that the names of those with AIDS should be made public; and believed that those who were infected through sex or drug use got what they deserved. More information about this measure is reported in Herek, Capitanio, and Widaman, *supra* note 21.

53. The variables listed in Table 1 were derived from a series of exploratory analyses with a larger number of variables. The variables of marital status, number of children, race, and political party affiliation displayed negligible correlations with AIDS stigma and were dropped from the analysis. A "negligible" correlation was operationally defined as $r < 0.10$ (i.e., the variable shared less than 1 percent of variance with the AIDS stigma index).

54. The coefficients can potentially range from –1.00 to +1.00, with values near zero indicating little or no association between the two variables and values near –1.00 or + 1.00 indicating a strong association. The sign of the coefficient indicates the direction of the relationship. A positive coefficient means that as values of one variable increased, values of the other also increased; a negative coefficient means that as values of one variable increased, values of the other decreased.

55. See generally T.W Adorno et al., *The Authoritarian Personality* (New York: Harper & Brothers, 1950); B. Altemeyer, *Enemies of Freedom: Understanding Right-Wing Authoritarianism* (San Francisco: Jossey-Bass, 1988).

56. A correlation coefficient less than r = 0.14 means that the variable shares only about 1 percent of its variance with AIDS stigma scores. These associations are statistically significant mainly because the sample for the survey was relatively large, but they have little substantive importance in the present analysis.

57. Like correlation coefficients, values for beta can potentially range from –1.00 to + 1.00, with values near zero indicating that the variable has little or no predictive power and values near –1.00 or +1.00 indicating that the variable helps to explain a substantial amount of variation in AIDS stigma scores. As with correlation coefficients, the sign of ß (positive or negative) indicates the direction of the relationship (see note 54, supra).

58. C.E. Rosenberg, *The Cholera Years: The United States in 1832, 1849, and 1866* (Chicago: University of Chicago Press, 1987).

59. *Id.* at 13–98.

60. *Id.* at 5, 101–225. See also C.E. Rosenberg, "Disease and Social Order in America: Perceptions and Expectations," in E. Fee and D.M. Fox, eds., *AIDS: The Burdens of History* (Berkeley: University of California Press, 1988): 12–32.

61. Herek, Capitanio, and Widaman, *supra* note 21.

62. G.M. Herek, "The HIV Epidemic and Public Attitudes Toward Lesbians and Gay Men," in M.P Levine, P. Nardi, and J. Gagnon, eds., *In Changing Times: Gay Men and Lesbians Encounter HIV/AIDS* (Chicago: University of Chicago Press, 1997): 191–218; Herek and Capitanio, *supra* note 26.

63. Herek and Capitanio, *supra* note 26, at 1140–42.

64. See generally S.B. Thomas and S.C. Quinn, "The Tuskegee Syphilis Study, 1932 to 1972: Implications for HIV Education and AIDS Risk Education Programs in the Black Community," *American Journal of Public Health*, 81 (1991): 1498–505; P.A. Turner, *I Heard It Through the Grapevine: Rumor in African-American Culture* (Berkeley: University of California Press, 1993).

65. G.M. Herek and J.P. Capitanio, "Conspiracies, Contagion, and Compassion: Trust and Public Reactions to AIDS," *AIDS Education and Prevention*, 6 (1994): 365–75, at 370–72.

66. S.W. Cole et al., "Elevated Physical Health Risk Among Gay Men Who Conceal Their Homosexual Identity," *Health Psychology*, 15 (1996): 243—51; S.W. Cole, M.E. Kemeny, and S.E. Taylor, "Social Identity and Physical Health: Accelerated HIV Progression in Rejection-Sensitive Gay Men," *Journal of Personality and Social Psychology*, 72 (1997): 320–35; G.M. Herek, "Why Tell If You're Not Asked? Self-Disclosure, Intergroup Contact, and Heterosexuals' Attitudes Toward Lesbians and Gay Men," in G.M. Herek, J. Jobe, and R. Carney, eds., *Out in Force: Sexual Orientation and the Military* (Chicago: University of Chicago Press, 1996): 197–225.

67. G.W. Allport, *The Nature of Prejudice* (Cambridge, Massachusetts: Addison-Wesley, 1954): at 261–82.

68 T.F. Pettigrew and L.R. Tropp, "Does Intergroup Contact Reduce Prejudice: Recent Meta-Analytic Findings," in S. Oskamp, ed., *Reducing Prejudice and Discrimination* (Mahwah, New Jersey: Lawrence Erlbaum, 2000): 93–114.

69. G.M. Herek and J.P. Capitanio, "'Some of My Best Friends': Intergroup Contact, Concealable Stigma, and Heterosexuals' Attitudes Toward Gay Men and Lesbians," *Personality and Social Psychology Bulletin*, 22 (1996): 412–24; G.M. Herek and E.K. Glunt, "Interpersonal Contact and Heterosexuals' Attitudes Toward Gay Men: Results from a National Survey," *Journal of Sex Research*, 30 (1993): 239–44; W. Schneider and LA. Lewis. "The Straight Story on Homosexuality and Gay Rights," *Public Opinion*, February–March 1984, at 16–20, 59–60.

70. B. Gerbert, J. Sumser, and B.T Maguire, "The Impact of Who You Know and Where You Live on Opinions About AIDS and Health Care," *Social Science and Medicine*, 32 (1991): 677–81;

K. Henry, S. Campbell, and K. Willenbring, "A Cross-Sectional Analysis of Variables Impacting on AIDS-Related Knowledge, Attitudes, and Behaviors Among Employees of a Minnesota Teaching Hospital," *AIDS Education and Prevention*, 2 (1990): 36–47; G.M. Herek and J.P Capitanio, "AIDS Stigma and Contact with Persons with AIDS: The Effects of Personal and Vicarious Contact," *Journal of Applied Social Psychology*, 27 (1997): 1–36; G.D. Zimet, "Attitudes of Teenagers Who Know Someone with AIDS," *Psychological Reports*, 70 (1992): 1169–70; G.D. Zimet et al., "Knowing Someone with AIDS: The Impact on Adolescents," *Journal of Pediatric Psychology*, 16 (1991): 287–94.

71. "From Hero to Crusader," *Newsweek*, November 18, 1991, at 69.

72. L. Montville, "Like One of the Family," *Sports Illustrated*, November 18, 1991, 44–45.

73. S.C. Kalichman et al., "Earvin 'Magic' Johnson's HIV Serostatus Disclosure: Effects on Men's Perceptions of AIDS," *Journal of Consulting and Clinical Psychology*, 61 (1993): 887–91.

74. W. Dannemeyer, *Shadow in the Land: Homosexuality in America* (San Francisco: Ignatius Press, 1989): at 217–23. Allan Brandt's study of the history of venereal disease in the United States probably offers a better model for symbolic AIDS stigma than Rosenberg's history of cholera. See A.M. Brandt, *No Magic Bullet: A Social History of Venereal Disease in the United States Since 1880* (New York: Oxford University Press, 1987).

75. Dannemeyer, *supra* note 74; P. Cameron, *Exposing the AIDS Scandal* (Lafayette, Louisiana: Huntington House, 1988). See also W.A. Bailey, "The Importance of HIV Prevention Programming to the Lesbian and Gay Community," in G.M. Herek and B. Greene, eds., *AIDS, Identity, and Community: The HIV Epidemic and Lesbians and Gay Men* (Thousand Oaks, California: Sage, 1995): 210–25.

76. M.R. Stevenson, "Promoting Tolerance for Homosexuality: An Evaluation of Intervention Strategies," *The Journal of Sex Research*, 25 (1988): 500–11; G.M. Herek, "Stigma, Prejudice, and Violence Against Lesbians and Gay Men," in J.C. Gonsiorek and J.D. Weinrich, eds., *Homosexuality: Research Implications for Public Policy* (Newbury Park, California: Sage, 1991): 60–80.

77. See generally Stevenson, *supra* note 76; Herek, *supra* note 76.

78. See *id.*

79. Herek and Capitanio, *supra* note 69.

80. Pettigrew and Tropp, *supra* note 68.

81. The stigma associated with injecting drug use is quite different from that associated with homosexuality. The American public shows growing acceptance of its gay and lesbian members and is increasingly willing to support their civil rights and liberties in many areas. Whereas homosexuality is widely considered to be irrelevant to an individual's ability to function effectively in society, injecting drug use is generally considered a social evil and IDUs are regarded very negatively. See Capitanio and Herek, *supra* note 26.

82. See generally S. Burris, "Studying the Legal Management of HIV-Related Stigma," *American Behavioral Scientist*, 42 (1999): 1229–43.

83. Burris, *supra* note 82, at 1235. Regarding ballot initiatives that would have severely curtailed the civil liberties of people with HIV, see N. Krieger and J.C. Lashof, "AIDS, Policy Analysis, and the Electorate: The Role of Schools of Public Health," *American Journal of Public Health*, 78 (1988): 411–15; G.M. Herek and E.K. Glunt, "Public Attitudes Toward AIDS-Related Issues in the United States," in J.B. Pryor and G.D. Reeder, eds., *The Social Psychology of HIV Infection* (Hillsdale, New Jersey: Lawrence Erlbaum, 1993): 229–61.

84. See, e.g., "Interventions to Prevent HIV Risk Behaviors," *NIH Consensus Statement*, 15, no. 2 (1997): 1–41; H.G. Miller, C.F. Turner, and L.E. Moses, eds., *AIDS: The Second Decade* (Washington, D.C: National Academy Press, 1990).

85. Burris, *supra* note 83; Bailey, *supra* note 75; C. Heredia, "S.F.'s HIV Fight May Be Too Sexy: Feds to Review City's Prevention Programs," *San Francisco Chronicle*, November 16, 2001, at A25; C. Ornstein, "Explicit Ads Prompt a Review of U.S. AIDS Prevention Grants," *Los Angeles Times*, January 4, 2002, at A1.

86. "Interventions to Prevent HIV Risk Behaviors," supra note 84; D.C. Des Jarlais, "Research, Politics, and Needle Exchange," *American Journal of Public Health*, 90 (2000): 1392–94.

87. For example, see S. Epstein, *Impure Science: AIDS, Activism, and the Politics of Knowledge* (Berkeley: University of California Press, 1996).

88. R.G. Parker, "Sexuality, Culture, and Power in HIV/AIDS Research," *Annual Review of Anthropology*, 30 (2001): 163–79.

89. Mann, *supra* note 1, at 3.

---

*Gregory M. Herek, Ph.D., is professor of psychology at the University of California, Davis. An internationally recognized authority on AIDS-related stigma, prejudice against lesbians and gay men, and antigay violence, he received the American Psychological Association's 1996 Award for Distinguished Contributions to Psychology in the Public Interest.

Gregory M. Herek, "Thinking about AIDS and Stigma: A Psychologist's Perspective," *The Journal of Law, Medicine and Ethics* 30, no. 4, (Winter 2002): 594–607.

DISCUSSION QUESTIONS

1. In this article Gregory Herek outlines the contours of social psychology in AIDS stigma that are based on the following three conditions: the fatality of the disease; its potential to be transmitted to others; and the assumption that contracting the disease was a result of the bearer's actions. Consequently, AIDS is likely to evoke stigma regardless of the social group affected. In the United States AIDS-related stigma is multilayered, due to its perceived association with "disliked sectors of the population." What do you think is the importance of this additional layer of stigma to the HIV and AIDS prevention efforts? Does this perception of HIV/AIDS as a disease closely associated with disliked sectors of the population exist in your country/community? What additional strategies could advocates employ to mitigate the impact of this additional layer of stigma?

2. The author distinguishes between "prejudice" and "stigma," albeit admitting that personal prejudice can be a manifestation of stigma. Is this distinction important for AIDS advocates, or does it merely serve a psycho-social purpose? Are there any other interconnections between prejudice and stigma?

3. Gregory Herek maintains that "when people are perceived to be personally responsible for having an undesirable condition, they generally are subjected to greater stigma than if their situation is perceived to be beyond their control." Do you think this is the case in your country/community? If yes, please suggest three key reasons why you think so.

4. Based on the analysis provided in Table 1, the author concludes that the following interventions can be effective in reducing AIDS-related stigma: conducting information campaigns; encouraging self-disclosure of serostatus; confronting the hostility directed toward disliked groups that have been linked with the epidemic; and enacting laws and policies that protect people living with HIV/AIDS and members of the "disliked groups" from the resulting discrimination. What are the pros and cons of each of the above-mentioned interventions for people living/affected by HIV and AIDS in your community/country? Would the above-mentioned strategies be effective on their own, or should they be integrated with other HIV/AIDS prevention, treatment and support strategies?

PART 2:
Experiences with Stigma

People living with HIV and AIDS (PLHA) in the Newly Independent States (NIS) of the former Soviet Union often face severe stigma and social alienation, evidenced by public opinion and further exacerbated by government policy. Over the past four years, Human Rights Watch issued four reports on rights violations and HIV and AIDS in the NIS.[1] These reports document numerous rights violations in Kazakhstan, Russia, and Ukraine, and provide an overview of the widespread and deep-rooted stigma against women, gay men, injection drug users, sex workers, and PLHA. Often the stigma associated with HIV is layered on top of a pre-existing negative public attitude toward traditionally marginalized populations. While more research must be conducted into stigmatization and rights violations related to HIV and AIDS in Central Asia, understanding the stigmatization and marginalization of some of the above-mentioned groups in other countries provides activists, professionals, and researchers with a glimpse into the everyday challenges these populations face.

This section offers two articles on experiences with stigma. In "Experiences of Social Discrimination Among Men Who Have Sex with Men in Shanghai, China," Jenny X. Liu and Kyung Choi report the results of a qualitative study they conducted in an attempt to characterize the experiences of "felt" and "enacted" stigma related to homosexuality in China, to identify the sources of stigma, and to describe how individuals react to instances of stigma and discrimination. They point to the importance of using the existing window of opportunity to prevent HIV- and AIDS-related stigma from firmly attaching itself to homosexuality. The authors suggest that stigma mitigation and prevention efforts among MSM should focus on creating supportive environments for this population that would encourage building social networks and boosting individual self-confidence.

In "Impact of HIV-Related Stigma on Health Behaviors and Psychological Adjustment Among HIV-Positive Men and Women," the authors discuss the impact of HIV-related stigma in the United States, analyzing the relationships between felt and enacted stigma and depression, disclosure, and sexual risk. Researchers have noted that although overt expressions of HIV- and AIDS-related discrimination has somewhat diminished over the past decade, in 2002 one in three Americans reported that he or she would actively avoid interacting with a person known to be living with HIV.[2] Perhaps the most important finding of the current study is the association of stigma with poorer treatment adherence and the impact of stigma on serostatus disclosure to sexual partners.

NOTES

1. See the following reports: "Fanning the Flames: How Human Rights Abuses Are Fueling the AIDS Epidemic in Kazakhstan" (June 2003); "Lessons Not Learned: Human Rights Abuses and HIV and AIDS in the Russian Federation" (April 2004); "Positively Abandoned: Stigma and Discrimination Against HIV-Positive Mothers and Their Children in Russia" (July 2005); "Rhetoric and Risk: Human Rights Abuses Impede Ukraine's Fight Against AIDS" (March 2006). Human Rights Watch, http://hrw.org/reports/2006/ukraine0306/ (accessed June 4, 2007).

2. G. Herek, J. Capitanio, and K. Widaman, "HIV-Related Stigma and Knowledge in the US: Prevalence and Trends, 1991–1999," *American Journal of Public Health* 92, no. 3 (2000): 371–377.

Experiences of Social Discrimination Among Men Who Have Sex with Men in Shanghai, China

by Jenny X. Liu and Kyung Choi*

Abstract

In China, men who have sex with men (MSM) are at increasingly high risk for HIV. However, prevention efforts targeting this population may be hindered because of the stigma associated with homosexuality in traditional Chinese culture. We conducted qualitative interviews with 30 MSM in Shanghai to better understand the types and sources of stigma and discrimination and how MSM respond to them. The stigma associated with homosexuality can be traced back to four culturally based factors: social status and relationships, the value of family, perceptions of immorality and abnormality, and gender stereotypes of masculinity. In particular, the centrality of the family and the importance of maintaining key relationships caused stress and anxiety, contributing to more frequent encounters with felt stigma. In response, MSM often evaded the scrutiny of family members through various tactics, even prompting some to leave their rural homes. Implications of these findings on HIV/AIDS prevention are discussed.

INTRODUCTION

Although estimates of the number of HIV infections in China have recently been reduced from 840,000 to 650,000 (CMS, 2006), the threat of a generalized epidemic still exists. While HIV/AIDS in China has been historically associated with isolated populations of intravenous drug users and former commercial blood donors, sentinel surveillance show that HIV/AIDS is beginning to spread into the general population (State Council AIDS Working Committee Office and UN Theme Group on HIV/AIDS in China [UN], 2004). Research suggests that men who have sex with men (MSM) in China may serve as a crucial bridge for HIV transmission between isolated groups and the general population. A survey of Beijing MSM revealed that 11% of participants had recent, unprotected sex with both men and women, and 85% believed that they were at little or no risk for HIV, while the rate of unprotected sexual intercourse with other men was 49% (Choi, Gibson, Han, & Guo, 2004). MSM survey in Harbin, Shenzhen, and Shenyang also had limited knowledge about HIV transmission routes and low rates of condom use (Gu, Qu, & Su, 2004; Wu, Bai, Liu, & Zhao, 2004; Zhu, Wang, Lin, & He, 2005). These factors may place MSM at high risk for HIV infection as HIV prevalence rates within these communities range from 1.0 to 3.1% (Choi, Liu, Guo, Mandel, & Rutherford, 2003; Wu et al., 2004; Zhu et al., 2005; Gu et al., 2004). In 2005, MSM accounted for 7.4% of all estimated HIV/AIDS cases in China (UN, 2006).

Despite the risk for HIV/AIDS, MSM in China may be especially difficult to reach due to existing stigma and discrimination—the "greatest barriers" to HIV/AIDS prevention according to the UN (Joint United Nations Programme on HIV/AIDS, 2002). According to the sociologist, Erving Goffman, stigma is associated with an undesirable attribute that is "deeply discrediting" and results in a "spoiled identity" that devalues the individual (1963). In China, as in other cultures around the world, homosexuality can be viewed as immoral and unacceptable as it runs counter to traditional values that emphasize lineage continuity and filial piety.

As a result, MSM in China experience rejection by family members and discrimination in employment, health care, education, housing, and other basic rights (Gill, 2002). However, outright acts of discrimination by family and other institutions represent only part of the negative consequence of stigma. According to Scambler's (1989) hidden distress model, felt stigma (shame and fear of discrimination) can prompt people to attempt to pass as a member of the non-stigmatized group to reduce the likelihood of experiencing enacted stigma (actual episodes of discrimination against people based solely on their socially unacceptable trait) (Jacoby, 1994; Scambler, 1989; Scambler & Hopkins, 1986). Therefore, even the mere perception of stigma can influence individual behavior, adding to chronic stress and detracting from physical and psychological well-being.

In terms of HIV/AIDS, however, stigma has been shown to contribute to negative self-images and low self-esteem (Herek & Capitanio, 1999; Meyer & Dean, 1998; Stokes & Peterson, 1998) and increased sexual risk behavior and/or decreased use of HIV prevention services (Diaz, Ayala, & Bein, 2004). In China, a study focusing on sexually transmitted diseases found that individuals who felt stigmatized were not only more likely to engage in with more sexual risk-taking behaviors, but also were less likely to notify spouses (Liu, Detels, Li, Ma, & Yin, 2002). A study of MSM in Beijing by Choi, Diehl, Guo, Qu, and Mandel (2002) suggests that stigma may detract from the ability of MSM to negotiate safer sex measures, and may ultimately lead to increased risk for HIV/AIDS. Moreover, current prevention efforts to reach MSM for voluntary testing have experienced setbacks as MSM may avoid seeking out health services to avoid stigma and discrimination (Jiangnan Times, 2004).

This study is aimed at gaining a greater understanding of the stigma and discrimination that MSM in China contend with so that HIV/AIDS prevention efforts could be better tailored to reach this population. The HIV/AIDS epidemic among MSM in China is only beginning to be understood and MSM were not added to China's HIV/AIDS national sentinel surveillance system until 2003 (He & Detels, 2005). To-date, only anecdotal evidence about stigma and discrimination against MSM has been reported. Because the conception of stigma is derived from social definitions of acceptable behaviors and attributes (Katz, 1979, 1981), we felt it important to research the different dimensions of stigma and discrimination facing MSM in Shanghai, China. In this qualitative study, we aimed to characterize the experiences of "felt" and "enacted" stigma related to homosexuality in China, identify the sources of stigma related to homosexuality in China, and describe how individuals react to instances of stigma and discrimination. We discuss the implications of our study findings for HIV/AIDS prevention efforts in China.

METHODS

From December 2003 to June 2004, we recruited 30 men who met three eligibility criteria: age 18 years or over, had ever had sex with a man, and was a Shanghai resident at the time. Volunteers for the Shanghai Tongzhi Hotline, which provides counseling, conducts research, and performs outreach in Shanghai's gay community, referred individuals interested in participating in this study to the research team. The study also recruited participants from MSM venues, such as bars. Four interviewers conducted in-depth interviews in Mandarin or the local Shanghainese dialect in private areas where the participant was recruited (e.g., bar, café) or at a location requested by the participant. Before each interview, participants were asked to read an information sheet that described the purpose of the study ("to identify AIDS-related concerns that tongzhi have") and the procedures outlined below. After verbal informed consent was given, interviewers asked a semi-structured series of open-ended questions following an interview guide. Individuals were asked about their migration experiences (if relevant), their life in general, social networks of friends or important individuals, venues that they frequent to meet other MSM, sexual partners, past sexual experiences, experiences with condoms, sex with women, and coming out as a MSM. Interviewers were instructed to probe for details in each of these areas and for experiences of "discrimination against being an MSM, an AIDS patient, or non-Shanghainese." Basic demographic data (birth date, occupation, education, ethnicity, and marital status) were also documented. Interviews were audio-recorded and then transcribed in Chinese. Each interview lasted an average of two hours. Each individual was offered 50 Chinese yuan ($6.50) as an incentive for participation and referrals to appropriate health and HIV prevention services were provided.

Two members of the research team who are fluent in both Chinese and English reviewed the transcriptions. For the purposes of this paper, we focused on segments of the interviews dealing with descriptions of experiences of stigma and discrimination. First, responses were coded by the type of stigma experienced and where it originated from (e.g., homosexuality, family values). Second, responses were categorized as felt stigma (referring to real or imagined fear of societal attitudes and potential discrimination arising from a particular attribute or association with a particular group or behavior) or enacted stigma (referring to the real experience of discrimination), according to definitions by Scambler (1989). Finally, drawing on Brewin's (1985) analysis of causal attributions, stigmatized participants' responses to the event (e.g., felt sorry for himself, walked away, got into an argument) were coded. All identified excerpts were then translated into English. It is important to note that text selections were interpreted from the perception of the respondent rather than the perpetrators. For example, others may have stigmatized an individual because he was not married, but from the viewpoint of the individual, he felt stigmatized because of an attribute related to homosexuality. Disagreements in coding were discussed among the coders along with a third research team member. Each coder was asked to support the identification with additional contextual evidence from the interview. Excerpts that lacked sufficient support were not included in the analysis. Coders were different members of the research team than interviewers in order to avoid interviewer recall bias.

The final set of transcription excerpts was grouped according to common themes under the three overall research aims of the study. Similar sub-categories (e.g, marriage, having children) were combined under more general categories (e.g, value of family) that encompassed the ideas expressed by interview participants. These categories were discussed amongst the three research team members, formulating precise definitions, with disagreements again requiring additional contextual support. Identified episodes were not required to be associated with a particular category if none was deemed appropriate.

RESULTS

Of the 30 participants interviewed, two were recruited from a bar frequented by MSM, another two were self-referred, and the remaining individuals were personal contacts of volunteer workers of the Shanghai Tongzhi Hotline. Nineteen respondents were aged 30 or under (mean age 29 years), while the age of all respondents ranged from 19 to 49. All but two men were ethnically Han Chinese, the dominant ethnicity in China. Five respondents were married or divorced; the remaining were single and never married. Twelve respondents were not officially registered residents of Shanghai (i.e, did not hold a Shanghai hukou—a household registration card required to access public services in urban settings). Half of all respondents had some college level education, while nine held a high school diploma, and six had not finished high school. Eight respondents were unemployed at the time of the interview, five of which were full-time college and graduate students. Twenty respondents self-identified as homosexual, seven as bisexual, and three as straight. Six participants reported being "money boys" (male sex workers).

A total of 97 descriptions of stigma and discrimination related to homophobia were documented. Each respondent reported at least one instance of stigma or discrimination related to homophobia. More instances of felt stigma than enacted stigma were noted (65 felt among 28 respondents compared with 31 enacted among 20 respondents). Respondents' experiences of stigma and discrimination could be traced to four different, but related sources: the importance of social status and relationships (36 episodes among 23 respondents), the value of family (20 episodes among 17 respondents), perceptions of immorality and abnormality (18 episodes among 14 respondents), and gender stereotypes (13 episodes among 10 respondents). In reaction to these experiences, four types of responses were documented: avoiding potentially stigmatizing situations (45 episodes among 24 respondents), rationalizing the behavior of others (32 episodes among 19 respondents), lying or pretending (12 episodes among 9 respondents), and disclosure of homosexuality (4 episodes among 4 respondents). The categories identified for sources of stigma and responses to stigma were not mutually exclusive as individuals' experiences sometimes exhibited multiple characteristics. We report on the results of each of the four sources of stigma, incorporating felt and enacted stigma and the different response types within each section.

The Importance of Social Status and Relationships

One of the primary sources of stigma related to homophobia involved the need to maintain the individual's social standing and social relationships. Many respondents experiences felt stigma that involved fear of being socially ostracized because of sexual orientation. For example, one respondent described his anxiety over how his homosexuality may affect his relationship with his parents:

> ... regarding homosexuality, it's a subject that can never be stirred ... it's like a piece of cloth, if you cut it, you can try all you want to sew it back up, but there'll always be holes. This is how it is with my parents. They certainly will not accept this. [Single, 30-year old, Shanghainese unemployed worker.]

In Chinese society, an individual's relationship to others can partially define one's identity and can also confer social status. Consequently, pressure to maintain key relationships can lead to internalized stress and constant fear, and can be especially salient in relationships with parents. Retaining the respect and trust of parents was cited as a decisive factor for not coming out, and when individuals did disclose their sexuality to others, peers, siblings, and other relatives were informed rather than parents.

While MSM may fear rejection from parents, actual social ostracism from more distant social ties could occurs.

> After I got divorced, I think my ex-wife told her family. Her family had all been very good to me [before this]. When I went to visit her family when her father fell ill ... I felt that they weren't that warm to me. Her relatives left one by one. [Divorced, 39-year old, junior high school-educated, Shanghainese clothing designer.]

Although divorce is not common in China, homosexuality was a reason for this respondent's divorce as well as an important factor in the dissolution of his social relationship with his former in-laws.

Because of the importance of maintaining good relationships, retaining one's reputation and the reputation of one's family is a corollary to preserving social respect and status. Subsequently, respondents also touched upon the need to "save face" and the social stigma attached to homosexuality that could cause one to "lose face."

> One the one hand, I worry that they won't be able to accept it. On the other, I have a sense of personal pride. If I tell them, it'll affect the way they think of me. [20-year old, high school educated, migrant Money Boy.]

Concerns over protecting one's reputation were especially common among migrants who stated that they would lose the respect of others in their native villages. Moreover, their homosexuality could also tarnish the reputations of their family and relatives within the village. Therefore, one's family could be stigmatized out of association, adding to the weight of felt stigma for MSM.

Perceptions of felt stigma influenced individuals' behavior in multiple ways. Most often, respondents indicated that they attempted to avoid potentially stigmatizing situations by either evading questions or comments even remotely related to their private sexual relations or "acting" in ways that appeared to be more respectable, such as the dilemma described here:

> When I socialize with people outside the gay circle, I really hold myself back …When going to work, it's time to be an ordinary, upright man. After work, it's another face. [Single, 44-year old, college-educated, Shanghainese business manager.]

Other respondents rationalized this type of behavior as the only way to protect against being socially ostracized, citing that society, individuals, and family members were either incapable of understanding homosexuality or unwilling to accept homosexuality.

> The people in my family … will reject this sort of thing, nor do I have the courage to test them out. [Single, 25-year old, college-educated, migrant communications salesman.]

In many cases, "coming out" was not a viable alternative as it could lead to disassociation from social groups significant to the individual. Therefore, the use of other coping strategies was essential to preserving the individual's important relationships.

Value of Family

Stigma related to homophobia also originated from the intense emphasis on creating a family, of great importance in traditional Chinese culture. Respondents recounted instances of both felt and enacted stigma related to pressures to marry and have children. For example, this respondent describes the distress he felt that centers on the individual's status as a single, male:

> ... many people will require you to get married! Such as siblings, parents, relatives, colleagues, usually this makes me fly into a rage of anger. [Single, 44-year old, college-educated Shanghainese supermarket manager.]

The practice of homosexuality was often described as being incompatible with the building of a family and viewed as a failure to fulfill the traditional male roles of son, husband, and father. The primacy of the family unit is a fundamental element in traditional Chinese culture where the continuity of one's paternal lineage is an undeniable duty for every man. Consequently, failure to fulfill one's obligations to one's parents, relatives, and ancestors can be viewed as an insult and a disgrace. Although respondents indicated that family members were among the most important people in their lives, the stigma associated with homosexuality also often came from family members. This respondent describes his mother's attitude toward his sexual orientation in an example of enacted stigma:

> She completely disagrees with it. No mother ever wishes her child to be homosexual. She, herself, got married and had a child, and wishes me to do the same. [Single, 33-year old, college-educated, human resources worker.]

This mother rejects homosexuality on the basis that it precludes the building of a family unit—a duty that she, herself, had fulfilled.

Normative expectations to fulfill family obligations such as marriage and raising a family also extended to the workplace. Respondents described situations in which they believed that their sexual orientation was under suspicion, possibly putting their jobs in jeopardy:

> If I go out and try to find a job now, people will ask me why I don't want to get married. This may make finding a job more difficult. The pressure will probably grow through the years. [Single, 33-year old, college-educated, human resources employee.]

For these men, being unmarried was perceived to lower chances of being hired and affecting work relationships. With social status so closely tied to marriage, being single was perceived as a failing.

Consequently, lying about their sexuality or habits was one way participants responded to stigma to elude suspicion.

If [my friends] ask me if I have a girlfriend, I'll always answer "yes." Lately, there's been this one girl that, if [my friends] tell me to bring a girl out, I'll ask her to make an appearance. [Single, 25-year old, college-educated, Shanghainese communications salesman.]

Other respondents lied about having girlfriends or asked women to pose as girlfriends while others excused themselves from dating or marrying because of being too busy with school or work, having physiological problems, or other life difficulties. Older married men, who reported not understanding their sexual orientation until later in life, rationalized their marriages in terms of duty to their parents and siblings. They explained that they had felt that it was "time to get married" and have a child.

Having sex with women wasn't because I wanted to. It's all because of social pressure to continue the lineage ... [Divorced, 47-year old, Shanghainese retiree.]

Given these societal expectations, many participants avoided stigmatizing situations by avoiding the topic or putting up a façade to deflect suspicions. In response to felt stigma, some respondents avoided the matter altogether by physically walking away, dropping or changing the subject, refusing to answer, or giving excuses.

When they talk about this, I just let the conversation die. If they bring up marriage or dating, I just leave, or just don't talk—that's my solution. [Single, 30-year old, Shanghainese unemployed worker.]

Respondents' attempts at evasion also reflected existing social divides and stereotypes of rural versus urban residents. Many rural migrants cited family traditions as their reason for moving to Shanghai:

If I didn't eventually get married, then I could face more and more pressure, so I left [my hometown]. [Single, 31-year old, migrant worker.]

Similarly, other respondents indicated that they preempted stigmatizing situations by avoiding going home or calling relatives. As most respondents preferred to use strategies that forestall stigma, "coming out" was an uncommon response. Only three respondents indicated that they tried to sway the views of others, only to be met with cool reception:

I told one of my cousins directly. I made a large effort to change her mind … Now she can understand it, but she still hasn't changed her attitude toward it and wishes that I could turn myself straight. [Single, 19-year old, Shanghainese college student.]

Consequently, perceptions that homosexuality lacks acceptance are realized in the negative reactions of individuals that respondents had confided in. Therefore, coping strategies that do not involve disclosure of one's status were reported as rational responses to the intense pressures associated with marriage and family. However, these tactics seemed not to prove as effective in the long-term as one respondent indicated that he would have to eventually give in to familial pressures, as disobeying parents was not a viable option for him.

PERCEPTIONS OF IMMORALITY AND ABNORMALITY

Participants' descriptions about stigma and discrimination could also be traced to popular perceptions about homosexuality as an immoral or abnormal condition. As conformity to cultural norms is highly valued, general beliefs about morality characterized anything contradicting cultural norms as abnormal or immoral. Furthermore, these constructs of what is upright behavior as opposed to "deviant" behavior are fueled by popular misconceptions about homosexuality. Respondents reported that the word "abnormal" was most commonly used by the public to describe homosexuality, relating to a defect in character of the individual:

I can feel that there's discrimination against homosexuals, as if other people were abnormal, this is what I've sensed over the years. [Married, 38-year old, migrant driver.]

Respondents rationalized popular beliefs that describe homosexuality as an "immoral" or "foul" practice as a product of Chinese philosophy and religion. Individuals cited principles of Taoism for propagating the necessity of yin-yang harmony between a man and a woman as in the following example:

The Chinese traditional ideology is about ying-yang harmony. Men with men, women with women are considered something else. [Single, 39-year old, college-educated, Shanghainese accountant.]

Furthermore, the interplay of religion and traditional values also suggested that lack of female companionship reflects some sort of "problem" with the individual, whether psychological or physical, causing abnormality to also be associated with being unmarried.

While respondents described attitudes related to immorality on the basis of felt stigma, popular misconceptions about homosexuality involved enacted stigma that reinforced beliefs that homosexuality represents a physical and mental defect. This respondent described his sister's reaction to his disclosure:

> I've told my sister … She asked me if this was a physiological problem. I said no. She then asked if it was psychological, said that I should go to see a doctor and have this problem beat back [into submission]. [Single, 25-year old, migrant, hair stylist.]

This and similar experiences of other respondents indicate that homosexuality is still perceived as a mental disease or a curable illness. Again, "coming out" is associated with negative reactions, and likely confronting the individual with charges of sexual deviancy and physical or mental conditions. Like conflicts involving family values, evading questions of morality was perceived to be necessary in certain situations. Respondents described being readily conscious of their actions and behaviors so as to conform to "normal" expectations:

> When socializing with my colleagues, I, of course, have to act very normal. [Divorced, 39-year old, junior high school-educated, Shanghainese clothing designer.]

Heightened sensitivity to the reactions of others to one's own actions and appearances kept some respondents at constant vigilance, not only among colleagues at work, but also among heterosexual friends and family and relatives.

GENDER STEREOTYPES OF MASCULINITY

Expectations to comply with established social constructs of masculinity and conform to gender stereotypes were also a source of stigma associated with homosexuality. This issue most often surfaced in relation to outward physical appearance that invited suspicion, provoked disapproval, and in some instances lead to police harassment. Respondents described a general disapproving public attitude toward men who do not act or appear to be masculine enough:

> When some of my friends outside of my gay group see my two best friends, they'll have a certain attitude, "How come your friends look like women?"… I think the way they dress themselves is rather clear. [Divorced, 39-year old, clothing designer.]

Furthermore, appearances need not be considered feminine to instigate stigmatizing comments. For example, this 33-year old respondent, who had already "come out" to his family, described his mother's reaction to meeting his friend:

> He is a very tall person ... My mom saw him and said, "This person is so tall, and yet he still acts insane." [Single, college-educated, Shanghainese human resources employee.]

Noteworthy is this mother's choice of words, using "insane" as a proxy for gay, reinforcing misconceptions of homosexuality as a psychological ailment or abnormality.

Associating with anyone or anything that is perceived to be peculiar can invite uncomfortable and probing questions, causing MSM to feel threatened. A subset of respondents blamed other MSM for contributing to the stigma of homosexuals as non-masculine by dressing or acting overly feminine:

> If a person is too feminine, then he can't be a part of my social network; he'll easily arouse suspicion. [Single, 25-year old, college-educated, Shanghainese real estate agent.]

Passing as a heterosexual can be very important as some respondents described instances where their appearances led to confrontations with police and public security officials:

> We were putting on a performance once and so we put on some women's clothes. There wasn't anything that was revealed or taken off ... someone called the police and we got arrested. We were locked up for seven days. [Single, 44-year old, college-educated Shanghainese supermarket manager.]

For these men, even engaging in seemingly innocent activities can lead to harassment as a result of violating behavior and appearance expectations. However, episodes involving police harassment were only relayed by older respondents in the study who had experienced these events at a younger age, suggesting that such police harassment may have declined in recent years.

DISCUSSION

A multitude of changes has occurred within Chinese society and culture in recent years as a result of rapid economic development and increased exposure of the country to transnational influences. Although alternative sexual identities have become more visible since the 1990s when MSM communities first began forming in large urban areas (Zhang & Chu, 2005), the experiences of social discrimination for MSM in our study indicate that same-gender sexual identities and practices are still not a part of mainstream culture in China. MSM are highly stigmatized, experiencing social discrimination from multiple people in their lives, such as family members, peers, colleagues, and employers. Even in Shanghai, a highly cosmopolitan city, MSM are feeling marginalized, experiencing forms of social discrimination that stem from tensions between traditional Chinese values and more contemporary influences.

Separate analysis of respondents' experiences of social discrimination according to Scambler's hidden distress model of felt and enacted stigma revealed that felt stigma is more prevalent in Shanghai. For the respondents in our study, their perceptions of stigmatization often related to fears that they would fail to meet their social and familial obligations. Scambler and Hopkins (1986) note that the occurrence of felt stigma can often originate from coaching by key individuals, such as parents. While this is true for many of the respondents interviewed, values of marriage, family, and familial duty are reinforced by many aspects of Chinese society as evinced by respondents' experiences of felt stigma with peers, colleagues, employers, and police.

Since Chinese social relations have traditionally been centered on the family, MSM often feared that their homosexuality would disrupt these important relationships. As obedience to one's parents and loyalty to one's family is highly valued, "coming out" was often not seen as a viable option. Instead, respondents coped with social discrimination by avoiding potentially stigmatizing situations through various elusive means, rationalizing away the attitudes of others, or hiding their activities behind lies and deception. Furthermore, family members were often characterized as being non-accepting, unable to comprehend, and misinformed about homosexuality, and thus more often a source of stress than support for MSM in China.

In addition to family, potential ostracism from other social groups, such as peers and colleagues, were also important considerations for our respondents. Since social status is defined in terms of one's relations to others in more traditional society, ostracism could damage an individual's reputation and integrity. For migrant respondents, their experiences with social discrimination indicated that the social status of their families was also at stake. Even as individual identities are emerging alongside more traditional collective identities that are centered on the family and emphasize an individual's responsibility to his family, traditional values may be stronger in rural areas. Some migrant MSM were deeply concerned about how their homosexuality would affect the social status of their families since an individual is linked to an extended family network. This was an important factor in some migrant respondents' decisions to leave their homes in the rural countryside as urban areas afforded increased anonymity and decreased intrusion into their personal affairs while preserving the integrity of their family name back home.

Even so, we find that individual identities are emerging alongside more traditional collective identities. While gender stereotypes dictate certain expectations of behavior and dress, violations of these expectations in respondents' descriptions of discrimination suggest that individuals may be expressing themselves more openly in contemporary China. The development of a personal identity, and not necessarily a homosexual one, may not wholly be accepted as anything different or strange invites comments and suspicions. Furthermore, a homosexuality identity is often misunderstood. Although homosexuality was officially de-listed as a psychological condition in 2001 by the Chinese Psychiatric Association (Chu, 2001), respondents' experiences suggest that popular misconceptions of homosexuality as a physical or mental abnormality still prevail.

Therefore, even though participants' different responses to social discrimination can be understood in terms of reducing their own exposure to discrimination, it may lead to potentially harmful behaviors that place them at increased risk for infectious diseases. Although this study does not explicitly link stigma and discrimination to risk for HIV/AIDS, evidence from other research has shown that MSM may engage in riskier sexual behavior because of stigma associated with homosexuality (Diaz et al., 2004). The use of avoidance mechanisms by MSM in this study suggests that few environments exist in which MSM feel they are able to make healthy decisions rather than feeling pressured to further hide their activities. To avoid the risk of discovery, MSM may be willing to forego safe-sex precautions, seek out health services, or be willing to accept outreach services, even if free. Given that the stigma of homosexuality is confounded with tensions between traditional Chinese culture and modern influences, public health educators will need to understand the risks associated with "coming out" in China and provide alternative coping methods for MSM and their families.

As a result, interventions will need to focus on two aspects to address the stigma facing MSM in China. First, interventions should work to create supportive environments for MSM that build social ties as well as individual self-confidence. As high levels of discrimination and low levels of conversation with family about discrimination have been associated with the highest levels of unprotected anal intercourse in other studies (Yoshikawa, Wilson, Chae, & Cheng, 2004), developing networks for social support from peers and other MSM may help reduce unsafe sex practices. These interventions can build on the importance social networks have in China and the influence that these networks may have on individuals' behaviors. Secondly, fostering safe and non-judgmental environments where MSM can openly discuss important issues and seek advice from others can help them to cope with pressures from their families, especially among migrant families. The positive effect on self-esteem of association with other similarly stigmatized persons (Crocker & Major, 1989; Jones et al., 1984; Postmes & Branscombe, 2002) can facilitate the making of health-promoting decisions (Strathde et al., 1998).

Because outreach may be especially difficult given the repressive social climate for gay men, current interventions that seek to advance HIV/AIDS awareness and disseminate information within this population will need to be sensitive to issues of stigma. Since HIV/AIDS in China has been associated more with intravenous drug use and commercial blood donation, the stigma associated with homosexuality is not automatically linked to HIV/AIDS stigma. However, as homosexuality becomes more visible and as the HIV/AIDS epidemic escalates in China, homosexuality may increasingly become associated with the disease. An opportunity exists to prevent this from occurring if HIV/AIDS interventions can be tailored to be sensitive to issues of stigma and discrimination against MSM. As shown in our study, even when an individual's homosexuality was not disclosed, enacted stigma could occur when attributes associated with homosexuality, such as being unmarried or dressing in peculiar ways, invited probing and intrusive questions. Therefore, interventions must also work to dispel misconceptions of homosexuality and stereotypes of gay men while propagating truthful and accurate HIV/AIDS information. Emphasizing awareness of HIV/AIDS among all members of the population, and not just high-risk groups, can help to sensitize individuals to issues regarding HIV/AIDS among MSM.

We recognize that our study has several limitations. The sample of men was not random and subsequently, the opinions and views expressed in the interviews may not be representative of MSM in Shanghai. Other types of stigma and discrimination may exist beyond those identified here and experiences of other individuals may differ in kind and intensity. Experiences of stigma may also differ in other parts of China as those reported here only attest to individual experiences in Shanghai. Since Shanghai is a densely populated city with increased exposure to Western influences and culture, cities elsewhere and smaller in size may be less tolerant of homosexuality. In addition, little insight is gained into stigma facing other ethnic groups in China as the men in our sample were predominately Han Chinese.

The conclusions drawn as a result of our study are intended to serve as a guide for better understanding of an issue facing HIV/AIDS prevention among MSM in China that has not been systematically documented before. To reduce investigator bias, we have taken a more descriptive approach to the presentation of results, as well as required consensus on coding and interpretation. Furthermore, because coders did not conduct actual interviews and only had access to taped recordings and transcripts, interpretation of interview responses may be limited without the benefit of nonverbal observation. All personal biases are unlikely to be wholly eliminated as the development of coding typologies is a subjective process. Further research, both qualitative and quantitative, is needed to explore this issue more in depth, as well as investigate how stigma and discrimination among MSM directly relate to HIV/AIDS risk.

Acknowledgements

We wish to thank Don Operario, Debbie Bain, and Nicolas Sheon for providing reviews of an earlier version of this paper. Their comments and suggestions were particularly insightful and constructive. In addition, we are grateful to Pierre Miege for his time and assistance in analysis and translation. This research was supported by NIMH Center Grant No. MH42459 (Center for AIDS Prevention Studies) and the Japanese Foundation for AIDS Prevention.

REFERENCES

Brewin, C. R. (1985). Depression and causal attributions: What is their relation? *Psychological Bulletin*, 98, 297–309.

China Ministry of Health (CMS), Joint United Nations Program on HIV/AIDS, and World Health Organization. (2006). *2005 update on the HIV/AIDS epidemic response in China*. Beijing, China: National Center for AIDS/STD Prevention and Control, China CDC.

Choi, K., Kumekawa, E., Dang, Q., Kegeles, S., Hays, R. B., & Stall, R. (1999). Risk and protective factors affecting sexual behavior among young Asian and Pacific Islander men who have sex with men: Implications for HIV prevention. *Journal of Sex Education and Therapy*, 24, 48–55.

Choi, K., Diehl, E., Guo, Y., Qu, S., & Mandel, J. (2002). High HIV risk but inadequate prevention services for men in China who have sex with men: an ethnographic study. *AIDS and Behavior*, 6, 3.

Choi, K., Liu, H., Guo, Y., Mandel, J. S., & Rutherford, G. W. (2003). Emerging HIV-1 epidemic in China in men who have sex with men. *The Lancet, 361*, 2125–2124.

Choi, K., Gibson, D., Han, L., & Guo, Y. (2004). High levels of unprotected sex with men and women among men who have sex with men: A potential bridge of HIV transmission in Beijing, China. *AIDS Education and Prevention, 16*, 19–30.

Chu, H. (2001, March 6). Chinese psychiatrists decide homosexuality isn't abnormal. *Los Angeles Times*, A1.

Crocker, J., & Major, B. (1989). Social stigma and self-esteem: The self-protective properties of stigma. *Psychological Review*, 96, 608–630.

Diaz, R. M., Ayala, G., & Bein, E. (2004). Sexual risk as an outcome of social oppression: Data from a probability sample of Latino gay men in three U.S. cities. *Cultural Diversity and Ethnic Minority Psychology, 10*, 255–267.

Gill, B. (2002, September 9). China's HIV/AIDS crisis: Implications for human rights, the Rule of Law and U.S.-China relations. Testimony before the Congressional-Executive Commission on China, Roundtable on HIV/AIDS.

Goffman, E. (1963). *Stigma: Notes on the management of a spoiled identity*. Englewood Cliffs, NJ: Prentice Hall.

Gu, Y., Qu, P., & Su, L. (2004). Survey of knowledge, attitude, behavior and practice related to STI/HIV among male homosexuality in Shenyang. *Chinese Journal of Public Health*, 20, 573–574.

He, N., & Detels, R. (2005). The HIV epidemic in China: history, response, and challenge. *Cell Research, 15*, 825–832.

Herek, G. M., & Capitanio, J. P. (1999). AIDS stigma and sexual prejudice. *American Behavioral Scientist, 42,* 1130–1147.

Jacoby, A. (1994). Felt versus enacted stigma: A concept revisited. *Social Science and Medicine, 38*(2), 269–274.

Jiangnan Times. (2004, February 15). Gay Clinic sees no patients on First Day. *China AIDS Info.* Available online at http://www.china-aids.org/english/News/News328.htm. Accessed on July 24, 2004.

Joint United Nations Programme on HIV/AIDS (UNAIDS). (2002). *A conceptual framework and basis for action: HIV/AIDS stigma and discrimination.* World AIDS Campaign 2002–2003. Geneva, Switzerland: UNAIDS.

Jones, E. E., Farina, A., Hastorf, A., Markus, H., Mella, D., & Scott, R. (1984). *Social stigma: The psychology of market relationship.* New York: Freeman and Company.

Katz, I. (1979). Some thoughts about the stigma notion. *Personality and Social Psychology Bulletin, 5,* 447.

Katz, I. (1981). *Stigma: A social psychological analysis.* Hillsdale, New Jersey: Erlbaum.

Liu, H., Detels, R., Li, X., Ma, E., & Yin, Y. (2002). Stigma, delayed treatment, and spousal notification among male patients with sexually transmitted disease in China. *Sexually Transmitted Diseases, 29,* 335–343.

Meyer, I. H., & Dean, L. (1998). Internalized homophobia, intimacy, and sexual behavior among gay and bisexual men. In G. M. Herek (Ed.), *Stigma and sexual orientation: Understanding prejudice against lesbians, gay men, and bisexuals* (pp. 160–186). Thousand Oaks, CA: Sage.

Postmes, T., & Branscombe, N. R. (2002). Influence of long-term racial environmental composition on subjective well-being in African Americans. *Journal of Personality and Social Psychology, 83,* 735–751.

Scambler, G. (1989). *Epilepsy.* London: Routledge.

Scambler, G., & Hopkins, A. (1986, March). Being epileptic: coming to terms with stigma. *Sociology of Health and Illness, 8,* 26–43.

State Council AIDS Working Committee Office and UN Theme Group on HIV/AIDS in China [UN]. (2004). *A joint assessment of HIV/AIDS prevention, treatment and care in China.* Beijing, China: State Council AIDS Working Committee, National Center for AIDS/STD Prevention and Control, China, UNAIDS China Office.

Stokes, J. P., & Peterson, J. L. (1998). Homophobia, self-esteem, and risk for HIV among African American men who have sex with men. *AIDS Education and Prevention, 10,* 278–292.

Strathde, S., Hogg, R., Martindale, S., Cornelisse, P., Craib, K., Montaner, J., et al. (1998). Determinants of sexual risk-taking among young HIV-negative gay and bisexual men. *Journal of Acquired Immune Deficiency Syndrome and Human Retroviruses, 19,* 61–66.

Wu, Y., Bai, L., Liu, Y., & Zhao, Z. (2004). Men who have sex with men and HIV/AIDS prevention in China. In Y. Lu & M. Essex (Eds.) *AIDS in Asia* (pp. 365–377). New York: Kluwer Academic/Plenum Publishers.

Yoshikawa, H., Wilson, P., Chae, D., & Cheng, J. (2004). Do family and friendship networks protect against the influence of discrimination on mental health and HIV risk among Asian and Pacific Islander gay men? *AIDS Education and Prevention*, 16, 84–100.

Zhang, B., & Chu, Q. (2005). MSM and HIV/AIDS in China. *Cell Research*, 15, 858–864.

Zhang, B., Liu, D., Li, X., & Hu, T. (2000). A survey of men who have sex with men: Mainland China. *American Journal of Public Health*, 90, 1949.

Zhu, T. F., Wang, C. H., Lin, P., & He, N. (2005). High risk populations and HIV-1 infection in China. *Cell Research*, 15, 852–857.

*Jenny X. Liu is with the School of Public Health, University of California, San Francisco, California.

Kyung Choi is with the Center for AIDS Prevention Studies, University of California, San Francisco, California.

J. Liu & K. Choi, "Experiences of Social Discrimination Among Men Who Have Sex With Men in Shanghai, China," *AIDS and Behavior*, published online (May 20, 2006).

Used by permission.

DISCUSSION QUESTIONS

1. Men who have sex with men (MSM) in China are difficult to reach with prevention messages due to the high levels of stigma in the society. This study surveyed 30 MSM in Shanghai and traced their experiences of stigma and discrimination to closely linked sources, including the value of family and gender stereotypes. What are the gender stereotypes that would lead to similar stigma and discrimination in your community/country? Can addressing these stereotypes have an effect on the AIDS epidemic? What is the role of family in addressing these stereotypes?

2. China's economy is growing rapidly. Can economic changes influence the society's perception of gender norms and sexuality? Is there a link between the rapidly growing economy and an increase in HIV infections?

3. In China, homosexuality is currently not automatically linked to HIV and AIDS stigma. The authors believe that this creates a window of opportunity to prevent another layer of stigma from developing toward this community. Would increased visibility of homosexuality more closely associate it with the HIV epidemic? Is preventing the development of HIV- and AIDS-related stigma possible without addressing the issues surrounding the stigma related to same-sex relationships?

Impact of HIV-Related Stigma on Health Behaviors and Psychological Adjustment Among HIV-Positive Men and Women

by Peter A. Vanable, Michael P. Carey, Donald C. Blair, and Rae A. Littlewood*

Abstract

HIV-related stigmatization remains a potent stressor for HIV-positive people. This study examined the relationships among stigma-related experiences and depression, medication adherence, serostatus disclosure, and sexual risk among 221 HIV-positive men and women. In bivariate analyses that controlled for background characteristics, stigma was associated with depressive symptoms, receiving recent psychiatric care, and greater HIV-related symptoms. Stigma was also associated with poorer adherence and more frequent serostatus disclosure to people other than sexual partners, but showed no association to sexual risk behavior. In a multivariate analysis that controlled for all correlates, depression, poor adherence, and serostatus disclosure remained as independent correlates of stigma-related experiences. Findings confirm that stigma is associated with psychological adjustment and adherence difficulties and is experienced more commonly among people who disclose their HIV status to a broad range of social contacts. Stigma should be addressed in stress management, health promotion, and medication adherence interventions for HIV-positive people.

INTRODUCTION

HIV remains a highly stigmatized illness in the United States and throughout the world. Although overt expressions of HIV-related stigma have declined in the past decade, nearly one in four Americans remain fearful of having direct contact with an HIV-positive person, and nearly one in three Americans reported that they would actively avoid interacting with a person they knew to be HIV-positive (Herek, Capitanio, and Widaman, 2002). Social discomfort, prejudice, and discrimination are experienced in response to a variety of medical and psychiatric illnesses (Angermeyer, Beck, Dietrich, and Holzinger, 2004; Rosman, 2004). However, stigmatizing attitudes and behaviors directed towards HIV-positive persons can be especially severe. HIV is highly stigmatized because of its historic association with subgroups of men and women who already experience marginalization within society, including gay men and injection drug users (Herek and Capitanio, 1999). Misinformation and fear also contribute to the persistence of HIV-related stigma. Forty percent of adults in a U.S. probability sample perceived some risk of HIV transmission through coughing, sneezing, or sharing a drinking glass, and those who were misinformed about transmission risks were also more likely to agree that persons with HIV "got what they deserved" (CDC, 2000).

Stigma directed towards HIV-positive people may perpetuate the epidemic in several ways. First, fear of being stigmatized leads some to avoid HIV testing (Chesney and Smith, 1999; Eisenman, Cunningham, Zierler, Nakazono, and Shapiro, 2003; Fortenberry et al., 2002; Stall et al., 1996). Lack of knowledge about one's serostatus may in turn lead to inadvertent transmission of the virus and delays in the initiation of treatment. Second, among those who have been tested and are HIV-positive, stigma constitutes a chronic stressor that may contribute to coping difficulties, inadequate self-care, and difficulties with safer sex negotiation and condom use.

Mental health may be jeopardized due to stigma (Major and O'Brien, 2005). Seropositive men and women are often shunned by family, friends, and intimate partners, and overt acts of discrimination in employment, health-care, and housing-related settings are not uncommon (Gostin and Webber, 1998). Further, findings from a U.S. probability sample indicate that an estimated 21% of women and 12% of MSM living with HIV have experienced physical violence since learning of their diagnosis (Zierler et al., 2000). Collectively, these stigma-related experiences may contribute to stress and adjustment difficulties among persons living with HIV (Clark, Lindner, Armistead, and Austin, 2003; Heckman et al., 2004; Lee, Kochman, and Sikkema, 2002). Indeed, findings from a two-city sample of HIV-positive men and women point to an association between internalized stigma and self-reported symptoms of depression, anxiety, and hopelessness (Lee et al., 2002).

Stigma may also interfere with health behavior adaptation and medical regimen adherence (Chesney and Smith, 1999), although few empirical studies have addressed this possibility. Experiences of social rejection, disapproval, and discrimination related to HIV may heighten a person's sense of shame regarding their illness and serve to lessen their motivation to maintain optimal health. Further, because HIV-positive men and women may respond to stigma by concealing their illness from others, concern about the consequences of inadvertent illness disclosure could interfere directly with self-care efforts. For example, lapses in adherence often occur when there is concern that an acquaintance may witness pill-taking or find pill bottles, leading to unwanted questions about a person's health and, potentially, an unexpected "outing" as being HIV-positive (Weiser et al., 2003).

Safer sexual practices may also be undermined by stigma-related experiences (Preston et al., 2004). Fear of rejection and intimate partner violence—exacerbated by past experiences of stigmatization—may lead some to hide their illness from sexual partners (Zierler et al., 2000). Similar concerns may inhibit condom use negotiation because discussions about the need for safer sex often lead to questions about a partner's serostatus. Although a few studies suggest an association between stigma and disclosure (Clark et al., 2003; van der Straten, Vernon, Knight, Gomez, and Padian, 1998), the association of stigma to condom use and negotiation has not yet been well characterized in the literature.

Several studies have begun to outline the effects of stigma on adjustment and health, and conceptual models of adjustment to HIV disease (Heckman, 2003; Schmitz and Crystal, 2000) increasingly recognize the importance of stigma. However, no study has investigated the relationship of stigma-related experiences across a broad spectrum of health behavior and coping domains among HIV-positive men and women. Therefore, in this study, we examined the role of stigma in relation to (a) current health status, (b) mental health, (c) medication adherence, and (d) sexual risk behavior, among 221 HIV-positive men and women receiving care at an infectious disease clinic. We first document the prevalence of stigma-related experiences and characterize the bivariate association of stigma-related experiences to demographic and health history variables. Next, we report results from multiple regression analyses that characterize the association of stigma to current health status, health behaviors, and mental health outcomes. We hypothesized that stigma-related experiences would be associated with poorer overall health, higher rates of depressive symptoms, decreased medication adherence, lower rates of serostatus disclosure, and higher rates of sexual risk behavior.

METHODS

Participants

Consecutive outpatients from a university-based Infectious Disease Clinic in central New York State were recruited on designated study days during a 16 month period beginning in July, 2001. A patient was eligible for the study if she or he was 18 years of age or older, HIV-positive, English speaking, and capable of providing informed consent based on medical and research staff observations.

A detailed overview of sample characteristics is provided in Table I. A total of 314 patients met eligibility criteria and were invited to participate. Among eligible participants, 76% consented to participate (N = 240). A subset of consenting participants failed to return for a scheduled interview appointment or had to leave the clinic prior to finishing their survey, yielding a final study N of 221 (44% female). Of these, 46% self-identified as White, 42% African-American, and 12% "other." The mean age of study participants was 40.4 (SD = 7.9), with 77% of participants falling between the ages of 30 and 49-years-old. Most participants were unemployed (67%) and impoverished (68% reporting incomes of less than $1000 per month). Thirty-eight percent had less than a high school diploma, 37% completed high school, and 20% had completed some college. Aggregate data from the entire clinic census (including non-participants) indicate that 38% of clinic patients were African-American, a majority (78%) were between the ages of 30–49-years-old, and 35% were female. Thus, the study sample includes a somewhat higher proportion of female patients, but is otherwise similar to the demographic profile of the clinic as a whole. Chart data indicated that 36% of participants had an undetectable viral load at their most recent clinic visit and 42% had experienced an AIDS-defining illness at the time of the interview. The average time since HIV diagnosis was 7.9 years (SD = 4.7). Among men in the sample, 65% self-identified as having previous sexual experiences with other men (not tabled). A majority of women (93%) identified as being exclusively heterosexual.

Measures

Data were obtained both by self-report and chart abstraction. The self-report battery included measures designed to assess demographics, medical history, safer sex attitudes, mental health, HIV-related stigma, sexual behavior, medication adherence, and substance use. Medical charts were reviewed for information concerning patients' current health status and attendance at clinic appointments (e.g., viral load for the most recent clinic visit, occurrence of AIDS defining illnesses).

Characteristic	(n)	(%)	M	SD
TABLE I. Sample Characteristics and Summary Statistics for Stigma, Adherence, Sexual Health, and Psychological Adjustment Variables (N = 221)				
Demographic variables				
Age (years)			40.4	7.9
Education (years)			11.7	2.2
Gender				
Male	124	56		
Female	97	44		
Ethnicity				
White	101	46		
African-American	93	42		
Other	27	12		
Currently unemployed	148	67		
Income below $1000 per month	150	68		
Stigma				
Frequency of stigma-related experiences (1–4)			1.9	0.85
Health status variables				
HIV-related symptoms (past month)			1.4	0.79
Years since HIV diagnosis			7.9	4.7
AIDS diagnosis	92	42		
Hospitalized for HIV-related illness	64	29		
Undetectable viral load (last clinic visit)	79	36		
Psychological adjustment variables				
Depressive symptoms, CES-D (0–30)			19.5	12.8
Psychiatric treatment (past year)	99	45		
Treatment adherence variables				
Medication adherence, past week (1–6)			4.6	1.3
Missed ≥ 1 clinic appointment, past year	48	22		
Sexual risk behavior and serostatus disclosure variables				
Unprotected anal/vaginal sex, 3 months	73	33		
Unprotected anal/vaginal sex with HIV-negative, or unknown serostatus partner	36	16		
Disclosure of HIV status to sexual partners (0–2)			1.6	0.68
Disclosure of HIV status, global index (0–2)			1.2	0.52

Demographic Information

Descriptive information, including age, gender, employment status, ethnicity, education, and income were assessed using standardized questions.

HIV-Related Symptoms

HIV-related symptoms were assessed using a validated self-report measure that includes both physical and cognitive symptoms associated with HIV disease (Justice et al., 2001). This questionnaire included a list of 20 common symptoms, and requires the patient to rate the degree to which each symptom has been bothersome to them within the last month on a 5-point Likert scale. An HIV symptoms score was computed based on participants' mean response across the 20 items.

Stigma-Related Experiences

This measure assessed the frequency with which specific stigma-related experiences occurred since being diagnosed with HIV. Five items drawn from previous work (Heckman, 2003; Heckman, Somlai, Kalichman, Franzoi, and Kelly, 1998) assessed the occurrence of negativity and discrimination related to being HIV-positive, including the experience of being mistreated due to being HIV-positive (e.g., "How often have you been treated badly by people because of your HIV/AIDS illness?") and the experience of social avoidance by others because of HIV (e.g., "How often do others avoid you after they learn of your HIV/AIDS status?"). Responses were rated on a 4-point frequency scale ("Never" to "Often"). A scale score was computed by averaging scores across the five items. The scale demonstrated excellent internal consistency in the current sample (alpha = 0.89).

Depressive Symptoms

Depressive symptoms were assessed using the 20-item Center for Epidemiological Studies Depression Scale (CES-D; Radloff, 1977). The CES-D has been used extensively in prior research with HIV-positive men and women (e.g., Ickovics et al., 2001; Moskowitz, 2003; Murphy et al., 2001). For the present study, a summary score on the CES-D was computed by summing the values across the 20-item measure. Coefficient alpha for the CES-D was 0.92.

Psychiatric Care

History of psychiatric treatment in the past year was assessed via a single self-report item that asked "Have you received treatment (medication or therapy) for depression, stress, or other psychological difficulties in the past year?"

Medication Adherence

Medication adherence was assessed using four-items adapted from previously validated measures (Catz, Kelly, Bogart, Benotsch, and McAuliffe, 2000; Chesney et al., 2000). Adherence difficulties were assessed based on a seven day recall period, consistent with other published reports (e.g., Heckman, Catz, Heckman, Miller, and Kalichman, 2004; Wilson, Tchetgen, and Spiegelman, 2001). Prior research confirms that a 7 day assessment interval provides a valid estimate of adherence that correlates with electronic (MEMS) monitoring data and is predictive of viral load (Arnsten et al., 2001). Participants indicated the frequency of (a) missed doses, (b) late doses, and (c) ignoring special instructions using a 6-point frequency scale ("more than once a day" to "never during the past week"). In addition, participants indicated when the last time was that they skipped taking any of their HIV medication using a 6-point frequency scale ("within the past week" to "never"). To reduce socially desirable responding, the instructions included text that normalized the fact that imperfect adherence was common and emphasized the importance of candid reporting. A summary adherence score was computed by averaging responses across the four items. The measure showed good reliability in the present sample (alpha = 0.80).

Missed Clinic Appointments

A measure of missed clinic appointments for the past year served as a second indicator of treatment adherence. Using chart data, a dichotomously coded variable was created to indicate whether participants had perfect attendance or missed one or more appointments in the previous year. Consistent attendance at medical appointments is essential for patients to fully benefit from the increasingly efficacious treatments available to them (Catz, McClure, Jones, and Brantley, 1999).

HIV Serostatus Disclosure

Fourteen items assessed the extent to which participants disclosed their HIV status, including disclosure to family, friends, sexual partners, neighbors, and heath care providers. For each item, participants were asked "To what extent have you told the following people about your HIV status?" Respondents rated each item on a three-point scale by indicating whether they had told "none of them," "some of them," or "all of them." In the present study, a global disclosure index was computed by averaging responses across the 14 items. In addition, a disclosure to sexual partners index was computed by averaging responses to two items assessing disclosure to steady and non-steady partners.

Sexual Risk Behavior

Sexual activity and condom use with steady and non-steady partners were assessed for behavior that occurred in the past three months using measures adapted from prior research (Vanable, Ostrow, McKirnan, Taywaditep, and Hope, 2000). The term "steady partner" was defined for participants as "someone you are emotionally close to and have sex with regularly." Non-steady partners were defined as "someone other than a steady partner" with whom the participant had had sex. Sexual risk behavior indices consisted of dichotomous indicators of any unprotected sex (vaginal or anal sex), and unprotected sex with an HIV-negative partner or partner of unknown serostatus during the previous three months.

Procedure

A clinic nurse informed patients about the study, and obtained verbal consent from the patient regarding his or her willingness to be introduced to a research assistant (RA). Patients who provided verbal consent were introduced to the RA, who informed the patient of the study goals and procedures. Patients were told that they would be asked to respond to questions about sexual activity, mental health, and substance use, and were informed that they would receive $10 for participation. Interested patients provided written consent.

Most participants ($n = 186$) responded to a self-administered questionnaire. To reduce survey administration difficulties related to reading difficulties (Kalichman and Rompa, 2000), data collection for low-literacy patients (those reading below the 9th grade level, $n = 35$) was completed using either an audio computer-assisted self-interview ($n = 21$; ACASI) or a face-to-face interview with an RA ($n = 14$). Interview administration was used in instances where the computer was unavailable (i.e., the assessment room was already being used).

Data Analyses

First, descriptive analyses characterize the frequency with which participants reported a range of stigma-related experiences. For descriptive purposes, items were coded as "agreed" if responses were 3 (sometimes) or 4 (often). Second, *t*-tests and chi-square analyses identify health history and demographic variables associated with stigma-related experiences. Third, a series of multiple regression analyses characterize the association of stigma history with current health status, health behaviors, and mental health functioning. To control for differences in the occurrences of stigma-related experiences related to demographic and health history differences (e.g., length of time since HIV diagnosis), background characteristics found to be associated with stigma history were entered in Step 1 of each regression analysis as covariates, followed by relevant criterion variables in Step 2. Finally, health status, health behavior, and psychological functioning variables identified as correlates of stigma history were entered simultaneously in a multiple regression analysis to characterize their independent contributions in predicting stigma history. Analyses of sexual risk behavior and serostatus disclosure to sexual partners excluded a subset of participants (*n* = 25) who were sexually inactive since learning that they were HIV-positive. Likewise, analyses involving medication adherence excluded participants who were not currently taking HAART (*n* = 42).

TABLE II. PREVALENCE OF STIGMA-RELATED EXPERIENCES AMONG HIV-POSITIVE MEN AND WOMEN [a]		
Questionnaire item	*n*	% Agreement
How often...		
... do people behave negatively toward you once they learned that you had HIV?	89	41
... have you been treated badly by people because of your HIV/AIDS illness?	65	30
... do others avoid you after they learn of your HIV/AIDS status?	64	29
... are you treated unfairly by others when they learn of your HIV/AIDS status?	63	29
... are you not invited to social events because of your HIV/AIDS status?	42	19

[a] Items were coded as "agreed" if responses were 3 (*sometimes*) or 4 (*often*).

RESULTS

Prevalence and Demographic Correlates of Stigma-Related Experiences

Stigma-related experiences were reported by a significant minority of participants in this diverse sample of HIV-positive men and women (see Table II), with agreement rates ranging from 19 to 41% across individual scale items. For example, 41% agreed that people often behaved negatively around them once they learned of their HIV status and 29% reported that people often avoid contact with them because they are HIV-positive. Stigma-related experiences were positively associated with time elapsed since HIV diagnosis ($r = 0.25$, $p < 0.01$) and occurred more frequently among participants who were currently unemployed, $t(219) = 3.06$, $p < 0.01$ and those reporting lower personal income ($r = -0.14$, $p < 0.05$). The occurrence of stigma-related experiences did not vary as a function of age, sexual orientation, gender, ethnicity, or education (all $ps > 0.15$).

Association of Stigma-Related Experiences to Current Health Status, Health Behaviors, and Psychological Adjustment

Primary study hypotheses concerning the association of stigma-related experiences to current health functioning, health behavior, and psychological adjustment were tested in a series of multiple regression analyses. Given the study's focus on the relation of stigma to current health status, health behaviors, and psychological adjustment, elapsed time since HIV diagnosis was included as a covariate to control for potential confounding effects related to differences in the length of time that participants have been living with HIV. Based on univariate findings, income and employment status were also included as covariates. Thus, years since HIV diagnosis, current income, and employment status were entered as covariates in Step 1 of each regression analysis, followed by relevant criterion variables in Step 2. Findings from Step 2 of each analysis are presented in Table III and summarized below.

Current Health Status

As hypothesized, HIV-related symptom severity emerged as a significant correlate of stigma-related experiences (see Table III). That is, patients reporting greater HIV-related symptomatology also reported more frequent stigma-related experiences. Current viral load was not associated with stigma-related experiences.

TABLE III. REGRESSION MODELS OF THE RELATIONSHIP OF STIGMA-RELATED EXPERIENCES TO HEALTH BEHAVIOR ADAPTATION AND PSYCHOLOGICAL ADJUSTMENT VARIABLES [a]

Predictor variable	β	ΔR^2	Cumulative R^2
Current health status			
Viral load (detectable vs. undetectable)	−0.07	0.01	0.10
HIV-related symptoms	0.29	0.08	0.17**
Psychological adjustment			
CES-D (depression)	0.38	0.13	0.22**
Psychiatric treatment, past year	0.18	0.03	0.12**
Treatment adherence			
HAART adherence, past week[b]	−0.24	0.06	0.16**
Clinic attendance[c]	0.17	0.03	0.12*
Safer sex and disclosure variables			
Unprotected anal/vaginal sex, 3 months (%)	0.07	0.01	0.10
Unprotected anal/vaginal sex, HIV-negative or unknown serostatus partner	0.07	0.01	0.08
Disclosure to sexual partners	0.10	0.01	0.09
Disclosure, global index	0.14	0.02	0.11*

[a]*Table summarizes the results from Step 2 of each regression analysis, with income, employment status, and time since HIV diagnosis entered at Step 1, followed by each relevant predictor variable at Step 2.*
[b]*The sample size was reduced (n = 179) for the medication adherence analysis because a subset of participants were not taking antiretroviral medications at the time of data collection. Higher scores on the adherence measure indicate better adherence.*
[c]*Clinic attendance is a dichotomous indicator of treatment adherence (100% attendance vs. <100% attendance).*
*p < 0.05; **p < 0.01

Psychological Adjustment

The hypothesized association of stigma to psychological adjustment was found for both indices of adjustment. As shown in Table III, mean scores on the CES-D were strongly related to stigmatization, indicating that participants reporting frequent stigma-related experiences were more likely to endorse items consistent with experiencing depressed mood. Similarly, psychiatric treatment in the previous year was positively associated with more frequent stigma-related experiences.

Treatment Adherence

The association of treatment adherence variables and stigma are summarized in Table III. Consistent with the hypothesis that stigma would be associated with more frequent lapses in treatment adherence, self-reported HAART adherence for the previous week emerged as a robust predictor of stigma-related experiences. Similarly, clinic attendance was significantly associated with stigma, indicating that patients who missed one or more clinic appointments in the previous year were more likely to report stigmatizing experiences.

Additional analyses were conducted to determine whether the association of missed clinic appointments to stigma was influenced by patient's current health status. Compared to patients with perfect attendance, those who missed one or more appointments in the previous year reported greater HIV-related symptomatology, $t(218) = 3.49$, $p < 0.01$, but did not differ in terms of their current viral load, $X^2(1, N = 221) = 0.16$ ns. With HIV-related symptoms and viral load included as additional covariates in the regression model, the association of missed clinic appointments to stigma was diminished, ($\beta = 0.11$, $\Delta R^2 = 0.01$, $p < 0.10$).

Sexual Risk Behavior and Serostatus Disclosure

Contrary to expectation, rates of unprotected sex (overall) and rates of unprotected sex with a partner who is HIV-negative or of unknown serostatus were not associated with stigma-related experiences. Likewise, serostatus disclosure to sexual partners was not associated with frequency report of stigmatization. Contrary to our hypothesis, stigma-related experiences were positively associated with scores on the global disclosure index that included disclosure to friends, family, co-workers, and other social contacts. That is, stigmatization was associated with higher overall rates of serostatus disclosure.

Multivariate Correlates of Stigma-Related Experiences

A final multiple regression analysis was conducted to characterize the independent associations of current health status, health behavior, and psychological adjustment variables to the occurrence of stigma-related experiences. Because medication adherence was included in the model, this analysis excluded a subset of patients who were not currently taking HAART ($N = 179$). The analysis controlled for background covariates by entering years since HIV diagnosis, current income, and employment status at Step 1, followed by inclusion of core study variables identified as bivariate correlates of stigma-related experiences in Step 2. The overall regression model was significant ($R^2 = 0.26$, $p < 0.01$). After controlling for relevant background variables, depressive symptoms ($\beta = 0.26$, $p < 0.01$), medication adherence ($\beta = -0.20$, $p < 0.01$), and serostatus disclosure (global index, $\beta = 0.15$, $p < 0.05$) remained as correlates of stigma-related experiences. Current HIV-related symptoms, psychiatric treatment status, and clinic attendance were not associated with stigma in the multivariate model (all $ps > 0.49$).

DISCUSSION

This study examined the impact of stigma-related experiences across a broad spectrum of health behavior and coping domains among HIV-positive men and women. Although a number of studies document that uninfected populations harbor stigmatizing views about persons living with HIV, this study advances the literature by characterizing the degree to which HIV-positive patients report experiencing stigma in their daily lives and by confirming that stigma contributes broadly to treatment adherence difficulties, psychological adjustment, and decisions about HIV serostatus disclosure. A substantial minority of participants reported that people behave negatively (42%), avoid being near them (29%), and exclude them from social events (20%), because of their HIV status. Although there are qualitative differences in the experience of living with HIV between men versus women (Hader, Smith, Moore, and Holmberg, 2001; Zierler et al., 2000), we found no gender differences in reporting of stigma, nor were there ethnic or age differences. Time since diagnosis was positively associated with having experienced stigmatization, as was lower personal income and employment status. Stigmatization was not associated with current viral load, but was associated with greater subjective reports of HIV-related symptoms. Such differences suggest that negativity, discomfort, and discrimination directed towards persons living with HIV may become more frequent as overt signs of illness emerge.

Results confirm that stigma contributes to psychological adjustment difficulties among HIV-positive men and women. In the multivariate analysis, current depressive symptoms emerged as a strong correlate of stigma frequency. Stigma was also associated with an increased likelihood of receiving psychiatric care in the previous year (bivariate analysis only). Although the cross-sectional design of this study precludes causal interpretations, it is reasonable to hypothesize that HIV-related stigma heightens vulnerability to depressed mood and other forms of distress rather than vice-versa. A link between stigma and poor psychological adjustment is consistent with recent empirical reports (Clark et al., 2003; Heckman et al., 2004; Lee et al., 2002) and conceptual models of adjustment to HIV disease (Heckman, 2003; Schmitz and Crystal, 2000). By increasing patients' vulnerability to depression, stigma may also effect longer term health outcomes, as depressive symptoms may further compromise immune functioning (Leonard, 2000) and contribute to more rapid progression to AIDS and mortality (Ickovics et al., 2001). Prospective studies can clarify the relationship between stigma and psychological functioning and explore the potential impact of recurrent stigmatization on disease progression.

Findings also confirm an association between stigma-related experiences and health behavior adaptation. Lapses in adherence to HAART regimens were associated with more frequent stigmatization in both the bivariate and multivariate models. Similarly, the bivariate analysis showed that patients who missed one or more HIV clinic appointments in the previous year were also more likely to report stigma-related experiences. However, the relationship between missed clinic appointments and stigma was diminished when the analysis included current health status indices as covariates. The mechanisms linking stigma to poor treatment adherence are not known. It may be that people who have experienced mistreatment in the past are less enthusiastic about seeking regular medical care, filling their prescriptions, and taking their medications because of concern about being inadvertently "outed" as HIV-positive. Alternatively, the relationship between stigma-related experiences and poor adherence may be explained by the association of stigma to decreased illness-related social support and mental health functioning. Indeed, a number of empirical reports (Catz et al., 2000; Gonzales et al., 1999) point to an association of decreased social support and depressed mood to adherence difficulties, and exploratory analyses with the present data set point to a bivariate association of CES-D scores to medication adherence ($r = -0.19$, $p < 0.05$). Thus, the association of stigma to adherence difficulties may be mediated by accompanying changes in depressed mood and social support. This hypothesis should be explored in future prospective studies.

Although the present study points to a cross-sectional association of stigma to both psychological adjustment and treatment adherence, we found no evidence of an association between stigma-related experiences and sexual risk behavior. Likewise, there was no association between stigma-related experiences and serostatus disclosure to sexual partners. Interestingly, findings from the global measure of serostatus disclosure showed that disclosure to people other than sexual partners was more rather than less common among participants reporting frequent stigma-related experiences. Although contrary to our original hypothesis, a plausible explanation is simply that frequent disclosure of HIV serostatus increases the likelihood that a person will eventually experience mistreatment and discrimination by allowing a broader range of people to be aware of a person's serostatus. Thus, avoiding serostatus disclosure may limit illness-related social support (Mansergh, Marks, and Simoni, 1995; Simoni et al., 1995), but may also lessen the likelihood that an HIV-positive person experiences overt acts of discrimination. Past experiences of discrimination may well reduce future disclosure of HIV status, an effect that is not detectable in the cross-sectional analyses presented in the present study. A prospective study would help to clarify what is likely a bidirectional relationship between disclosure decisions and stigmatization.

Strengths of this study include the fact that we report on the impact of stigma across a broad spectrum of health-related domains, using psychometrically reliable and valid measures, the inclusion of both men and women, and the use of a behaviorally oriented index of stigma-related experiences. Study limitations include the use of a cross-sectional design, sampling from a single outpatient clinic, reliance upon self-report, and our use of face-to-face interviews for a subset of low-literacy participants. In addition, our sample included a large percentage of patients with fairly advanced HIV disease. Findings may not generalize to HIV+ men and women with more recent HIV diagnoses. Future research should establish the generalizability of findings to other domestic and international samples of HIV-positive men and women and employ prospective studies that seek to clarify the mechanisms linking stigma to poor adherence, depressed mood, and decisions regarding serostatus disclosure.

Interventions to reduce the negative impact of stigma on the lives of persons living with HIV should be pursued on several fronts. First, risk reduction, adherence, and coping interventions should address HIV-positive patients' concerns about stigmatization. At a minimum, interventions should provide a supportive environment for discussing the ways in which stigma interferes with mood management, medication adherence, and sexual partner communication. Although a more daunting challenge, a second focus for intervention research is the advancement of effective strategies for reducing stigmatization at the societal level. Several small-scale interventions have been shown to be effective in reducing negativity directed towards persons living with HIV (Brown, Macintyre, and Trujillo, 2003), but many gaps remain in determining the most effective means of producing lasting change. Finally, as research continues to illuminate the social and cultural context for HIV-related stigma, public health policy, legislative initiatives, and mass media content related to HIV disease should be guided by the goal of reducing or eliminating HIV-related stigma. In the short term, this research serves to remind medical, mental health, and social service professionals that, for many HIV patients, stigma remains a barrier to adjustment and positive health outcomes.

Acknowledgments

This work was supported by the National Institute of Mental Health Grant R21-MH65865. The authors thank the staff at University Hospital for their support of this work. Special thanks are extended to Missy Albert, Linda Bartlett, Mary Beth Cavalieri, Kelley Flood, Lois Needham, Paul Preczewski, Pamela Wickham, Judy Rees, Craig Withers, Jennifer Lewis, and Jennifer Brown for their assistance.

REFERENCES

Angermeyer, M., Beck, M., Dietrich, S., and Holzinger, A. (2004). The stigma of mental illness: Patients' anticipations and experiences. *International Journal of Social Psychiatry*, 50, 153–162.

Arnsten, J. H., Demas, P. A., Farzadegan, H., Grant, R. W., Gourevitch, M. N., Chang, C. J., et al. (2001). Antiretroviral therapy adherence and viral suppression in HIV-infected drug users: Comparison of self-report and electronic monitoring. *Clinical Infectious Diseases*, 33, 1417–1423.

Brown, L., Macintyre, K., and Trujillo, L. (2003). Interventions to reduce HIV/AIDS stigma: What have we learned? *AIDS Education and Prevention*, 15, 49–69.

Catz, S. L., Kelly, J. A., Bogart, L. M., Benotsch, E. G., and McAuliffe, T. L. (2000). Patterns, correlates, and barriers to medication adherence among persons prescribed new treatments for HIV disease. *Health Psychology*, 19, 124–133.

Catz, S .L., McClure, J. B., Jones, G. N., and Brantley, P. J. (1999). Predictors of outpatient medical appointment attendance among persons with HIV. *AIDS Care*, 11, 361–373.

Centers for Disease Control and Prevention [CDC] (2000). HIV-related knowledge and stigma— United States. *Morbidity and Mortality Weekly Report*, 49, 1062–1064.

Chesney, M. A., Ickovics, J. R., Chambers, D. B., Gifford, A. L., Neidig, J., Zwickl, B., et al. (2000). Self-reported adherence to antiretroviral medications among participants in HIV clinical trials: The AACTG adherence instruments. *AIDS Care*, 12, 255–266.

Chesney, M. A., and Smith, A. W. (1999). Critical delays in HIV testing and care: The potential role of stigma. *American Behavioral Scientist*, 42, 1162–1174.

Clark, H. J., Lindner, G., Armistead, L., and Austin, B. J. (2003). Stigma, disclosure, and psychological functioning among HIV-infected and non-infected African-American women. *Women and Health*, 38, 57–71.

Eisenman, D. P., Cunningham, W. E., Zierler, S., Nakazono, T. T., and Shapiro, M. F. (2003). Effect of violence on utilization of services and access to care in persons with HIV. *Journal of General Internal Medicine*, 18, 125–127.

Fortenberry, J. D., McFarlane, M., Bleakley, A., Bull, S., Fishbein, M., Grimley, D. M., et al. (2002). Relationships of stigma and shame to gonorrhea and HIV screening. *American Journal of Public Health*, 92, 378–381.

Gonzales, V., Washienko, K. M., Krone, M. R., Chapman, L. I., Arredondo, E. M., Huckeba, H. J., et al.(1999). Sexual and drug-use risk factors for HIV and STDs: A comparison of women with and without bisexual experiences. *American Journal of Public Health*, 89, 1841–1846.

Gostin, L. O., and Webber, D. W. (1998). The AIDS Litigation Project: HIV/AIDS in the courts in the 1990s, Part 2. *AIDS Public Policy Journal*, 13, 3–19.

Hader, S. L., Smith, D. K., Moore, J. S., and Holmberg, S. D. (2001). HIV infection in women in the United States: Status at the millennium. *Journal of the American Medical Association*, 285, 1186–1192.

Heckman, B. D., Catz, S. L., Heckman, T. G., Miller, J. G., and Kalichman, S. C. (2004). Adherence to antiretroviral therapy in rural persons living with HIV disease in the United States. *AIDS Care*, 16, 219–230.

Heckman, T. G. (2003). The chronic illness quality of life (CIQOL) model: Explaining life satisfaction in people living with HIV disease. *Health Psychology*, 22, 140–147.

Heckman, T. G., Anderson, E. S., Sikkema, K. J., Kochman, A., Kalichman, S. C., and Anderson, T. (2004). Emotional distress in nonmetropolitan persons living with HIV disease enrolled in a telephone-delivered, coping improvement group intervention. *Health Psychology*, 23, 94–100.

Heckman, T. G., Somlai, A. M., Kalichman, S. C., Franzoi, S. L., and Kelly, J. A. (1998). Psychosocial differences between urban and rural people living with HIV/AIDS. *Journal of Rural Health*, 14, 138–145.

Herek, G. M., and Capitanio, J. P. (1999). AIDS stigma and sexual prejudice. *American Behavioral Scientist*, 42, 1130–1147.

Herek, G. M., Capitanio, J. P., and Widaman, K. F. (2002). HIV-related stigma and knowledge in the United States: Prevalence and trends, 1991–1999. *American Journal of Public Health, 92,* 371–377.

Ickovics, J. R., Hamburger, M. E., Vlahov, D., Schoenbaum, E. E., Schuman, P., Boland, R. J., et al. (2001). Mortality, CD4 cell count decline, and depressive symptoms among HIV-seropositive women: Longitudinal analysis from the HIV Epidemiology Research Study. *Journal of the American Medical Association, 285,* 1466–1474.

Justice, A. C., Holmes, W., Gifford, A. L., Rabeneck, L., Zackin, R., Sinclair, G., et al. (2001). Development and validation of a self-completed HIV symptom index. *Journal of Clinical Epidemiology, 54,* S77–S90.

Kalichman, S. C., and Rompa, D. (2000). Functional health literacy is associated with health status and health- related knowledge in people living with HIV-AIDS. *Journal of Acquired Immune Deficiency Syndrome, 25,* 337–344.

Lee, R. S., Kochman, A., and Sikkema, K. J. (2002). Internalized stigma among people living with HIV-AIDS. *AIDS and Behavior, 6,* 309–319.

Leonard, B. (2000). Stress, depression and the activation of the immune system. *World Journal of Biological Psychiatry, 1,* 17–25.

Major, B., and O'Brien, L. T. (2005). The social psychology of stigma. *Annual Review of Psychology, 56,* 393–421.

Mansergh, G., Marks, G., and Simoni, J. M. (1995). Self-disclosure of HIV infection among men who vary in time since seropositive diagnosis and symptomatic status. *AIDS, 9,* 639–644.

Moskowitz, J. T. (2003). Positive affect predicts lower risk of AIDS mortality. *Psychosomatic Medicine, 65,* 620–626.

Murphy, D. A., Durako, S. J., Moscicki, A. B., Vermund, S. H., Ma, Y., Schwarz, D. F., et al. (2001). No change in health risk behaviors over time among HIV infected adolescents in care: Role of psychological distress. *Journal of Adolescent Health, 29,* 57–63.

Preston, D. B., D'Augelli, A. R., Kassab, C. D., Cain, R. E., Schulze, F. W., and Starks, M. T. (2004). The influence of stigma on the sexual risk behavior of rural men who have sex with men. *AIDS Education and Prevention, 16,* 291–303.

Radloff, L. S. (1977). The CES-D Scale: A self-report depression scale for research in the general population. *Applied Psychological Measurement, 1,* 385–401.

Rosman, S. (2004). Cancer and stigma: Experience of patients with chemotherapy-induced alopecia. *Patient Education and Counseling, 52,* 333–339.

Schmitz, M. F., and Crystal, S. (2000). Social relations, coping, and psychological distress among persons with HIV/AIDS. *Journal of Applied Social Psychology, 30,* 665–683.

Simoni, J. M., Mason, H. R., Marks, G., Ruiz, M. S., Reed, D., and Richardson, J. L. (1995).

Women's self-disclosure of HIV infection: Rates, reasons, and reactions. *Journal of Consulting and Clinical Psychology, 63,* 474–478.

Stall, R., Hoff, C., Coates, T. J., Paul, J., Phillips, K. A., Ekstrand, M., et al. (1996). Decisions to get HIV tested and to accept antiretroviral therapies among gay/bisexual men: Implications for secondary prevention efforts. *Journal of Acquired Immune Deficiency Syndrome, 11,* 151–160.

Vanable, P. A., Ostrow, D. G., McKirnan, D. J., Taywaditep, K. J., and Hope, B. A. (2000). Impact of combination therapies on HIV risk perceptions and sexual risk among HIV-positive and HIV-negative gay and bisexual men. *Health Psychology, 19,* 134–145.

van der Straten, A., Vernon, K. A., Knight, K. R., Gomez, C. A., and Padian, N. S. (1998). Managing HIV among serodiscordant heterosexual couples: Serostatus, stigma and sex. *AIDS Care, 10,* 533–548.

Weiser, S., Wolfe, W., Bangsberg, D., Thior, I., Gilbert, P., Makhema, J., et al. (2003). Barriers to antiretroviral adherence for patients living with HIV infection and AIDS in Botswana. *Journal of Acquired Immune Deficiency Syndrome, 34,* 281–288.

Wilson, I. B., Tchetgen, E., and Spiegelman, D. (2001). Patterns of adherence with antiretroviral medications: An examination of between-medication differences. *Journal of Acquired Immune Deficiency Syndrome, 28,* 259–263.

Zierler, S., Cunningham, W. E., Andersen, R., Shapiro, M. F., Nakazono, T., Morton, S., et al. (2000). Violence victimization after HIV infection in a US probability sample of adult patients in primary care. *American Journal of Public Health, 90,* 208–215.

---

*Peter A. Vanable, Michael P. Carey and **Rae A. Littlewood** are with the Department of Psychology and Center for Health and Behavior, Syracuse University, Syracuse, New York.

Donald C. Blair is with the Department of Medicine, SUNY Upstate Medical University, Syracuse, New York.

P. Vanable, M. Carey, D. Blair, R. Littlewood, "Impact of HIV-Related Stigma on Health Behaviors and Psychological Adjustment Among HIV-Positive Men and Women", *AIDS and Behavior,* published online (April 08, 2006).

Used by permission.

DISCUSSION QUESTIONS

1. As was demonstrated in the previous articles, HIV- and AIDS-related stigma can have a strong impact on the effectiveness of prevention, treatment, care, and support interventions. Furthermore, the stigma also negatively affects individuals through depression, which has been linked to increased sexual risk and poor adherence to medication regiments. What interventions are needed to lessen the impact of stigma in the following settings: sexual health clinics, public schools, and AIDS treatment centers?

2. One of this study's findings is that frequent disclosure of a person's HIV status to people other than his or her sexual partners was associated with frequent stigma-related experiences and discrimination. Based on what you have learned about stigma and its consequences, what might be the potential relationship between disclosure and stigma in your community/country?

3. This study suggests that people living with HIV and AIDS might be more likely to experience discrimination as the overt signs of illness emerge. Discuss why this might be so. Do you think information and media campaigns could help prevent such discrimination?

4. Has your community/country developed interventions that aim to reduce HIV/AIDS stigma at the societal level? Do you think they are effective? If your community/country has no such interventions, suggest some that might be appropriate.

PART 3:
Stigma, Law, and Human Rights

This section addresses the relationship between stigma and the law from a human rights perspective. To be effective, laws build on existing community standards and norms, balancing out the interests of the individual and the public. But laws and policies also have the power to shape community standards and norms by punishing acts, allocating services, and providing benefits. Laws and government policies have a particular role to play in providing a successful response to the HIV and AIDS epidemic because they help shape access to resources and treatment as well as the community's response to discrimination.

The following five articles explore whether laws can be a factor in preventing or reducing the effects of stigma, and examine when and why laws can be hurdles to effective HIV prevention. The section begins with Scott Burris's overview of the relationship between law and stigma. Criminalization of HIV transmission and some types of personal behavior, such as prostitution, drug use, or sex between people of the same gender render people living with or affected by HIV and AIDS further vulnerable to discrimination from the public and the authorities. While according to UNAIDS, in 2006 84% of countries surveyed introduced equality laws, and many of them prohibited discrimination based on one's HIV/AIDS status,[1] as Burris rightly points out, legal protection against stigma is limited.

In "HIV and the Law: Integrating Law, Policy, and Social Epidemiology," Zita Lazzarini and Robert Klitzman explore the potential role of law in exacerbating an individual's vulnerability to HIV. While law can alter some conditions that render an individual extremely vulnerable to HIV—including the power to prohibit and effectively punish instances of HIV-related discrimination—it has certain limitations in addressing the wide spectrum of vulnerabilities. The practicalities of legal implementation and varied understanding of laws by different communities, as well as trust in governmental authority are among these limitations. While this article focuses specifically on the United States, some issues raised—for example, the need for policy makers to rely on evidence-based approaches when designing public health laws and policies and to address stigma and discrimination—are appropriate in Central Asia as well.

The final three articles discuss how often contradictory or outdated laws and government regulations, as well as aggressive policing, have impacted the AIDS epidemic in Kazakhstan and Russia, exacerbating existing stigma and creating an environment conducive to the spread of HIV. In "HIV/AIDS and Human Rights in Kazakhstan," Andrei Andreev describes how laws and government policies often catalyze HIV- and AIDS-related discrimination, and emphasizes the importance of effective implementation of existing laws.

Sex workers often face discrimination because of their profession, even in countries that do not prohibit sex work. In Kazakhstan, the law does not directly ban sex work, yet sex workers still remain vulnerable to rights violations or discrimination. Vera Sergunina, from the Women's Rights Center in Almaty, Kazakhstan, points out that in Kazakhstan the implementation of a law frequently contradicts the primary objective of that law, and that the absence of clear legal norms positioning sex work as a profession opens the door for rights abuses and discrimination. Inefficient policies are barriers to the effective legal protection of sex workers' rights, but the reluctance of the Kazakh government to legalize sex work, paired with the increase in HIV/AIDS and the overall stigmatization of sex workers, further increases their vulnerability to the epidemic.

Drug users represent another population that faces severe stigma and discrimination. They are often subject to numerous rights violations, especially in the countries where, until recently, drug use was a crime. "Street Policing, Injecting Drug Use and Harm Reduction in a Russian City: A Qualitative Study of Police Perspectives" surveys police attitudes toward injection drug users (IDUs) in the effort to highlight the underlying reasons for excessive policing and ongoing discrimination of IDUs in Togliatti, a city in the Samara region of Russia. The widespread portrayal of drug users as potential criminals and a source of risk, as well as overall misinformation about drug use, has contributed to aggressive street policing and pervasive IDUs surveillance that has undermined HIV and AIDS prevention efforts. The authors conclude that better police training and sensitization is needed to help Togliatti combat the AIDS crisis.

NOTE

1. As cited by Dr. Mandeep Dhaliwal, "Stigma and Discrimination: The Undoing of the Universal Access," Presentation at the XVI International AIDS Conference, Toronto, http://www.kaisernetwork.org/health_cast/hcast_index.cfm?display=detail&hc=1837 (accessed September 3, 2006).

Stigma and the Law

by Scott Burris*

There are three broad areas where law affects the operation of stigma in society. Law can be a means of preventing or remedying the enactment of stigma as violence, discrimination, or other harm; it can be a medium through which stigma is created, enforced, or disputed; and it can play a role in structuring individual resistance to stigma. For the individual with a stigmatised health condition, acceptance of society's views and self-stigmatisation may lead to concealment to avoid discrimination. But an anti-stigma activism is also possible. For many stigmatised diseases (epilepsy, for example[1]), the consequences of concealment may often be more severe than those of resistance. In both cases the individual faces status loss and discrimination, but, depending on the nature and incidence of enacted stigma, people who adopt resistance strategies may actually face less stigma, experience less social harm, and be better able to cope with any discrimination. At the same time they avoid the life-long hidden distress and unhappiness experienced by people who conceal.

LEGAL PROTECTION AGAINST THE ENACTMENT OF STIGMA

Law is most commonly seen as a tool for blunting the effects of stigma by protecting health information and prohibiting discrimination based on a health condition. Legal protection can deter harmful conduct and can provide recompense when harm has been done. But law is limited. It addresses behaviour, but does not necessarily change the attitudes that produce the behaviour. Moreover, most enacted stigma is not forbidden by law, and many of the effects of stigma will not take the form of overt acts. If a Bible company fires a salesman because he has HIV, that is discrimination under the law. But if customers refuse to deal with him, it is called choice. There is no legal protection against being ostracised by one's family, rejected by one's spouse, shunned by one's neighbours. Furthermore, in America, discrimination laws are tied to the notion of intent. In most cases, judges demand proof that a person actively disliked somebody and wanted to do harm, in order to show discrimination. That is why we continue to have glass ceilings and why we continue to have differences in earnings between women and men, and between black and white employees. Additionally, legal remedies are often not substantial or certain enough to deter the enactment of stigma or, more importantly, to reassure persons with stigmatised conditions that they can run the risk of going public or openly resisting the stigma.

Stigma is a potent form of social control precisely because it can be integrated into social structures, effecting the kind of structural discrimination described by Link and Phelan[2] (when, for example, treatment facilities for stigmatised conditions are located in poor or isolated neighbourhoods). Equally important is the fact that stigma is as often as not enforced by its victims. Their shame and guilt can result in a self-discrimination that limits life's opportunities: they avoid situations (from making friends to applying for a job) in which their secret could be discovered or in which they might experience stigma. Structural discrimination and self-stigmatisation are extremely powerful forces, not covered by law.

For law to protect civil rights, nations must also have a legal system in place that can effectively enforce rules against discrimination. Enforcement infrastructure is lacking not only in some developing countries, but also in wealthy nations like the USA, where research has shown that most disability discrimination complaints are never investigated by government enforcement agencies.[3] Even where legal systems work, marginalised populations often do not regard the legal system as a source of protection and many are priced out of the system, even when they have a meritorious claim. Law can also be part of the problem by enforcing stigma, as it has in prohibiting people with HIV from being soldiers, or preventing people with epilepsy from obtaining a driver's licence.

LAW AND THE PROPAGATION OF STIGMA

Discussion so far has focused on the proximal role of law as an instrument for dealing directly with enacted stigma. We need as well to understand the expressive role of law as it applies in the development or the undermining of stigma at the social level.

The oldest view in legal sociology, now largely rejected, is that law reflects norms; it never changes social attitudes. Law clearly is a medium to define and protect social status. It can be used deliberately to assert low status, as it was in the Helms amendment, which prohibited the portrayal of homosexuality in safe sex brochures funded by the US government.[4] Senator Jesse Helms argued that including such portrayals would send the message that the government endorsed homosexuality. Senator Helms represented a constituency who were troubled by the open emergence of homosexuality and wanted to gain the endorsement value of legislation to show that the USA officially regarded homosexual acts as bad. Opposition to the Helms Amendment was, in turn, one way to challenge the stigma, and to demonstrate that many Americans accept the equality and dignity of gay men and lesbians. In this way law was a medium for dispute about social values.

Senator Helms' use of law to promote stigma is not unusual. Indeed, law is deliberately used in public health to enforce so-called good stigma. It has been deployed, for example, to add to the stigma of smoking by forcing smokers outside, prohibiting them from lighting up at work or in public places to protect non-smokers from the harmful effects of second-hand smoke. Sensitivity to the way stigma operates, particularly through self-lacerating shame and self-discrimination, invites reflection on whether it is morally acceptable to use stigma as a means of social control, even for public-health purposes.[5]

LAW AND INDIVIDUAL RESISTANCE TO STIGMA

Finally, we need to consider how law affects the day-to-day experience of stigma at the individual level, specifically whether law affects whether individuals accept or resist a "spoiled identity," and the ways they can resist. Presumably, law can promote resistance by reducing the absolute level of bad enacted stigma ("presumably" because there are few data on how effectively law does this). Even if enacted stigma is reduced, however, people do not make decisions based on what happens, but on their perceptions of what happens. Hence the important questions include: Can law promote resistance by reducing the perceived risks of resistance and by changing self-conception? Can law facilitate activism by acting against discrimination and providing a script to guide social interactions? Can it mobilise collective action? Clearly, resistance to stigma needs to become more prominent in any thinking about how law can address the problem.

Some insights may be forthcoming from studies of the Americans with Disabilities Act. Researchers are looking at how people with disabilities integrate a new protective law into their long-term coping strategies.[6] The "disabled" label may make things worse in some ways—e.g. reinforcing separate status or victimhood. Prohibition is also permission; the Act forbids discrimination against a person with a disability who can do a job with no more than minimal changes in procedures or job environment, but therefore authorises discrimination against those who need more.

Stigma exemplifies the fact that law is more than just words on paper. "Laws on the books" are transformed in the course of implementation into social practices and attitudes that must be accounted for in any consideration of law's relation, good and bad, to stigma. The stigma research agenda thus demands greater integration of health, science, and law.

REFERENCES

1. Scambler G. Epilepsy. London: Routledge, 1989.

2. Link B, Phelan J. Conceptualizing stigma. *Annu Rev Sociol* 2001; 27: 363–85.

3. Moss K, Burris S, Ullman M, Johnsen MC, Swanson J. Unfunded mandate: an empirical study of the implementation of the Americans with Disabilities Act by the Equal Employment Opportunity Commission. *Kansas Law Rev* 2001; 50: 1–110.

4. Burris S. Education to reduce the spread of HIV. In: Burris S, Dalton HL, Miller JL, eds. AIDS law today: a new guide for the public. New Haven and London: Yale University Press 1993: 82–114.

5. Burris S. Disease stigma in US public health law. *J Law Med Ethics* 2002; 30: 179–90.

6. Engel DM, Munger FW. Rights of inclusion: law and identity in the life stories of Americans with disabilities. Chicago: University of Chicago Press, 2003.

*Scott Burris is a professor at Temple University's Beasley School of Law. He has written extensively in the areas of HIV and public health law.

Reprinted from *The Lancet*, vol. 367, Burris, S., "Stigma and the law," pp. 529–531, ©2006, with permission from Elsevier.

DISCUSSION QUESTIONS

1. Scott Burris asserts that laws have a particular role to play in the AIDS epidemic. Laws can shape access to resources, deny or allow access to treatment, and respond to discrimination. Since the beginning of the epidemic, HIV transmission has been primarily associated with individual behavior. Can laws affect personal behaviors, especially those that increase or reduce the risk of HIV and AIDS? How do laws and policies link with risk?

2. Discrimination is often the result of stigma. Does your country have laws that punish HIV- and AIDS-related discrimination? Are they effective? What is needed for laws targeting discrimination to be effective in your community/country?

3. Can laws contribute to AIDS-related stigma and discrimination by actually re-enforcing stigma? Can you think of any examples from your own community/country?

HIV and the Law: Integrating Law, Policy, and Social Epidemiology

by Zita Lazzarini and Robert Klitzman*

In the foundational piece in this issue of the journal, "Integrating Law and Social Epidemiology," Burris, Kawachi, and Sarat present a model for understanding the relationship between law and health.[1] This article uses the case of a specific health condition, the human immunodeficiency virus (HIV) infection, as an opportunity to flesh out this schema and to test how the model "fits" the world of the HIV pandemic. In applying the model to this communicable disease, we hope to illustrate the multitude of ways that laws affect the course of the pandemic as well as the course of an individual's vulnerability or resilience to the disease, and how the complexities of an individual's life dealing with the virus interface with the world of laws and legal institutions. Ultimately, we believe that in the case of HIV infection we will learn something about the nature of the connections between law and health.

We give a brief overview of the epidemiology of HIV infection that is particularly relevant from the perspective of the role of law. By epidemiology we mean both the more common analysis that focuses on geographic, risk behavior, age, gender, and temporal distribution of disease, including what we know of incidence and prevalence data, as well as social epidemiology, specifically the relationships between HIV infection and social determinants such as socioeconomic status, education, race, social cohesion, and social capital. This integrated framework sets the stage for the next step, seeking evidence of how law might act either as a pathway to disease or how it might structure the social determinants for disease that have been identified.

At its core, the HIV pandemic involves the deceptively simple act of the virus passing directly or indirectly from the body of one individual to the body of another. Laws, however, may affect many of the variables that determine when and how transmission occurs; whether condoms are used, needles are shared, blood is tested; and even whether an infected person is likely to be on effective antiretroviral treatment that may reduce his or her risk of infecting others. At a deeper level, poverty, stigma, and discrimination are associated with increased vulnerability to HIV and a wide range of laws can exacerbate or mitigate each of these social conditions.

HIV is not transmitted through the air or through casual contact. Transmission requires some intimate connection, which, once identified, should be easy to prevent. Yet, interruption of transmission has proven difficult for many reasons. At times, law and policy may be ill suited to directly interrupting HIV transmission because they often fail to address the larger social context in which the behavior takes place.

This article will consider first how laws in the United States could plausibly act as pathways, or mechanisms, by which deeper social determinants affect health, specifically HIV risk and resilience. Next, it will address the role of law in shaping those determinants themselves. For each example, we will ask the following questions: (1) how do law and policy link with risk; (2) what evidence supports this link; (3) what conclusions can we draw from the relationship between law/policy and risk; and (4) based on these conclusions, what policy options or research questions can we identify that will enhance the use of law/policy as a structural intervention.

The article does not specifically address the role of law in HIV in the developing world, where the vast majority of the estimated 40 million people currently living with HIV reside.[2]

EPIDEMIOLOGY OF HIV

Epidemiology

Acquired immunodeficiency syndrome (AIDS) was first identified in 1981. Shortly after discovery of the first cases, epidemiologists from the Centers for Disease Control and Prevention (CDC) identified the major risk factors for AIDS and issued recommendations for the prevention of sexual, drug-related, and occupational transmission of the disease.[3] The incidence of AIDS and deaths associated with AIDS increased in the United States during the 1980s, peaked in the early 1990s, and began declining in 1996 due to the effects of new antiretroviral therapies, treatments to prevent opportunistic infections, and decreases in the incidence of the HIV infection which leads to AIDS.[4] As of December 2000, 774,467 persons had been reported with AIDS in the United States, and of these 448,060 are known to have died.[5]

In the United States, AIDS primarily affects men who have sex with men and racial/ethnic minorities; minority men who have sex with men are the most affected. Although men who have sex with men make up the largest group of persons affected by HIV and AIDS, rates have increased dramatically among women and minorities since the start of the epidemic. Reported AIDS cases among women increased from approximately 8 percent of all cases in 1981 to 23 percent in 2000.[6] During the same time period, the proportion of reported AIDS cases among African-Americans increased from 25 percent to 45 percent of all cases, and among Hispanics from 14 percent to 20 percent of all cases.[7] Rates among white, non-Hispanic Americans decreased from 60 percent to 34 percent of all cases by 2000.[8]

In the period from 1988 to 1999, rates of death from AIDS were consistently associated with poverty; the lower the income for a county, the higher the rate of death.[9] In addition, death was associated with race; in 1999, rates of death among African-Americans were nearly 11 times higher than among whites.[10] Although death rates from AIDS began to decrease after 1996, this decrease was disproportionately smaller among minorities, women, and residents of poorer areas of the country. African-American women and women from southern U.S. states showed the smallest decreases in rates of death.[11]

AIDS diagnoses also decreased starting in 1993, but the rate of decrease was smallest among minorities and residents of poorer geographic areas.[12] Since 1995, AIDS diagnoses have been highest among African-Americans, who now represent almost half of all new cases. In 1999, diagnoses among the poor accounted for more than 40 percent of new cases.[13]

HIV incidence reached approximately 150,000 per year by the mid-1980s, then declined and remained level at an estimated 40,000 per year starting in 1992.[14] Approximately 900,000 Americans are now living with HIV infection.[15] Rates of new infections are highest among men who have sex with men and injection drug users (IDUs), and among African-Americans compared with other racial/ethnic groups.[16]

Since the start of the epidemic in the United States, HIV transmission has been primarily associated with behavior—high-risk sexual behaviors, including male-to-male and unprotected sex, and injection drug use. Increasingly, HIV and AIDS are linked to economic disadvantage—minority status, being female, and low income.[17]

Social Epidemiology

The patterns of disease in a society reflect its social conditions. As stated in Burris, Kawachi, and Sarat ... social epidemiology searches for "societal characteristics that promote (or inhibit) health."[18] The epidemiology of AIDS in the United States and globally gives substance to this association. Perhaps more than many other diseases, HIV is a "biologic expression of inextricably connected social experience."[19] HIV compels public health experts to examine broad social determinants of health as well as more proximal structural factors associated with health.[20]

HIV is linked with the behaviors of high-risk sex and injection drug use, and associated with societal conditions. The work of social epidemiologists illustrates the social and structural correlates and determinants of HIV. Social determinants include poverty, race, and gender, and are expressed as under- or unemployment, homelessness, poor education, racism, discrimination, gender inequality, and stigmatization. Structural factors that facilitate or inhibit infection with HIV, and progression from HIV to AIDS, may be expressed through access to economic resources, policy supports, societal attitudes, and organizational structures and functions; they may be implemented by governments, businesses, faith communities, justice systems, the media, educational systems, and other sectors that form or implement policies or procedures.[21]

Measures of disease and risk of disease by "race" appear in both epidemiology and social epidemiology, but with differing emphases. For social epidemiologists, "race" has complex meanings, since it describes a system of distinctions often relying on ideology, privilege, and politics for its continued justification.[22] Overall, "race" is considered a social construct often based on superficial physical characteristics or common heritage, but poorly supported by biologic and medical distinctions. Social epidemiological research appears to show that there is something about "race" that affects health status and risk entirely independent of the identifiable physical differences—perhaps it is best explained as the effects of "racism." Here, when we measure diseases by "race," we may actually be measuring the effects of "racism" or the negative physical consequences of discrimination and stigma over a lifetime.[23]

Social epidemiology aims to describe these broad social determinants and more proximal structural factors that influence HIV/AIDS: how they relate to the disease, and the mechanisms by which they impact the disease. The basic premise of this paper is that law both acts as a pathway for social determinants that impact HIV and helps to establish or change those social determinants themselves. Ultimately, we ask if and how laws and policy may facilitate or prevent HIV infection and AIDS among individuals.

How Does Law Act as a Pathway from Social Determinants of Health to HIV/AIDS?

One way to conceptualize the relationship between laws and HIV is to describe how social determinants act through the pathway or mechanism of law to influence HIV risk or resilience in individuals and populations. This section briefly describes a variety of ways that law might be a pathway, and then discusses a few examples at more length.

There is limited research on the mechanisms through which law impacts HIV/AIDS. Most prevention research has focused on the impact of interventions on individual behavior rather than on the role of law or policy in those interventions. However, we can identify a few areas in which research has revealed some insights into the way law works and possible ways to use law to reduce HIV risk and facilitate care and treatment for those already infected.

First, we can deduce the mechanisms through which laws affect behaviors by observing existing laws. Laws may establish programs that make health care or public health services available (e.g., HIV-testing sites); create duties for health-care providers (e.g., mandated reporting of patients with AIDS); direct health officials to use information to target services or interventions (e.g., partner notification); punish prohibited acts (e.g., criminal HIV exposure/transmission laws); interpret community norms (e.g., anti-sodomy laws); establish criteria for health education (e.g., specifying HIV-education activities); or control access to means of prevention (e.g., syringe exchange or over-the-counter sale laws). Laws appear to function by prohibiting and punishing acts (deterrence), allocating (or denying) services, shaping community standards and norms, signifying social acceptance (or disapproval), incapacitating wrongdoers, and providing benefits, among others.[24]

These mechanisms may operate proximally, as where law either does or does not require that blood products be tested for HIV and other pathogens; at an intermediate level, where law increases or decreases poor people's access to safe and stable housing; or more distally, by influencing social determinants, which in turn increase or decrease vulnerability to HIV.

Access to Treatment

Since the United States has no system to guarantee universal access to health care, ability to pay for care or entitlement to insurance through employment or other status is a necessity. For those with the fewest financial resources, the poor, uninsured, and underinsured, a complex web of laws governing eligibility to various public programs acts as one mechanism mediating the effects of low socioeconomic status on their health.

Comprehensive access to high quality care is vital for the individual well-being of persons with HIV disease. The current recommendations for HIV care involve careful monitoring of immune status, prophylactic treatment to prevent opportunistic infections, and combination antiretroviral therapy to delay or prevent progression of HIV disease to AIDS.[25] Persons with HIV who are poor, uninsured, or dependent on government insurance (Medicaid) may be less likely to receive antiretroviral treatment than those with private insurance.[26] Some studies have shown that access to treatment and health outcomes also vary by race and gender.[27] In some states, persons with HIV have to wait until they are eligible for treatment through state AIDS drug assistance programs (ADAPs). Delays may mean that damage to their immune systems has already occurred.[28] Delays in care and treatment may mean that untreated persons will develop high viral loads and will be more likely to transmit the virus to others.[29] Those who develop opportunistic infections, such as tuberculosis, pose a risk to others with HIV, to their friends and families, and to the public as a whole.[30] In the simplest sense, law, in the form of budgetary allocations and specific rules on eligibility for Medicaid and state ADAPs, may act as a pathway through which poverty can lead to restricted access to care for HIV disease. Although these programs serve the vital purpose of providing some funding for care, their limitations ensure that not all needy patients get the full range of HIV services. Because minorities with HIV depend disproportionately on Medicaid and state ADAPs, law may also act as a pathway through which race[31] can lead to poorer health care for HIV.

Law may also act as a pathway when it fails, as when the legal system does not provide remedies or promote equity. In this context, commentators have noted that very limited and ineffective legal remedies are available for claims of unfairness against Medicaid programs (e.g., claims for discrimination due to race or denial of services that match those of non-state insurance).[32] In a larger sense, having 40.4 million Americans uninsured[33] also represents a pathway through which the failure of law negatively affects health, including the health of those with HIV.

Methadone Treatment

Law can also act as a barrier to or a facilitator of public health measures. The presence or absence of laws restricting access to sterile syringes, laws permitting syringe exchange programs, and federal regulations on the prescription and use of methadone illustrate this point. Other articles in this issue[34] discuss the laws related to syringe availability at some length. Here we turn to methadone availability.

An obvious means to reduce IDUs' likelihood of contracting HIV is to stop or reduce their frequency of injection. Opiate substitutes, including methadone, have been found to be effective in reducing injections and other HIV-risk behaviors,[35] and to allow many IDUs to stabilize their lives in other ways. In the United States, while use of methadone for treatment of addiction is legal, its use for this purpose is limited to federally licensed clinics and subject to strict prescription limitations.[36] Strict regulation has resulted in a "treatment gap" of up to 600,000 persons who are addicted to opiates but not in treatment.[37]

While restrictive regulation may help decrease abuse of methadone, limitations also exacerbate the overall shortage of drug treatment opportunities for many IDUs and contribute to stigmatization of IDUs as clients of methadone clinics.[38] In this way, the law acts as a pathway for stigma, which in turn limits the number of IDUs willing to use methadone clinics and may negatively affect IDUs' attitudes toward themselves. Easing restrictions on methadone prescription and treatment could provide wider access to methadone maintenance and decrease related stigma.[39] A consensus statement of a National Institute of Health panel in 1997 recommended both loosening restrictions on the use of methadone and requiring coverage of methadone maintenance for all public and private insurance programs.[40] Such modification could "mainstream" methadone treatment, making it both more accessible and acceptable.

Drug Control Laws

Ideally, criminal law and law enforcement are tools through which society ensures public safety and health and strengthens communities by reinforcing norms of noncriminal behavior. Unfortunately, criminal law and law enforcement can act as pathways for determinants that negatively impact health. Police use of racial profiling illustrates one way in which law enforcement practices related to criminal laws act as a pathway for racism to play out in the daily experience of many African-Americans and other minorities.[41] How might such racial bias in the application of criminal laws impact HIV and HIV risk? We know that HIV and AIDS increasingly concentrate in minority communities, particularly African-American communities. (See "Epidemiology of HIV," above.) Consequently, the possible role of law, and particularly criminal law, in increasing (or decreasing) exposure to HIV for African-Americans and other minorities carries some epidemiological urgency. The design and enforcement of drug control laws in the United States is one possible means through which race and racial bias can influence health outcomes, here leading to increased HIV risk.

The evidence that U.S. drug control laws act as a mechanism for reinforcing the unequal experience of race and racism in the United States is substantial. In the last two decades, the implementation and enforcement of U.S. drug control laws has led to increased arrests and incarcerations for drugrelated offenses.[42] The United States incarcerates its population at a rate (greater than 600/100,000 population) that is second only to Russia (690/100,000 population) worldwide.[43] Most European countries have rates at or below 100/100,000 population.[44] The majority (80 percent) of growth in the U.S. federal prison population between 1985–1995 was due to drug convictions.[45] The number of women incarcerated for drug offenses grew by an astonishing 888 percent during this time, while those women incarcerated for nondrug offenses increased 129 percent.[46] These statistics demonstrate a clear national trend toward strict, incarceration-focused drug laws. When these rates are disaggregated by race and sex, however, the disparate impact emerges. In 2000, white women in the United States were incarcerated at a rate of 63/ 100,000, white men at 683/100,000, Hispanic women at 117/100,000, Hispanic men at 1,715/100,00, African-American women at 380/100,000, and African-American men at 4,777/100,000.[47]

The National Household Survey on Drug Abuse in 2000 estimated that 24.5 million Americans have used illicit drugs. Of these, 18.2 million (74 percent) were white, 2.7 million (11 percent) were African-American, and 2.4 million (10 percent) were Hispanic.[48] In other words, Americans use illegal drugs in about equal proportions to their representation in the population. Rates of arrest, conviction, and incarceration for racial minorities, however, remain significantly higher than the rates for whites. African-Americans make up 38 percent of those arrested for drug offenses and 59 percent of those convicted.[49] African-Americans serve an average federal drug sentence that is 49 percent longer than that imposed on whites.[50]

Specific drug control laws that appear racially neutral may have a disproportionate impact on minorities due to differing patterns of drug use. For example, crack cocaine has been sold predominantly in inner cities and marketed on the streets in minority neighborhoods. Mandatory sentencing guidelines impose disproportionately harsher penalties for crack versus powder cocaine, including mandatory minimum sentences for simple possession of crack, even by first-time offenders.[51] Although approximately two-thirds of crack users are white or Hispanic, in 1994, 84.5 percent of those convicted of possession of crack were African-American.[52]

As drug control laws are currently enforced, their health impact, particularly in terms of HIV risk, is particularly problematic. To the degree that arrest or incarceration results in drug users stopping drug use or entering treatment, they could have health benefits. However, drug treatment slots in prison are inadequate to the need, and drug use often continues in prison. Incarceration exposes inmates to risky sex and drug use, since condoms and clean needles are largely unavailable in prison and sex may be coerced.[53] Additionally, disruption of social networks among drug users, sex workers, and other marginalized groups can change mixing patterns for drug use and sex work, exposing more individuals to infected partners and making it more likely that drug use or sex will occur in the most high-risk settings. Disruption of networks also decreases social supports. Each of these represent ways that frequent arrests and/or prosecutions can increase HIV risk in those communities.[54]

Laws designed to prevent commercial sex work or illicit drug use may also disproportionately affect the homeless. Homelessness, like race, makes an individual more likely to be arrested under certain kinds of laws, and exposes the homeless to incarceration much more frequently than the general population. For drug- and sex-related crimes, this is at least partly because homeless persons may trade sex for money or a place to sleep or use abandoned buildings or street settings to use illegal drugs. Some local ordinances, referred to as antihomeless laws, ban camping, loitering, or panhandling, all or some of which are typically done by the homeless.[55] Many behaviors related to homelessness put people at greater risk of HIV, including elevated rates of substance abuse and mental illness, multiple sexual partners, trading sex for money or shelter, and unsafe injection practices.[56] Unfortunately, some of the laws intended to address homelessness or to prevent illegal drug use, sex work, or petty crime work only to increase the risks of the homeless.[57] (See "Housing," below.)

Of course drug control laws were intended to protect the public health and welfare by decreasing dangerous activities—the use of illegal drugs and the criminal activity that often accompanies it. Some proponents of strict drug control laws, those which emphasize incarceration of offenders, have claimed they will primarily benefit African-American communities.[58] To the degree that a policy of strict enforcement of drug laws and incarceration of offenders actually decreases drug use and related crime, and supports social organization of communities, such a policy might actually benefit minorities.[59]

From a theoretical perspective, there are at least three possible mechanisms through which these laws could work to shape individuals' behavior: deterrence, norm setting, and incapacitation. Deterrence, or an instrumentalist-based approach, suggests that individuals respond to laws based on their rational consideration of the penalties or the incentives in place to comply with the law.[60] Another approach holds that individuals respond less to the instrumental effects of laws than to their normative effects. In other words, we are more likely to obey specific laws when they comport with what we think is right, fair, or moral.[61] According to this model, our beliefs in the fairness and legitimacy of the legal system, the norms of our neighbors, how we fit into society, and how society treats us become very important. Finally, criminal law can work by incapacitating those who have violated the law (through incarceration) and thus prevent or delay subsequent violations.

Some commentators, however, worry that incarceration is unlikely to decrease drug use or make communities notably safer. They note that incarceration can only incapacitate a small proportion of active users.[62] Consequently, the possibility that tough sentences will deter individuals remains low, since the risk of arrest for any single incident of law breaking is so small.[63] Moreover, the racially disproportionate enforcement might actually increase community distrust of law enforcement and undermine community members' attitudes toward the legitimacy of law. Since studies suggest that people are less likely to obey laws they feel are unfairly applied or lack legitimacy,[64] the net effect of a policy of strict enforcement and incarceration may be to make fewer people likely to obey drug control laws.[65]

Criminal HIV Exposure/Transmission Laws

In recent years, state legislatures have devoted substantial effort to drafting and adopting HIV-specific exposure/transmission criminal provisions.[66] Twenty-seven states currently have some provision criminalizing HIV exposure or transmission, and many states have more than one provision.[67] Although these provisions have generated extensive commentary,[68] whether and how these laws actually influence behavior has not been rigorously studied.

Currently, research is underway to test a model for measuring how laws influence individual decisions to engage in risky behavior.[69] However, for this article the key question is whether these laws act as pathways for one or more social determinants or shape those determinants in some way. For example, do they contribute to stigmatization of persons with HIV or reinforce racist stereotypes? If either of these were true, the laws might have unintended health consequences, such as deterring those at risk from being tested and contributing to individual and social vulnerability in other ways.

Although we know that a substantial minority of the general public holds at least some stigmatizing attitudes toward people with HIV or AIDS,[70] we know little about the actual impact of HIV-specific exposure/transmission laws on AIDS-related stigma. We might theorize that by criminalizing otherwise legal acts (consensual sex) by a person with HIV, such laws could cast all persons with HIV as criminals in the eyes of the general public. Or, from the perspective of the person with HIV, criminalizing a normal and pleasurable part of life could alienate that individual from the rest of society. In either case, fear of being stigmatized has been associated with individual reluctance to acknowledge risk and to seek testing or other preventive and care-related services.[71]

Another issue is whether these laws are actually a mechanism for racism. As we can see from the example of drug control laws, equally important to what the law says is how vigorously it is implemented and en forced. Overall, enforcement of criminal penalties for HIV exposure appears rare. One study found only 316 distinct prosecutions over 15 years of the epidemic (1986–2001).[72] Although the investigators were not able to determine the race of all the defendants, the most notorious case in terms of media coverage involved an African-American man suspected of exposing more than forty white women and infecting thirteen of them.[73] The media coverage of the case revealed many deep-seated stereotypes related to race and sexuality.[74] Arguably then, either the law or the public attention surrounding its enforcement served as a mechanism for racism. But does this response increase or decrease HIV risk in either the African-American or white communities? Although incapacitation of individuals who continue to expose others to HIV could have a positive impact by reducing the overall risk of individuals being exposed, such risk reduction may have a high price. If enforcement of HIV-specific criminal laws magnifies or legitimizes expression of underlying racial fears, they could contribute to the larger adverse impact of race in our society.

How Does Law Shape Social Determinants of Health?

Fundamental determinants of health are distinct from specific causes of disease. This helps explain some failures of specific interventions to improve overall health status. Among groups with negative determinants of health, such as poverty, specific interventions to prevent or treat one disease may succeed, but other diseases associated with poverty might remain stable or increase. Thus, it would be erroneous to think that public health could define the perfect set of interventions to prevent HIV/AIDS without addressing fundamental determinants, and also wrong to think that interventions aimed at fundamental determinants would have an impact on only one disease. Recognizing the fundamental role of social determinants means that some interventions likely to reduce HIV risk will not necessarily appear HIV-specific. Consequently, this section shifts the focus of analysis to consider how law(s) might actually shape or restructure the environment, particularly broad social determinants of health, which in turn are important factors in HIV risk and resilience.

Social epidemiology demonstrates that in the United States elevated risk of HIV infection is associated with poverty and minority race/ethnicity. More rapid progression to AIDS and elevated AIDS death rates are associated with lower socioeconomic status, minority race/ethnicity, and female gender.[75] (See "Epidemiology" and "Social Epidemiology," above). We will examine the ways, known or proposed, that law and policy shape resources closely linked to social determinants housing and education—as well as several determinants: income inequality, race/racism, and social cohesion/human capital.

Housing

Housing could perhaps more accurately be called a resource, or an "intermediate factor," than a fundamental determinant of health. Housing, however, is closely linked to socioeconomic status, social cohesion, and other more fundamental determinants. It is also both clearly linked to HIV risk (and adherence to treatment) and shaped by law.

Even laws meant to provide housing can actually perpetuate instability, poor living conditions, and homelessness. Laws, regulations, and policies influence who, among the homeless or unstably housed, is eligible for housing. For example, the Department of Housing and Urban Development (HUD) defines a homeless person in very specific terms, and some programs exclude persons who are in substandard or crowded housing or living with friends or relatives.[76] State and federal governments provide a variety of programs to help persons who lack shelter, but in some cases individuals may be ineligible for housing supports because of behavioral problems such as drug use or criminal records.[77] Those who have recently arrived in a city may be excluded from local housing and social services because they do not meet residency requirements or because they lack necessary knowledge of local procedures for accessing services. This problem will be even greater for homeless persons, who lack neighborhood networks and sources of local information, and who must attend to housing needs before seeking other services. When these new arrivals are HIV-infected, they may delay accessing prevention and treatment services.[78]

Availability of housing influences risk of or resilience to HIV infection. This is partly because lack of housing covaries with poverty and with related behaviors such as trading sex for money and drug use.[79] Housing also offers hygiene, safety, and shelter; it supports the maintenance of nurturing relationships; and because it provides a stable mailing address, it enables access to various health and social services that help to maintain or improve health behaviors and health status. The homeless, like those infected with HIV, are often stigmatized as unproductive members of society, dangerous or unpredictable, and culpable for their situation.[80] By contrast, having housing confers some status and affirms membership in society.

Housing has a particular impact on risky behaviors leading to HIV infection, and on the status and care of persons who are infected with HIV or who have AIDS. Studies have found high rates of HIV infection and high rates of HIV risk behaviors among homeless youth,[81] among adults who are homeless,[82] and among those who are homeless and substance users and/or mentally ill.[83] In addition, research has documented that for persons with HIV, those with housing are significantly more likely to access appropriate health care and to adhere to medications than those without housing.[84]

Poverty and Income Inequality

On a global scale, the United States is far from being a poor country.[85] The benefits of our national wealth are far from equally distributed, however. Income inequality in the United States is markedly greater than in many other developed countries[86] and is worse now than 30 years ago.[87] Research has documented that it is income inequality, not absolute level of income, which is most closely associated with disparities in health.[88]

How does law help create, maintain, or change the degrees of income inequality in the United States and thus the determinants of HIV? One way that law might influence or shape income inequality is through debtor-creditor law. These laws could increase income inequality by exacerbating the problems of debt, making it more difficult for consumers to get out of debt, and promoting loss of assets by persons who temporarily lose their income. Debtor-creditor-related law may actually predispose some households to adverse health effects.[89] Studies demonstrate the relationship between low income and HIV.[90] An interesting question, unanswered by the current data, is whether debtor-creditor law has a direct effect on HIV-related risk behaviors or states (substance abuse, depression), or whether it acts more indirectly, by decreasing household income, increasing income inequality, and contributing to economic instability for those individuals and families in or near bankruptcy.

We can readily identify other types of laws that contribute to increasing income inequality. As discussed elsewhere in this issue,[91] the current tax code and modifications in the last two decades have contributed to greater income disparities in the United States. To the degree that income inequality contributes to ill health, the tax code could be viewed as having potentially negative impacts on health and HIV risk in particular.

Welfare laws also shape poverty and income inequality, yet the nature of that relationship is complex. Until 1996, welfare in the United States was a federal entitlement program providing some level of guaranteed income support to a large number of persons who were unemployed. Public support for welfare eroded as critics argued that rather than helping recipients to get out of poverty, welfare actually perpetuated dependence and reinforced the gap between the gainfully employed and those on public assistance.[92]

In 1996, Congress eliminated the federal entitlement to welfare and replaced it with a mandated job training program to be implemented at the state level. State "welfare to work" programs imposed a 5-year lifetime cap on the length of time any individual could receive benefits.[93] The goals of these reforms were to get the poor off welfare and into work, with the presumption that this would reduce poverty and dependence. In the first years of the new program, most states showed sharp declines in the number of persons receiving public benefits.[94] These years coincided, however, with the longest peacetime expansion of the U.S. economy in the twentieth century. Overall unemployment levels reached all-time lows and the availability of entry-level jobs facilitated the transition to work for many former welfare recipients. Whether "welfare to work" programs will be as successful during economic downturns remains unknown.[95] From the perspective of this article, the key question is whether such programs reduce income inequality, leave it largely untouched, or make it worse.

Previous antipoverty programs have been shown to have some positive benefits, though not directly related to health or HIV. Preschool programs, such as Head Start, that prepare poor preschoolers to enter kindergarten with the same skills as middle-class children, have been shown to increase readiness for school, enhance school performance in the early grades, and raise high school completion rates.[96] Job training programs, such as the Comprehensive Employment and Training Act (CETA), led to marked improvements in the wages of the women who participated. Yet neither Head Start nor CETA has received sustained political support (CETA was discontinued in 1982) or funding adequate to enroll all those eligible at any one time.[97]

Unfortunately, law can also interfere with programs intended to help poor men and women maintain an adequate standard of living and satisfy their basic income and nutritional needs. One section of the 1996 welfare reform act passed by Congress bars anyone convicted of a state or federal felony involving the sale or use of drugs from ever receiving cash assistance or food stamps.[98] Notably, convictions for violent crimes, including murder, do not carry the same ban on federal assistance. Currently, an estimated 92,000 women, many with children, in twenty-three states are covered by this ban.[99] This deprives women of a key source of income support, which may help them keep stable housing, provide nutritious food for their families, and avoid illegal means to supplement their incomes. Additionally, the lifetime ban seems poorly related to the overall goals of the welfare or food stamps programs.[100] To the degree that such policies increase or decrease income inequality, they may work on a much deeper level to affect the health of populations.

If we take seriously the epidemiologists' findings linking income inequality to health and to risk of specific diseases including HIV, laws that could affect income inequality and HIV risk or resilience are natural targets for potential policy change. If we know law shapes the determinant, and we know the determinant is associated with HIV risk, this information can provide us with guidance for identifying and promoting policy options.

Race and Racism

How does the law structure race and racism in this country? Since the repeal of laws that discriminated explicitly on the is of race, this question has been more difficult to answer.

The role of the law in supporting stigmatization and isolation of African-American men who have sex with men is subtle. Problems may have to do with a lack of laws or policies, or a failure to enforce them. For example, state health policies may fail to offer active and targeted prevention services to minority groups because limited resources are used for surveillance, testing, or contact tracing. School districts may not offer HIV-prevention education.[101] Policies may endanger persons in minority neighborhoods by failing to address deterioration and urban decay.[102] Health officials may fail to enforce laws against revealing the names of infected persons during contact investigations, thus contributing to mistrust of service and prevention agencies among minorities.[103]

Discrimination against African-Americans by other racial groups, and stigmatization and isolation of African-American men who have sex with men, may lead to highly risky behaviors and to sexual and drug-use mixing patterns that put young men who have sex with men in contact with partners who are likely to be infected.[104] A recent study of HIV infection among groups of young men who have sex with men who were tested between 1994 and 1996 in seven cities revealed 14 percent HIV prevalence among young African-Americans in this group, compared to 7 percent of Hispanics and 3 percent of whites.[105] The incidence rate among African-Americans was 4 percent per year compared with 1.8 percent among Hispanics and 2.4 percent among whites.[106]

Earlier this paper examined drug control laws as a mechanism or pathway for racism with impacts on health. But here we consider how these and other laws shape race and racism itself. The highly disparate impact of the enforcement of drug laws on minorities, and African-Americans in particular, and their high rates of incarceration have created a widespread perception of an association among African Americans, drug use, criminal activity, and dangerousness. This stigmatization of all African-Americans has led Tracy Meares to label incarceration as a "race-making factor." By a "race-making factor" she means "a physical construct [similar to ghettos] that sustain[s] and nourish[es] an African-American identity that is in opposition to "mainstream" American identity."[107] Not only does this stigma reinforce false stereotypes among the non-African-American population in ways that perpetuate racist attitudes (and behavior, and potential health effects), but it can also have a more profound effect. This stigma may encourage African-Americans who have neither been incarcerated nor used drugs to assume that "mainstream" American identity and values do not apply to them.

Community Social Organization

The concept of community social organization is a sociological theory of determinants of low crime rates; it bears a striking resemblance to social epidemiology's view of determinants of population levels of disease. The concept of community social organization maintains that it is the characteristics of the community, rather than its individual members, that predisposes the community to lower rates of crime, delinquency, and feelings of safety and security.[108] Factors social epidemiologists consider important, including social capital, social cohesion, education, and socioeconomic status, fit well with this model. Thus, social determinants of disease may also support characteristics of a community that contribute to stability, safety, and lower levels of crime. Ultimately, strong community social organization, to the degree that it includes improved social determinants, ought to produce better health status, including lower levels of HIV infection and a more supportive environment for those already infected.

Social Capital and Social Cohesion

Drug control laws and their enforcement negatively affect each of these determinants in a variety of ways. Because of the disenfranchisement provisions of many states' laws, approximately 13 percent of African-American men are currently unable to vote.[109] By some estimates, this proportion will grow to more than 30 percent in coming decades. Voting is a powerful measure of social participation and it is closely linked to other measures of social participation, including membership in civic groups and participation in community improvement activities.[110] Depriving such a large portion of minority residents of a key element of civic involvement decreases the social capital of everyone in the community, limits the community's voice in municipal, state, and national elections, and discourages other community-building activities. Additionally, the identity of "convict," which adheres to former prisoners, makes it difficult for them to invest in building individual social capital through education or gainful employment. Because former prisoners are not usually considered good candidates for educational opportunities, good jobs, or close relationships with other community members, they are also less able to contribute to the social capital of the community.[111]

High rates of incarceration also decrease social cohesion by disrupting social networks of families, friendships, and organized community life. For example, the Bureau of Justice Statistics indicates that 2.8 percent of all children under 18 have at least one parent incarcerated. This breaks down to 1 in 40 with an inmate father and 1 in 359 with an inmate mother.[112] One study found that "Black children (7.0 percent) were nearly 9 times more likely to have a parent in prison than white children (0.8 percent). Hispanic children (2.6 percent) were 3 times as likely as white children to have an inmate parent."[113] Incarceration of parents deprives children and adolescents of adult supervision, and when many parents in a community are incarcerated, it can drastically decrease the number of adults available to supervise children.[114] Adult supervision is one means of reducing risky behaviors by adolescents, such as smoking, alcohol and other drug use, vandalism, mischief, and petty crime.

Education and Socioeconomic Status

Incarceration is associated with a long-term decline in socioeconomic status for those who have been incarcerated.[115] These reduced prospects may be due to several factors. Being identified as a former "convict" can directly limit job opportunities,[116] since many employers will not hire someone with a criminal, especially felony, record. Conviction for a drug offense can also indirectly affect long-term earning prospects by decreasing educational opportunities, since educational level is closely associated with income and socioeconomic status. Federal law now bars students who have been convicted of a drug offense from receiving federal student loans.[117] Given the disproportionate impact of drug law enforcement, this burden falls heavily on minority young people.

Families where the father or husband is absent are closely associated with poverty,[118] so incarcerating one parent increases the likelihood that children will experience poverty.[119] Single-parent families headed by young women are also less likely to be able to send children to college. Even where children of such families are accepted to college, there may be fewer parental or family resources to help them. By limiting the educational opportunities of the next generation, incarceration of parents for drug crimes perpetuates the problems of low socioeconomic status from generation to generation.[120]

Low socioeconomic status and lower levels of education are both associated with increased HIV/AIDS risk.[121] Although not the sole factor, laws that perpetuate low socioeconomic status and limit education for those convicted of drug offenses and their children arguably shape important determinants of disease.

POTENTIAL STRUCTURAL INTERVENTIONS TO DECREASE HIV RISK

Whether and how laws actually work to influence behavior, make environments safer, and facilitate public health are important questions to those interested in HIV prevention and control. Key aspects of our public health and clinical interventions are authorized, required, permitted, funded, or shaped by laws. Laws form the foundation of public health work; they articulate the mission, set the agenda, and establish policy priorities.[122] In this section, we discuss future directions for the law as a structural intervention to reduce HIV, and the limitations to this approach.

Policy Options

Consideration of the impact of proposed laws on social determinants (such as income inequality) deserve a place in the routine analysis of public health and other policy initiatives. Much like the various "human rights impact assessments" that have been developed[123] (see also the articles by Watchirs, and O'Keefe and Scott-Samuel, in this issue[124]), such an analysis could assist in the design of policies most likely to be effective against a certain disease or health condition, while giving preference to policies that are likely to benefit social determinants.

Strengthening some laws could have an immediate impact on HIV risk and resilience. Examples include expanding laws that provide methadone as an opiate replacement or improving access to comprehensive HIV care, such as through Medicaid. In fact, provisions that would increase access to HIV thera-py have been estimated to produce net economic benefits through reduced hos-pital costs and improved retention of HIV-infected workers.[125] Increased legal emphasis on prevention and treatment of drug use might help to reduce drug-related incarcerations and associated HIV risk. In addition, eliminating manda-tory sentences and restoring discretion to judges in sentencing for all forms of drug offenses could reduce the negative effects of incarceration for many first-time or nonviolent offenders. Judges could reserve prison time for those offend-ers for whom prosecutors strongly support incapacitation.

Law might assist with much longer term approaches to HIV prevention by influencing underlying social determinants, such as the level of community social organization or access to important resources such as education and housing. For example, city planning that seeks to promote mixed housing with access to public transportation and employment for all economic class-es and races might reverse some of the concentrating effects that urban, innercity communities are having on the HIV/AIDS epidemic. Changes in the drug control laws and law enforcement practices could help to decrease stigmatization of minorities as dangerous drug users, and reduce disruption of social networks, loss of social cohesion, and diminution of social capital that flows from labeling so many community members as "drug felons" or "con-victs." Changes in laws that restrict the access of ex-prisoners to education-al loans, public assistance, food stamps, or public housing would promote access to important resources that are closely linked to improving social determinants.

Efforts to change fundamental determinants might seem frustratingly slow and indirect in the face of a serious epidemic like HIV/AIDS. However, these interventions can be coupled with those that will have more immediate effects, especially where those effects are tailored to supporting social systems. Meares describes this approach to building community social organizations in commu-nities with high levels of drug abuse and related crime. In contrast to some social scientists who discuss only interventions aimed at poverty and aspects of social organization, she emphasizes the importance of including law enforce-ment in any effort to decrease the harms of drug abuse.[126] She writes that polic-ing ought to promote a sense of safety among community members, encourage civic participation, and build trust among neighbors and between the commu-nity and law enforcement.[127]

Possible Limitations of Law as a Structural Intervention

Whether and how laws are implemented and enforced will have an impact on their ultimate efficacy. For example, some laws may seek to regulate behavior that is so private or so intimate that the law proves a poor tool for change. Commentators have noted that sodomy, adultery, and fornication have all been prohibited at times, but few claim the laws were effective in abating the behaviors.[128] Other laws, including those criminalizing HIV exposure/transmission, are so rarely enforced that their practical importance may be questioned.[129]

Individuals and communities also understand laws differently, depending on their knowledge, familiarity with the legal system, and trust in governmental authority. Empirical studies reveal that many people harbor misperceptions about laws, including those related to HIV.[130] Where laws are perceived as illegitimate, they may be less likely to shape behavior, norms, or a sense of engagement in the process of disease prevention and health promotion.[131]

Policymaking

Although both medicine and public health increasingly rely on "evidence-based" approaches, public health laws and policies are not subjected to similar scrutiny. This absence is apparent both in the occasional failures of policymakers to rely on sound science in making policy, and in the general dearth of literature empirically evaluating the impact of public health laws, regulations, or policies. Specific to HIV interventions, a national conference convened at the National Institutes of Health (NIH) in 1997 to look at interventions to prevent HIV risk behaviors concluded that "the gap between science and public policy is frightening."[132] This gap between science and policy may persist if legislators lack adequate access to scientific information or must consider competing policy priorities. However, the nature of the law and the legal system itself may also contribute to this gap. Scientists and lawyers often speak different languages. Public health officials, medical clinicians, and behavioral scientists speak in terms of "probability," "risk," and "associations" between behaviors and disease; whereas lawyers use terms such as "proof," "guilt," "innocence," "right," and "wrong." In fact, one commentator notes that, in addition to a general disregard for empirical research, the law and lawmakers exhibit a very low level of understanding of human behavior. The law is, he states, "every bit as sociologically impoverished as it is psychologically impoverished."[133]

Where lawmakers are reluctant to use science and scientists rarely study the empirical effects of laws, our knowledge of the impact of laws on health is limited. This poses a serious problem. If we as a society impose burdens on health agencies to provide services, track cases, and provide interventions, and we demand that individuals change intimate and/or pleasurable behaviors and sometimes punish them if they fail to do so, then we ought to know that the law works to produce its desired outcomes and minimizes unintended negative consequences.

CONCLUSION

Although previous research has often described or analyzed areas of law related to HIV prevention and control, considering law's role as a pathway or shaper of social determinants is somewhat new. This article reviews evidence from the scientific and legal literature on the potential role of law in relation to social determinants and illustrates an approach to integrating law and social epidemiology. We also hope that it has identified specific areas of HIV law and policy ripe for additional research, reform, or intervention.

Existing research suggests that law affects HIV risk and resilience at many levels, in many situations, both directly and indirectly, and that it does so through a rich variety of mechanisms. Understanding these effects and their mechanisms in more detail will allow policymakers, if they choose to rely on the research, to shape policy in a more positive way. Much more research is needed to clarify both effects and mechanisms at all levels. Policymaking, because it happens in the political arena, will inevitably be influenced by non-scientific considerations. Providing sound research is probably only one part of the solution. Another facet may be to consider whether health policy can be made more responsive to scientific information.

HIV serves as a rich case study. Nationally and globally, HIV is concentrated among the marginalized who face prior stigma and discrimination and also bear a disproportionate burden of other diseases. HIV-related policy and law may act as sensitive indicators of both population vulnerability and society's responsiveness to public health needs precisely because HIV so heavily affects marginalized groups. To the degree that law and policy can alter the equation of vulnerability and of risk and resilience, they promise to be key public health interventions.

Acknowledgments

Work on this article was supported in part by CDC Grant No. R62/CCR317863, "A Structural Analysis of the Role of Law and Human Rights in Preventing HIV," and by a grant from the American Foundation for AIDS Research, "Health, Law and Human Rights: Exploring the Connections." The opinions and information expressed in the article are those of the authors and not of the Centers for Disease Control and Prevention or of the American Foundation for AIDS Research. The authors would like to acknowledge Esther Sumartojo, Ph.D., for her work on the project and her significant contributions to the article. We would also like to acknowledge research assistance from Lorilyn Rosales, Jennifer McSweeney, Amy Hozer, and Jonathan von Kohorn. Thank you to Theo Ungewitter for her assistance in preparation of the manuscript.

NOTES

1. S. Burris, I. Kawachi, and A. Sarat, "Integrating Law and Social Epidemiology," *Journal of Law, Medicine & Ethics*, 30, no. 4 (2002): 510–21.

2. Centers for Disease Control and Prevention, *AIDS Epidemic Update—December 2001*, UNAIDS, available at <http://www.unaids.org/epidemic_update/report dec01/index.html>.

3. Centers for Disease Control and Prevention, "HIV and AIDS—United States 1981–2000," *Morbidity Mortality Weekly Reports*, 50, no. 21 (2001): 430–34.

4. Centers for Disease Control and Prevention, "U.S. HIV and AIDS Cases Reported Through June 2001," *HIV/AIDS Surveillance Report*, 13, no. 1 (2001): 1–36.

5. Centers for Disease Control and Prevention, *HIV/AIDS Surveillance Report*, 12, no. 2 (2000): at 5.

6. Centers for Disease Control and Prevention, *supra* note 3, at 431 (Table 1).

7. *Id.*

8. See Centers for Disease Control and Prevention, *supra* note 2.

9. J.M. Karon et al., "HIV in the United States at the Turn of the Century: An Epidemic in Transition," *American Journal of Public Health*, 91 (2001): 1060–68.

10. *Id.*

11. *Id*

12. *Id.*

13. *Id.*

14. See Centers for Disease Control and Prevention, *supra* note 2.

15. Centers for Disease Control and Prevention, "World AIDS Day—December 1, 2000," *Morbidity Mortality Weekly Reports*, 49, no. 47 (2000): 1061.

16. See Centers for Disease Control and Prevention, *supra* note 2.

17. *Id.*

18. Burris, Kawachi, and Sarat, *supra* note 1, at 511.

19. S. Zierler and N. Krieger, "Reframing Women's Risk: Social Inequalities and HIV Infection," *Annual Review of Public Health*, 18 (1997): 401–36, at 425.

20. E. Sumartojo and M. Laga, eds., "Structural Factors in HIV Prevention," AIDS, 14, suppl. 1 (2000): S1–S72.

21. E. Sumartojo, "Structural Factors in HIV Prevention: Concepts, Examples, and Implications for Research," *AIDS*, 14, suppl. 1 (2000): S3–S10.

22. N. Krieger, "A Glossary for Social Epidemiology," *Journal of Epidemiology and Community Health*, 55 (2001): 693–700.

23. N. Krieger, "Discrimination and Health," in L. Berkman and I. Kawachi, eds., *Social Epidemiology* (New York: Oxford University Press, 2000): 36–75.

24. S. Burris, "Introduction: Merging Law, Human Rights, and Social Epidemiology," *Journal of Law, Medicine & Ethics*, 30, no. 4 (2002): 498–509.

25. United States Public Health Service, *Guidelines for the Use of Antiretroviral Agents in HIV-Infected Adults and Adolescents* (February 4, 2002), available at <http://www.hivatis.org/guidelines/ adult/May23_02/AAMay23.pdf>; *2001 USPHS/IDSA Guidelines for the Prevention of Opportunistic Infections in Persons Infected with HIV* (November 28, 2001), available at <http:// www.hivatis.org/guidelines/other/Ols/OIGNov27.pdf>.

26. J. Levi and J. Dates, "HIV: Challenging the Health Care Delivery System," *American Journal of Public Health*, 90, no. 7 (2000): 1033–36.

27. B.D. Smedley, A.Y Stith, and A.R. Nelson, eds., *Unequal Treatment: Confronting Racial and Ethnic Disparities in Health Care* (Washington D.C.: National Academy Press, 2002): at 5 (summarizes findings of studies showing unequal access by race to HIV care [African-Americans receive less and lower quality care than whites], and negative impact on survival rates); R.D. Moore et al., "Racial Differences in the Use of Drug Therapy for HIV Disease in an Urban Community," *N. Engl. J. Med.*, 330, no. 11 (1994): 763–68; M.F. Shapiro et al., "Variations in the Care of HIV-Infected Adults in the United States: Results from the HIV Cost and Services Utilization Study," *JAMA*, 281 (1999): 2305–15 (negative impact on sur-

vival for African-Americans); C.L. Bennett et al., "Racial Differences in Care Among Hospitalized Patients with Pneumocystis Carinii Pneumonia in Chicago, New York, Los Angeles, Miami, and Raleigh-Durham," *Archives of Internal Medicine*, 155, no. 15 (1995): 1586–92; K.H. Anderson and J.M. Mitchell, "Differential Access in the Receipt of Antiretroviral Drugs for the Treatment of AIDS and Its Implications for Survival," *Archives of Internal Medicine*, 160, no. 20 (2000): 3114–20.

28. L. DeSimione, "Guaranteeing Treatment Access," GMHC *Treat Issues*, 13, no. 4 (April 1999): 10–11.

29. M.A. Pedraza et al., "Heterosexual Transmission of HIV1 Is Associated with High Plasma Viral Load Levels and a Positive Viral Isolation in the Infected Partner," *Journal of Acquired Immune Deficiency Syndrome*, 21, no. 2 (June 1, 1999): 120–25; H. Chakraborty et al., "Viral Burden in Genital Secretions Determines Male-to-Female Sexual Transmission of HIV-1: A Probabilistic Empiric Model," *AIDS*, 15, no. 5 (March 30, 2001): 621–27; M. Hisada et al., "Virus Load and Risk of Heterosexual Transmission of Human Immunodeficiency Virus and Hepatitis C Virus by Men with Hemophilia. The Multicenter Hemophilia Cohort Study," *Journal of Infectious Disease*, 181, no. 4 (April 2000): 1475–78.

30. Centers for Disease Control and Prevention, "Prevention and Treatment of Tuberculosis Among Patients Infected with Human Immunodeficiency Virus: Principles of Therapy and Revised Recommendations," *Morbidity and Mortality Weekly Reports*, 47, no. RR-20 (1998): 1–58.

31. Smedley, Stith, and Nelson, *supra* note 27, at 5, and other studies cited in note 27 above.

32. S.D. Watson, "Race, Ethnicity and Quality of Care: Inequalities and Incentives," *American Journal of Law & Medicine*, 27 (2001): 203–24, at 217–20.

33. *Coalition Forms to Reverse Rising Trend of Uninsured Americans*, Out of Many, One; Seniors USA (February 9, 2002) (reporting estimates of at least 40.4 million uninsured as of January 31, 2002, with approximately 2 million having lost insurance during the preceding 13 months), at <http://senrs.com/coalition_forms_to_reverse_rising_trend_of_uninsured_americans.htm>.

34. Burris, Kawachi, and Sarat, *supra* note 1; Kim M. Blankenship and S. Koester, "Criminal Law, Policing Policy, and HIV Risk in Female Street Sex Workers and Injection Drug Users," *Journal of Law, Medicine & Ethics*, 30, no. 4 (2002): 548–59.

35. R.L. Hubbard et al., "Treatment Outcome Prospective Study (TOPS): Client Characteristics and Behaviors Before, During and After Treatment," in F.M. Tims and J.P Ludford, eds., *Drug Abuse Treatment Evaluation Strategies Progress and Prospects* (Rockville, Maryland: National Institute on Drug Abuse, 1984): at 60; *Effective Medical Treatment of Opiate Addiction*, NIH Consensus Statement, 15, no. 6 (November 17–19, 1997): 1–38, at 4 (panel concluded that "methadone maintenance treatment is effective in reducing illicit opiate drug use, in reducing crime, and in enhancing social productivity, and in reducing the spread of viral diseases such as AIDS and hepatitis"); M. Farrell et al., "Effectiveness of Drug Dependence Treatment in Prevention of HIV Among IDUs," Abstract No. A8 88, *13th International Conference on*

Reduction of Drug Related Harm, Ljubljana, Slovenia, March 3–7, 2002 (summarizes meta-analyses of the efficacy of drug treatment programs, including methadone maintenance, in reducing HIV-risk behavior; overall finding that methadone maintenance has a significant benefit on risk behavior, although some data inconsistent); M.W. Tyndall et al., "The Impact of Initiating Methadone Maintenance Treatment on Patterns of Drug Use and Other Risk Behaviors in Vancouver, Canada," Abstract No. Al 86, *13th International Conference on Reduction of Drug Related Harm*, Ljubljana, Slovenia, March 3–7, 2002 (reporting "marked reduction in non-fatal over-doses, sex trade work, and incarcerations with modest reduction in overall drug use"); E. Gottheil, R.C. Sterling, and S.P Weinstein, "Diminished Illicit Drug Use as a Consequence of Long-Term Methadone Maintenance," *Journal of Addictive Diseases*, 12, no. 4 (1993): 45–57.

36. National Institute of Drug Abuse, *Buprenorphine Update: Questions and Answers*, at <http://165.112.78.61/Bupupdate.html> (last updated January 30, 2001).

37. *Id.*

38. D.A. Feillan et al., "Methadone Maintenance in Primary Care: A Randomized Controlled Trial," *JAMA*, 286 (2001): 172431, at 1724.

39. B.J. Rounsaville and T.R. Kosten, "Treatment of Opioid Dependence: Quality and Access," *JAMA*, 283 (2000): 1337–39; M. Weinrich and M. Stuart, "Provision of Methadone Treatment in Primary Care Medical Practices: Review of the Scottish Experience and Implications for U.S. Policy," *JAMA*, 283 (2000): 1343–48.

40. *Effective Medical Treatment of Opiate Addiction, supra* note 35, at 2.

41. D.A. Harris, *Driving While Black: Racial Pro filing on Our Nation's Highways*, American Civil Liberties Union Special Report June 1999), available at <http://www.aclu.org/profiling/report/>; American Civil Liberties Union, "Is Jim Crow Justice Alive and Well in America Today?," at <http://www.aclu.org/profiling/> (last visited May 11, 2002).

42. U.S. Department of Justice, Bureau of Justice Statistics, Prisoners in 1996 (Washington D.C.: U.S. Department of Justice, 1997).

43. M. Mauer, *Americans Behind Bars: U.S. and International Rates of Incarceration, 1995* (Washington, D.C.: The Sentencing Project, 1997).

44. E. Currie, *Crime and Punishment in America* (New York: Metropolitan Books, Henry Holt and Company, 1998): at 15.

45. U.S. Department of Justice, *supra* note 42.

46. M. Mauer, C. Potler, and R. Wolf, *Gender and Justice: Women, Drugs, and Sentencing Policy* (Washington, D.C.: The Sentencing Project, 1999).

47. A.J. Beck and J. Karberg, Bureau of Justice Statistics, *Prison and jail Inmates at Midyear 2000* (Washington D.C.: U.S. Department of Justice, March 2001): at 9.

48. Substance Abuse and Mental Health Services Administration, U.S. Department of Health and Human Services, *Summary of Findings from the 2000 National Household Survey on Drug Abuse* (Rockville, Maryland: SAMHSA, 2001): at 124 (Table EA), 132 (Table F.2), and 144 (Table F.14), available at <http:// www.samhsa.gov/oas/NHSDA/2kNHSDA/lot.htm>.

49. "Race and the War on Drugs," *Drug Policy Alliance*, Online Library, Focal Point (March 2001), available at <http:// www.lindesmith.org/library/focal_race2.html> (last visited June 5, 2002).

50. M.R. Durose and P.A. Langan, Bureau of Justice Statistics, *State Court Sentencing of Convicted Felons, 1998 Statistical Tables* (Washington, D.C.: U.S. Department of Justice, December 2001): at Table 2.5, available at <http://www.ojp.usdoj.gov/bjs/abstract/scsc98st.htm>; B.S. Meierhoefer, *The General Effect of Mandatory Minimum Prison Terms: A Longitudinal Study of Federal Sentences Imposed* (Washington, D.C.: Federal Judicial Center, 1992): at 20.

51. "Crack Cocaine Sentencing Policy: Unjustified and Unreasonable," The Sentencing Project, available at <http://www.sentencingproject.org/brief/pub1003.htm> (last visited June 5, 2002). (The federal law mandates similar sentences for quantities of crack: powder cocaine of 1:100, and mandatory prison sentences for simple possession of crack, even for first-time offenders. This means that someone caught with five grams of crack will be sentenced to 5 years in prison, while possession of five grams of powder cocaine will probably receive probation.)

52. *Id.*

53. "U.S. Prisons Fail to Adopt Proven Prevention Measures, Experts Say," *AIDS Policy Law*, 12, no. 6 (April 4, 1997): 1, 9–10.

54. See Blankenship and Koester, *supra* note 34.

55. D. Lee et al., "HIV Risks in a Homeless Population," *International Journal of STD & AIDS*, 11, no. 8 (2000): 509–15; L.M. Takahashi, "The Socio-Spatial Stigmatization of Homelessness and HIV/AIDS: Toward an Explanation of the NIMBY Syndrome," *Social Science & Medicine*, 45, no. 6 (1997): 903–14.

56. D.A. Zanis et al., "HIV Risks Among Homeless Men Differentiated by Cocaine Use and Psychiatric Distress," *Addictive Behaviors*, 22, no. 2 (1997): 287–92; A.H. Kral et al., "Prevalence of Sexual Risk Behavior and Substance Use Among Runaway and Homeless Adolescents in San Francisco, Denver and New York City," *International Journal of STD & AIDS*, 8 (1997): 109–17.

57. P. Bourgois, "The Moral Economies of Homeless Heroin Addicts: Confronting Ethnography, HIV Risk, and Everyday Violence in San Francisco Shooting Encampments," *Substance Use & Misuse*, 33, no. 11 (1998): 2323–51.

58. Attorney General William Barr has been quoted as asserting that African-Americans would benefit disproportionately from increased incarcerations (of African-Americans) for drug offenses; M. Tonry, *Malign Neglect: Race, Crime, and Punishment in America* (New York: Oxford University Press, 1995): at 36. But see Drug Czar Barry McCaffery's description of our current

incarceration policy: "We must have law enforcement authorities address the [drug use] issue because if we do not, prevention, education, and treatment messages will not work very well. But having said that, I also believe that we have created an American gulag." Gen. Barry R. McCaffrey (USA Ret.), Director, Office of National Drug Control Policy, Keynote Address, Opening Plenary Session, *National Conference on Drug Abuse Prevention Research*, National Institute of Drug Abuse, Washington, D.C., September 19, 1996, available at <http://165.112.78.61/MeetSum/CODA/Keynote2.html>.

59. T.L. Meares, "Social Organization and Drug Law Enforcement," *American Criminal Law Review*, 35 (1998): 191–227, at 191, 198–205.

60. F.E. Zimring and G.J. Hawkins, *Deterrence: The Legal Threat in Crime Control* (Chicago: University of Chicago Press, 1973); G. Becker, "Crime and Punishment: An Economic Approach," *Journal of Political Economy*, 76 (1968): 169–217.

61. T. Tyler, *Why People Obey the Law* (New Haven: Yale University Press, 1990); T.R. Tyler, "Public Trust and Confidence in Legal Authorities: What Do Majority and Minority Group Members Want from the Law and Legal Institutions?," *Behavioral Sciences & the Law*, 19 (2001): 215–35.

62. See Meares, *supra* note 59, at 212.

63. See *id.* at 210–14.

64. See Tyler, *supra* note 61.

65. See Meares, *supra* note 59.

66. S.F. Morin, "Early Detection of HIV: Assessing the Legislative Context," *Journal of Acquired Immune Deficiency Syndromes*, 2, suppl. 2 (2000): 5144–50.

67. Z. Lazzarini, S. Bray, and S Burris, "Evaluating the Impact of Criminal Laws on HIV Risk Behavior," *Journal of Law, Medicine & Ethics*, 30, no. 2 (2002): 239–53.

68. For discussions in the legal literature, see J.G. Hodge and L.O. Gostin, "Handling Cases of Willful Exposure Through HIV Partner Counseling and Referral Services," *Women's Rights Law Reporter*, 23 (2001): 45–62; K. Sullivan and M. Field, "AIDS and the Coercive Power of the State," *Harvard Civil Rights-Civil Liberties Law Review*, 23 (1988): 139–97; C.M. Shriver, "State Approaches to Criminalizing the Exposure of HIV: Problems in Statutory Construction, Constitutionality and Implications," *Northern Illinois University Law Review*, 21 (2001): 319–53; J. Mosiello, "Why the Intentional Sexual Transmission of Human Immunodeficiency Virus (HIV) Should Be Criminalized Through the Use of Specific HIV Criminal Statutes," *New York Law School Journal of Human Rights*, 15 (1999): 595–624; D.L. Chambers, "Gay Men, AIDS, and the Code of the Condom," *Harvard Civil Rights–Civil Liberties Law Review*, 29 (1994): 353–85; D.H.J. Hermann, "Criminalizing Conduct Related to HIV Transmission," *Saint Louis University Public Law Review*, 9 (1990): 351–78; G.P. Schultz and C.A. Parmenter, "Medical Necessity, AIDS, and the Law," Saint Louis University Public Law Review, 9 (1990): 379–419; L. Gostin, "The Politics of AIDS: Compulsory State Powers,

Public Health, and Civil Liberties," *Ohio State Law Journal*, 49 (1989): 1017–58; G. Schultz, "AIDS: Public Health and the Criminal Law," *Saint Louis University Public Law Review*, 7 (1988): 65–113; M.L. Clown et al., "Discussion: Criminalization of an Epidemic: HIV-AIDS and Criminal Exposure Laws," *Arkansas Law Review*, 46 (1994): 921–83; M. Markus, "A Treatment for the Disease: Criminal HIV Transmission/Exposure Laws," *Nova Law Review*, 23 (1999): 847–79.

69. Zita Lazzarini, Principle Investigator, "Influence of Criminal Law on HIV Sexual Risk Behavior," supported by CDC grant numbers R06/CCR118660-01 and H400-898-2021.

70. See Centers for Disease Control and Prevention, "HIV—Related Knowledge and Stigma—United States, 2000," *Morbidity and Mortality Weekly Reports*, 49, no. 47 (2000): 1062–64.

71. See M. Chesney and A. Smith, "Critical Delays in HIV Testing and Care: The Potential Role of Stigma," *American Behavioral Scientist*, 42 (1999): 1162–74; G. Herek, "AIDS and Stigma," *American Behavioral Scientist*, 42 (1999): 1106–16.

72. See Lazzarini, Bray, and Burris, *supra* note 67.

73. See Centers for Disease Control and Prevention, "Cluster of HIV-Positive Young Women—New York. 1997–1998," *Morbidity and Mortality Weekly Reports*, 48, no. 20 (1999): 413–16.

74. See J. Wypijewski, "The Secret Sharer," *Harper's Magazine*, 297, no. 1778 (July 1, 1998): at 35, for consideration of local response to issues of sex, race, and denial around the HIV epidemic.

75. See Centers for Disease Control and Prevention, *supra* note 3; Karon et al., *supra* note 9; Centers for Disease Control and Prevention, *supra* note 2; Zierler and Krieger, *supra* note 19; K.G. Castro, "Distribution of Acquired Immunodeficiency Syndrome and Other Sexually Transmitted Diseases in Racial and Ethnic Populations, United States; Influences of Life-style and Socioeconomic Status," *Annals of Epidemiology*, 3 (1993): 181–84.

76. See U.S. Department of Housing and Urban Development's website for these definitions, available at <http://www.hud.gov>.

77. *Department of Housing and Urban Development v. Rucker*, No. 00-1770, 2002 U.S. LEXIS 2144 (U.S. March 26, 2002).

78. See LD. Montoya et al., "Barriers to Social Services for HIV-Infected Urban Migrators," *AIDS Education and Prevention*, 10, no. 4 (1998): 366–79.

79. See Lee et al., *supra* note 55.

80. See Takahashi, *supra* note 55.

81. See R.W. Pfeifer and J. Oliver, "A Study of HIV Seroprevalence in a Group of Homeless Youth in Hollywood, California," *Journal of Adolescent Health*, 20, no. 5 (1997): 339–42; K. Clements et al., "A Risk Profile of Street Youth in Northern California: Implications for Gender-Specific Human Immunodeficiency Virus Prevention," *Journal of Adolescent Health*, 20, no. 5 (1997): 343–53; M.C. Clans et al., "Correlates and Distribution of HIV Risk Behaviors

Among Homeless Youths in New York City: Implications for Prevention and Policy," *Child Welfare League of America*, LXXVII, no. 2 (1998): 195–207; S.L. Bailey, C.S. Camlin, and S.T. Ennett, "Substance Use and Risky Sexual Behavior Among Homeless and Runaway Youth," *Journal of Adolescent Health*, 23, no. 6 (1998): 378–88; Kral et al., *supra* note 56.

82. See A.M Somlai et al., "Patterns, Predictors, and Situational Contexts of HIV Risk Behaviors Among Homeless Men and Women," *Social Work*, 43, no. 1 (1998): 7–20.

83. See G.A.D. Smereck and E.M Hockman, "Prevalence of HIV Infection and HIV Risk Behaviors Associated with Living Place: On-the-Street Homeless Drug Users as a Special Target Population for Public Health Intervention," *American Journal of Drug and Alcohol Abuse*, 24, no. 2 (1998): 299–319; Zanis et al., *supra* note 56.

84. See A.A. Aidala et al., *Housing, Health & Wellness Study: Final Report* (October 4, 2000); PS. Arno et al., "The Impact of Housing Status on Health Care Utilization Among Persons with HIV Disease," *Journal of Health Care for the Poor and Underserved*, 7, no. 1 (1996): 36–49.

85. The World Bank Group, United States Data Profile, at <http://devdata.worldbank.org/external/CPPProfile.asp?SelectedCountry=USA&CCODE= USA&CNAME=United+States &PTYPE=CP> (last visited February 6, 2002) (with a gross domestic product [GDP] per capita of $34,000 [2000], the United States consistently rates in among the highest standards of living in the world and among the highest per capita GDP). Only seven countries had higher per capita GDP than the United States in 1999. These countries were Bermuda, Denmark, Japan, Liechtenstein, Luxembourg, Norway, and Switzerland. United Nations Statistics Division—Social Indicators, *Indicators on Income and Economic Activity*, at <http://www. un.org/Depts/unsd/ social/inc-eco.htm> (last visited February 7, 2002).

86. See A.B. Atkinson, L. Rainwater, and IM. Smeeding, *Income Distribution in OECD Countries: Evidence from the Luxembourg Income Study* (Paris: Organisation for Economic Co-operation and Development, 1995) (the United States is one of the richest countries, and one with the most unequal distribution of income and wealth).

87. See U.S. Census Bureau, *Income Inequality* (March Current Population Survey) (Washington, D.C.: Government Printing Office, 1997) (inequality of income distribution in the United States is getting worse); E. Wolff, *Top Heavy: A Study of the Increasing Inequality of Wealth in America* (New York: 20th Century Fund, 1995).

88. I. Kawachi, "Income Inequality and Health," in L. Berkman and I. Kawachi, eds., *Social Epidemiology* (New York: Oxford University Press, 2000): 76–94; B.P. Kennedy, I. Kawachi, and D. Prothrow-Stith, "Income Distribution and Morality: Cross Sectional Ecological Study of the Robin Hood Index in the United States," *BMJ*, 312 [1996]: 1004–07 (see also important correction, *BMJ*, 312 [1996]: 1194) (Analyzed age-adjusted death rates and income inequality in all fifty U.S. states, finding a strong correlation between greater degrees of income inequality and elevated death rates. Together, income inequality and poverty accounted for 25 percent of differences between state mortality rates, and over half of differences in

homicide rates); J.W Lynch et al., "Income Inequality and Mortality in Metropolitan Areas of the United States," *American Journal of Public Health*, 88 (1998): 1074–80 (cities with low per capita income and high inequality had excess deaths of nearly 150 per 100,000 when compared to cities with relatively higher income and lower inequality).

89. M. Jacoby, "Does Indebtedness Influence Health? A Preliminary Inquiry," *Journal of Law, Medicine & Ethics*, 30, no. 4 (2002): 560–71.

90. See Centers for Disease Control and Prevention, *supra* note 3.

91. Burris, Kawachi, and Sarat, *supra* note 1.

92. See J.S. Lehman, "To Conceptualize, to Criticize, to Defend," *Yale Law Journal*, 101 (1991): 685–727 (public support for Aid to Families with Dependent Children decreased as concern grew that the program perpetuated dependence); T.R. Marmor, J.L. Mashaw, and PL. Harvey, *America's Misunderstood Welfare State: Persistent Myths, Enduring Realities* (New York: Basic Books, 1990); H. Heclo, "Poverty Politics," in S.H. Danziger, G.D. Sandefur, and D.H. Weinberg, eds., *Confronting Poverty: Prescriptions for Change* (New York: Russell Sage Foundation, 1994): 396–437.

93. See Personal Responsibility and Work Opportunity Reconciliation Act of 1996, Pub. L. No. 104-193 (August 1996) (Congress eliminated Aid to Families with Dependent Children and adopted The Personal Responsibility and Work Opportunity Reconciliation Act, which put a 5-year lifetime limit on benefits, food stamps included).

94. U.S. Department of Health and Human Services, *Indicators of Welfare Dependence*, 2002 annual report to Congress: at Chapter II, "Indicators of Dependence," Figure IND3a, available at <http://aspe.hhs.gov/hsp/indicators02/index.htm>.

95. See J.S. Heymann, "Health and Social Policy," in L. Berkman and I. Kawachi, eds., *Social Epidemiology* (New York: Oxford University Press, 2000).

96. N. Zill, G. Resnick, and R.H. McKey, *What Children Know and Can Do at the End of Head Start and What It Tells Us About the Program's Performance, paper presented at Emerging Views of Children in Poverty: The Health Start Family and Child Experiences Survey (FACES)*, the Society for Research in Child Development Biennial Meeting, Albuquerque, New Mexico, April 16, 1999, available at <http://www.2acf.hdhhs.gov/programs/hsb/hsreac/faces/albqfinl2.doc> (finding that children in Head Start achieve significant gains in preparedness for kindergarten and improvement in academically and socially related skills); E. Graces, D. Thomas, and J. Currie, *Longer Term Effects of Head Start*, DRU2439-NICHD/NSF, Labor and Population Program, Working Paper Series 00-20 (December 2000), available at <http:// www.rand.org/labor/DRU/DRU2439.pdf> (showing higher rate of high school graduation among Head Start participants).

97. See G. Burtless, "Public Spending on the Poor: Historical Trends and Economic Limits," in S.H. Danziger, G.D. Sandefur, and D.H. Weinberg, eds., *Confronting Poverty: Prescriptions for Change* (New York: Russell Sage Foundation, 1994) (Comprehensive Employment and

Training Act (CETA) of 1973 benefited poor through job training, with 25–75 percent gains in wages of adult women who were trained).

98. Section 115 (a) of the Personal Responsibility and Work Opportunity Reconciliation Act of 1996, Pub. L. No. 104-193.

99. P Allard, *Life Sentences: Denying Welfare Benefits to Women Convicted of Drug Offenses* (Washington, D.C.: The Sentencing Project, February 2002).

100. See *id.*

101. See B.M.J. Rotheram, "Expanding the Range of Interventions to Reduce HIV Among Adolescents," *AIDS*, 14, suppl. 1 (2000): 533–40.

102. See D. Cohen et al., "Broken Windows and the Risk of Gonorrhea," *American Journal of Public Health*, 90, no. 2 (2000): 230–36.

103. See B. Lichtenstein, "Secret Encounters: Black Men, Bisexuality, and AIDS in Alabama," *Medical Anthropology Quarterly*, 14, no. 3 (2000): 374–93.

104. See J.L. Peterson, "AIDS-Related Risks and Same-Sex Behaviors Among African American Men," in MY Levine, PM. Nardi, and J.H. Gagnon, eds., *Changing Times: Gay Men and Lesbians Encounter HIV/AIDS* (Chicago: University of Chicago Press, 1997): 283–301; Lichtenstein, *supra* note 103.

105. See L.A. Valleroy et al., "HIV Prevalence and Associated Risks in Young Men Who Have Sex with Men," *JAMA*, 284, no. 2 (2000): 198–204.

106. Centers for Disease Control and Prevention, "HIV Incidence Among Young Men Who Have Sex with Men—Seven U.S. Cities, 1994–2000," *Morbidity and Mortality Weekly Reports*, 50, no. 21 (2001): 440–44.

107. See Meares, supra note 59, at 213; D. James, "The Racial Ghetto as a Race-Making Situation," *Law & Society Inquiry*, 19 (1994): 407, 420–28; E. Anderson, *Streetwise: Race, Class and Change in an Urban Community* (Chicago: University of Chicago Press, 1990): at 208.

108. See C. Shaw and H. McKay, *Juvenile Delinquency and Urban Areas* (Chicago: University of Chicago Press, 1969): at 321.

109. J. Fellner and M. Mauer, *Losing the Vote: The Impact of Felony Disenfranchisement Laws in the United States* (Washington, D.C.: Human Rights Watch, The Sentencing Project, 1998): at 8 (In 1998, approximately 1.4 million black men were disenfranchised, compared to a total of 4.6 million black men who voted in 1996. U.S. Census Bureau, *Voting and Registration in the Election of November 1996* [July 1998]: at 20–504).

110. See Meares, *supra* note 59. See generally S. Verba et al., *Voice and Equality: Civic Voluntarism in American Politics* (Cambridge: Harvard University Press, 1996).

111. See Meares, *supra* note 59, at 209–10.

112. L.A. Greenfield and T.L. Snell, Bureau of Justice Statistics, *Women Offenders* (Washington, D.C.: U.S. Department of Justice, 1999): at 8, Table 18.

113. C. J. Mumola, Bureau of Justice Statistics, *Incarcerated Parents and Their Children* (Washington, D.C.: U.S. Department of Justice, 2000): at 5.

114. See Meares, *supra* note 59, at 207.

115. M. Mauer, *Intended and Unintended Consequences: State Racial Disparities in Imprisonment* (Washington, D.C.: The Sentencing Project, 1997): at 1 ("research has documented that a first-time arrest for a property crimes results in a 7% decline in incomes.").

116. See Meares, *supra* note 59, at 209–10.

117. S. Sekaran, *New Policy with a Familiar Consequence: African Americans and the Higher Education Act*, Drug Policy Alliance (February 27, 2002), available at <http://www.alternet.org/ story.html?StoryID=12501> (Higher Education Act (HEA) of 1998 delays or prohibits granting federal financial aid to any student convicted of nonviolent drug offenses, including misdemeanors.).

118. J. Dalaker, "Current Population Reports," *Poverty in the United States: 2000* (Washington, D.C.: U.S. Government Printing Office, September 2001): at Table A; R. Blank, *It Takes a Nation: A New Agenda for Fighting Poverty* (Princeton: Princeton University Press, 1997); C. Jenks, *Rethinking Social Policy: Race, Poverty, and the Underclass* (New York: Harper Perennial, 1993).

119. See Meares, *supra* note 59, at 207.

120. C. Haney and P Zimbardo, "The Past and Future of U.S. Prison Policy. Twenty-Five Years After the Stanford Prison Experiment," *American Psychologist*, 53, no. 7 (1998): 709–27, at 716.

121. See Allard, *supra* note 99.

122. L.O. Gostin, S. Burris, and Z. Lazzarini, "The Law and the Public's Health: A Study of Infectious Disease Law in the United States," *Columbia Law Review*, 59 (1999): 99–128.

123. L.O. Gostin and J.M. Mann, "Towards the Development of a Human Rights Impact Assessment for the Formulation and Evaluation of Public Health Policies," *Health and Human Rights*, 1, no. 1 (1994): 58–80; L.O. Gostin and Z. Lazzarini, *Human Rights and Public Health in the AIDS Pandemic* (New York: Oxford University Press, 1997): at 57–67.

124. H. Watchirs, "Review of Methodologies Measuring Human Rights Implementation," *Journal of Law, Medicine & Ethics*, 30, no. 4 (2002): 716–33; E. O'Keefe and A. Scott-Samuel, "Human Rights and Wrongs: Could Health Impact Assessment Help?," *Journal of Law, Medicine & Ethics*, 30, no. 4 (2002): 734–38.

125. D.P. Goldman et al., "The Impact of State Policy on the Costs of HIV Infection," *Medical Care Research and Review*, 58, no. 1 (2001): 31–53, 54–59 (discussion).

126. See Meares, *supra* note 59, at 217–20.

127. See *id.* at 219–20.

128. K. Strader, "Criminalization as a Response to a Public Health Crisis," *John Marshall Law Review*, 27 (1994): 435–47, at 437.

129. See Lazzarini, Bray, and Burris, *supra* note 67.

130. R. Klitzman et al., "Views of HIV-Related Policies Among HIV Positive Men and Women: HIV Named Reporting, Partner Notification, and Criminalization of Non-disclosure" (2002, in review).

131. See Tyler, *supra* note 61.

132. EM. Rowe, "Commentary: Changing the Risk Behavior of Politicians," *Lancet*, 349, no. 9051 (1997): 520.

133. H. Dalton, "Law and Responsibility Lecture Series: Shaping Responsible Behavior: Lessons from the AIDS Front," *Washington & Lee Law Review*, 56 (1999): 931–52, at 934.

---

*Zita Lazzarini, J.D., MTH., teaches health law and bioethics at the University of Connecticut Health Center and the Harvard School of Public Health, and directs the Division of Medical Humanities at the University of Connecticut Health Center. She has co-authored *Human Rights and Public Health in the AIDS Pandemic*, published by Oxford University Press in 1997.

Robert Klitzman, M.D., is the co-director of the Center for Bioethics and assistant professor of clinical psychiatry in the College of Physicians and Surgeons and the Mailman School of Public Health at Columbia University.

Z. Lazzarini, R. Klitzman, "HIV and the Law: Integrating Law, Policy and Social Epidemiology," *Journal of Law, Medicine and Ethics*, 30 (2002): 533–547.

DISCUSSION QUESTIONS

1. There is a growing understanding that HIV/AIDS is linked to social and economic disadvantages, often known as the social determinants of health. What are the social determinants of health in your community/country?

2. In the United States, rates of HIV and AIDS are often the highest among men who have sex with men, intravenous drug users, and African Americans. What communities in your country have the highest HIV and AIDS rate? Does this have any implication for HIV- and AIDS-related stigma? Can the law can play a role in mitigating the HIV and AIDS epidemic among these communities? What is the stigma surrounding these communities?

3. A human rights framework for HIV and AIDS prevention forms the basis of an effective prevention strategy. National laws not only must include clauses protecting the rights of people living with HIV/AIDS and the vulnerable populations, but also contain a mechanism for effective enforcement. What are some of the conditions for an effective enforcement system?

4. What are the areas in which law can have impact on HIV and AIDS? In what way can the law have a positive impact on the issues surround HIV- and AIDS-related stigma and discrimination?

5. How can AIDS advocates work effectively with policy makers to ensure laws have a positive impact in confronting stigma?

HIV/AIDS and Human Rights in Kazakhstan

by Andrei Andreev*

HIV/AIDS has a number of complex social, psychological, emotional and legal consequences for a person living with HIV/AIDS and his/her friends, relatives, doctors, colleagues and all those who work to prevent this epidemic.

Many people still believe that only injection drug users can get HIV; others blame gay men and sex workers for the ongoing epidemic. When voicing their opinions about people living with AIDS (PLHA) many people speak negatively not only about the infection and the disease it causes, but about the people who have it. The discrimination stems from the lack of understanding of the infection and its transmission. For many people, HIV/AIDS closely associates with death, and this leads to fear of infection, and as a result—negative attitude towards PLHA.

Discrimination is closely tied in with the denial of basic human rights. HIV/AIDS-related discrimination does not only contribute to human suffering of PLHA but also further exacerbates the spread of HIV/AIDS. Such discrimination makes people "shut down" and avoid opening up about their infection, their life and feelings. This represents a barrier to seeking treatment and counseling, and leads to the patient's inability to access full and true information about HIV/AIDS, hence limiting efforts towards effective HIV/AIDS prevention, including the government prevention programs. Rights violations of PLHA threaten their very life. Fears and prejudices, related to the perceived low morale of the PLHA, are especially effective in encouraging discrimination. HIV/AIDS-related discrimination exacerbates people's vulnerability to HIV/AIDS.

The definition of discrimination itself implies limitation of human rights and freedoms based on certain criteria (gender, nationality, social status, political opinions, sickness, and other). The Constitution of the Republic of Kazakhstan has a separate legal norm that prohibits all forms of discrimination. However, in practice, this constitutional norm is not properly implemented, especially around the issues related to HIV/AIDS.

The law "On AIDS Prevention" (October 5, 1994) is the key legal document regulating legal status of PLHA. It is interesting to note that the law doesn't provide a definition for the term "HIV infection," defining AIDS as follows: "AIDS—the Acquired Immune Deficiency Syndrome—is a dangerous infectious disease related to the Human Immune Deficiency Virus." Despite the lack of the definition for HIV in this law and in the name of the state institution tasked with working on the related issues, the Republican Center on AIDS Prevention and Control distinguishes clearly between HIV and AIDS in its monthly epidemiological statements. It is obvious that for medical professionals HIV and AIDS are separate. At the same time, the inability of the law to take this into account seriously complicates its interpretation and implementation.

Twelve years after the law was adopted, most of its articles are out of date today and do not reflect the realities of the epidemic and neither do they correspond with the internationally adopted standards and other laws and policies adopted in Kazakhstan. This situation is strange, to say the least, as according to the national Law "On Normative and Legal Acts" (adopted on March 24, 1998), the laws of higher hierarchy then governmental policies or ministerial decrees automatically cancel out the norms of the above-mentioned policies that contradict the law.

The article 6 of the Law "On AIDS Prevention" foresees compulsory and voluntary testing for AIDS.[1] This article prescribes for foreigners, people without citizenship and citizens of Kazakhstan to undergo "testing for AIDS" when there are enough reasons to believe that they can be infected with the human immune deficiency virus.

At the same time, the law does not identify these "reasons" that should be the grounds for testing. According to the above-mentioned law, in case a foreigner avoids being tested, or tests positive for AIDS, they are deported from the territory of Kazakhstan.

According to the Rules of medical assistance to foreigners and people without citizenship, permanently or temporary residing in Kazakhstan (approved by the Decree of the Public Health Agency of Kazakhstan on January 15, 2000), any foreigner or person without citizenship, refugee claimant and such, if infected with infectious diseases, such as tuberculosis, AIDS, sexually transmitted diseases and other infections have to undergo treatment as prescribed by the state government institutions. In case they deny or avoid treatment they are deported from the territory of Kazakhstan.

The Government's Decree from June 19, 2001 No. 836 re-affirms the Rules determining the quota and conditions to allow employers to hire foreigners to work in Kazakhstan. Article 4 of these Rules mandates that a document stating the HIV status of the potential employee be submitted to the local authority that issues work permits. This means that if a foreigner wants to work in Kazakhstan, he or she must go through HIV-testing. In Kazakhstan, most foreign labor comes from the neighboring states of the Commonwealth of Independent States (CIS). The 1998 Agreement on Collaboration in the Field of HIV-Infection (signed by the heads of CIS states in Moscow on November 25th, 1998), in its article 9 guarantees the citizens of CIS countries a right to entry the other CIS state's territory without a certificate stating one's immune status.

The Law "On AIDS Prevention" refers the reader to the "Public Health Law of Kazakhstan" for the process of testing and treatment. However, the current "Public Health Law of Kazakhstan" (adopted in May 19th, 1997) does not contain any explanation of the above-mentioned processes.

In 2002, the Decree of the Public Health Minister of Kazakhstan (issued on June 11, 2002), affirmed the Rules for Medical Testing for Human Immune Deficiency Virus. According to these rules, the following types of testing were introduced in Kazakhstan:

- Voluntary testing—anonymous or confidential;

- Obligatory testing—confidential consensual testing. The consent is given only after all information about the test has been disclosed. Blood and other donors are obliged to go through compulsory HIV-testing every time they make a donation;

- Compulsory testing—when testing is performed in accordance with a decision of a law-enforcement agency. The Rules hereby mention that such testing can only be done in accordance with the laws of Kazakhstan, however the current laws do not provide any guidance on this matter.

The current stigma around HIV/AIDS is further exacerbated by the recent Government's Decree No. 468 (adopted on March 30, 2000), where the Government of Kazakhstan affirms a list of so-called "socially meaningful" infectious diseases, dangerous for others. Included in this list along with sexually transmitted diseases are people infected with HIV, and patients with AIDS. Note that if in case of other diseases, the disease was mentioned, then in case of HIV/AIDS, this list includes people, not the disease itself, but people who are infected. This presentation of HIV/AIDS as an infectious disease not only doesn't serve its very purpose—underlying the importance of its prevention and treatment, but names people living with HIV/AIDS as dangerous to the society.

The current laws of Kazakhstan still have norms that foresee liability for avoiding medical testing and treatment of people who were in contact with PLHA, people with TB and drug users. The mere existence of this norm also demonstrates that not only blood and plasma donors have to undergo HIV-testing, but that there is a vaguely-defined group of people who can be forced to undergo HIV testing, and in case they refuse, they will be liable under the Administrative Code of Kazakhstan.

1. Continuing avoidance of the medical testing and treatment for people who have been in contact with HIV-infected, people with AIDS, sexually transmitted diseases, tuberculosis, if lasting for three months after a written warning, issued by a public health institution, leads to a fine of five monthly salaries.

2. In a case a person who is suspected to use drugs and psychotropic substances without medical prescription, avoids medical testing and treatment, this person will be fined up to 10 times of a monthly salary.

Article 326 of the Administrative Code of Kazakhstan
(adopted on January 30, 2001, N. 155 – II).

Article 19th of the Public Health Law mandates that special centers, labs and treatment facilities be created for confidential treatment and testing of sexually transmitted diseases, including HIV/AIDS. At the same time, the law mentions that those avoiding testing and treatment in these institutions are liable in accordance with the laws of the Republic of Kazakhstan.

The Law on AIDS Prevention states in its article 7 that citizens of Kazakhstan who are infected with HIV, are eligible to receive free medication, hospital and out-patient treatment in state medical institutions, as well as reimbursements of their travel expenses to and from the medical institution where they are treated. Furthermore, the decree of the Public Health Minister No. 891 (issued on December 27, 2004), entitled "Affirming the List of Diseases and Populations Eligible for Free Medications During their Out-Patient Treatment" mentions anti-retroviral therapy for PLHA. The Governmental Decree No. 1348 (adopted on December 21, 2004) further foresees PLHA receiving free medical care. Despite all these guarantees for free treatment and medications, found in the national laws and policies, in practice, doctors often refuse to provide medical care to PLHA only because of their diagnosis. To add to this, the current public health care system of Kazakhstan is also poorly equipped to serve the needs of PLHA. For example, in Almaty, there is only one delivery ward that accepts pregnant women with HIV/AIDS. There are numerous reports from PLHA when they were turned away from gynecologists, dentists, surgeons and other medical professionals who refused to treat them for the fear of infection. As it pertains to reimbursement of the travel expenses, this issue although found in law, is not regulated by any decree or explained by guidelines, and hence, there is practically no reimbursement of these expenses.

It is important to mention that the legislation of Kazakhstan doesn't foresee liability for rejecting PLHA right to work, housing, social security, education, etc., although all these actions should be regarded as discrimination, and as such they need to be prosecuted by law.

To conclude, I would like to note that at the moment this article is written, the Republic of Kazakhstan is yet to ratify a single international human rights document, including the International Covenants of 1966.

Contradicting legal norms, lack of explanatory decrees and guidelines, gaps between laws and their practical implementation; legal norms referring to non-existent laws and policies, delayed ratification of international human rights documents—these factors further aggravate the epidemiological situation with HIV/AIDS in Kazakhstan, and contribute to the spread of HIV/AIDS and rights violations of PLHA. To illustrate this, one should only look at the statistics of the epidemic. On December 1, 2000 there were 1,275 PLHA registered in Kazakhstan (34 people had AIDS), and already on September 1, 2005, this number grew 5 times—there were 5,275 PLHA in Kazakhstan with 299 people with AIDS. According to medical officials, this is not a realistic description of current HIV/AIDS epidemic in Kazakhstan. To get a better idea of the real proportions of the epidemic, they suggest multiplying these numbers by not less then 10.

Kazakhstan still has a lot to do to improve its situation with HIV/AIDS prevention, treatment and support, as well as amending current laws and policies, and adopting a holistic approach to public health legislation and the mechanisms for its implementation.

NOTE

1. It would be correct to say "testing for antibodies to the HIV infection" (editorial comments). As the law in question does not mention HIV infection and refer to the testing as "testing for AIDS," this language remains in the text of this article.

---

*Andrei Andreev is the Director of Legal Initiative, a non-governmental rights-based organization working out of Almaty, Kazakhstan. This article has been translated by A. Alexandrova.

A. Andreev, "HIV/AIDS and Human Rights in Kazakhstan," Legal Initiative, in "Drug Policy, HIV/AIDS and Human Rights," eds. K. Malinowska-Sempruch, S. Gallagher (Almaty, 2006).

Used by permission.

DISCUSSION QUESTIONS

1. Andrei Andreev believes that AIDS-related discrimination in Kazakhstan generally stems from the lack of understanding of the infection and its transmission. Given the context of the epidemic as described in this article, can pre-existing prejudice toward drug users, women, men who have sex with men, and sex workers worsen AIDS-related stigma and discrimination? Can one effectively eliminate stigma by addressing only its top layer (i.e., that related to the disease) without addressing the issues underlying the stigmatization of populations and communities particularly vulnerable to HIV and AIDS?

2. The author alludes to linkages between stigma and human rights. What is the relationship between AIDS-related stigma and human rights?

3. Laws and policies built on evidence and best practices can be effective tools in mitigating the impact of AIDS-related stigma. At the same time, out-of-date policies can impede HIV prevention efforts and contribute to increased stigma and discrimination. Given the legal and political situation, what can the Kazakh government do to ensure the effectiveness of its existing laws and policies regarding HIV and AIDS?

Kazakh Laws Pertaining to Commercial Sex Work: An Overview

by Vera Sergunina*

The law in Kazakhstan does not punish commercial sex work. At the same time, the law does neither officially recognize commercial sex work, not does it regulate this profession.

While the Government of Kazakhstan admits that commercial sex work exists in Kazakhstan, there is no recognition of commercial sex work as a profession, and no regulation of sex work. Instead of legalizing commercial sex work and ensure its proper taxation, protection of the workers' rights, etc., the Government of Kazakhstan views commercial sex work as an anti-social activity. In light of the lack of legal clarity on the commercial sex work, and the past record of police rights violations, commercial sex workers (CSWs) find themselves outside of the legal domain, despite the lack of legal liability for engaging in commercial sex work. Their uncertain legal status often opens a door for rights violations from those controlling the business and the police.

The Criminal Code of the Republic of Kazakhstan foresees criminal liability for involving someone into prostitution by using force or a threat of force, the person's dependent position, blackmail or deceit. The law also punishes prostitution den-running, and pimping.

According to the official statistics, in 2004 there were 357 crimes registered that were related to prostitution den-running and keeping and pimping. This data is only the very tip of the iceberg of commercial sex work in Kazakhstan.

Recently, the criminal law of Kazakhstan has undergone through some positive changes due to its ratification of the United Nations Convention on Transnational Organized Crime in 2000. The national criminal law was amended to reflect the positions of the Convention and the Protocol pertaining to human trafficking. The policy-makers introduced criminal liability for abduction for the purposes of exploitation; exploitation, recruitment, transportation, and other actions committed to exploit a human being. In this case, the term "exploitation" is understood to include using forced labor or services, prostitution of others, slavery or practices similar to slavery and servitude. While these changes are timely and important, special attention needs to be focused on the proper implementation of these norms and aligning them with appropriate policies. At the same time, these improvements did not resolve the issue of legal vacuum around commercial sex work.

Despite the fact that CSWs are not regulated by the labor laws, the Government of Kazakhstan has attempted to pay special attention to this population on a somewhat ad hoc basis. Primarily, this attention is due to the HIV/AIDS epidemic, and the implementation in Kazakhstan of diverse regional health and HIV/AIDS prevention programs. These documents often contain data on CSWs, and document rights violations of this community. These rights violations are often related to lack of proper legal protection for CSWs. Furthermore, CSWs are often exposed to violence and are often at risk of diseases.

Despite CSWs' vulnerability to violence and disease, and a high demand for their services, the Government is unwilling to entertain a possibility to legalize prostitution and define the legal status of CSWs in the Republic of Kazakhstan.

---

*Vera Sergunina is the director of the Women's Rights Center, an NGO in Almaty, Kazakhstan, that promotes the rights of women and girls. The Center is also a member of the Sex Workers' Advocacy Rights Network in Central and Eastern Europe and Central Asia.

V. Sergunina, Women's Rights Center, "Laws Pertaining to Commercial Sex Work in Kazakhstan: An Overview," *Novosti, Pravo, Obschestvo* 67, (June, 2006).

DISCUSSION QUESTIONS

1. Does the Kazakh government's position that sex work is an anti-social activity exacerbate the stigma surrounding sex workers? Do you think this position affects HIV and AIDS prevention efforts in Kazakhstan?

2. The author mentions the absence of legal clarity surrounding sex work. What are the links between the ambiguous legal status of sex work and sex workers' ability to access services, including health care? How do you think this ambiguity affects the HIV and AIDS situation in the country?

3. What are some key factors that contribute to the stigmatization of sex workers in Kazakhstan? Think of potential strategies that rights advocates and AIDS activists could employ to address these factors.

Street Policing, Injecting Drug Use and Harm Reduction in a Russian City: A Qualitative Study of Police Perspectives

by Tim Rhodes, Lucy Platt, Anya Sarang, Alexander Vlasov, Larissa Mikhailova, and Geoff Monaghan*

INTRODUCTION

Public health research and intervention among socially marginalised populations requires appreciation of how social environmental factors mediate individual and community capacity for risk avoidance.[1-5] In Russia, as elsewhere in eastern Europe, large scale social and economic changes associated with political transition may have contributed to the creation of environments conducive to HIV epidemics.[6-8] There is growing appreciation of the critical role of social structural factors in the production and reduction of HIV risk among injecting drug users (IDUs), including in relation to legal restrictions placed on the availability, distribution and exchange of needles and syringes.[9-15]

There is substantial evidence noting the potential for negative health effects among IDUs of intensive street policing initiatives.[9, 16-23] Some view anti-drug policing as a potential "public health menace."[24] Studies have associated intensive street policing, and police "crack-downs" in drug market areas, with market displacement or disruption rather than eradication, little effect on drug prices and related revenue-raising crime levels, reduced access among IDUs to health services and clean injecting equipment, elevated levels of health risk including overdose and bacterial infections or vascular damage associated with hurried injection, and increased HIV risk including linked to syringe sharing.[9, 16-19, 23, 25] A perceived fear of police arrest among IDUs can be associated with reluctance to carry needles and syringes, reluctance to access pharmacies or syringe distribution points, and increased risk of syringe sharing at the point of drug use or sale.[14, 19, 20, 22, 26]

The HIV epidemic in Russia remains predominately associated with IDU, with explosive outbreaks reported in some cities.[27, 28] The majority of IDUs in Russia are reliant upon pharmacies for their access to clean needles and syringes.[29, 30] There are approximately 70 syringe exchanges throughout the Federation, which according to crude estimates, have low levels of coverage of local IDU populations.[28] While pilot syringe exchanges since 1998 have been technically operable within Federal laws,[31] the legality of syringe exchange remains under some dispute. Article 230 of the 1996 Criminal Code makes "inclining to consumption" of illegal narcotics an offence, which some have interpreted as including actions judged to be facilitative of another person's use of drugs.[32] While there are no documented examples of harm reduction projects being prosecuted in relation to this article, such a policy context has not facilitated collaboration between law enforcement and harm reduction initiatives.[32,33] An explanatory note to Article 230 was added in 2003 giving formal recognition to the distribution of drug injecting equipment for the purposes of HIV prevention.[34]

Research in Russia, as elsewhere, suggests that reluctance among IDUs to carry needles and syringes, or to access syringe exchanges or pharmacies for clean equipment, may be linked with a fear of detention or arrest.[22, 30] Prior to 2004, such fears of arrest were not unfounded given that the Criminal Code enabled the possession of very small amounts of street heroin (up to 0.005 g) to be punishable by incarceration. These laws were repealed in December 2003 (Article 228, Russian Criminal Code, 1996), in effect decriminalising possession of small quantities of illegal drugs, in a move rationalised to reduce overcrowding in Russian prisons.[33, 34] Article 228 was once again revised in February 2006, in effect recriminalising possession of 0.5 g and above of heroin as "large scale" and 2.5 g and above as "especially large scale."

The research we report below was undertaken in Togliatti, a city in Samara region in which 2.7% of the adult population are estimated to be IDUs.[35] An explosive outbreak of HIV was reported in the city in 2001, with 56% of 423 community-recruited IDUs found HIV positive and 87% found HCV positive.[27, 36] The same study found that 15% of IDUs had had their needles and syringes confiscated by police in the last 4 weeks, and that 83% (345) had experienced police arrest or detainment. Increased odds of receptive sharing in the city were associated with history of detention for drug-related offences.[37]

The negative effects of law enforcement have been found to coincide with other structural forces which together intensify not only health risk but social and economic vulnerability among IDUs.[9, 3, 38–43] Consequently, the impact of behavioural interventions are relative and context dependent.[1,2,26,44] Conscious that most published research focusing on the links between street policing, injecting drug use and HIV prevention have drawn upon studies of IDUs, we sought to explore police officer perspectives.[45, 46]

MATERIALS AND METHODS

Sampling

We undertook qualitative interviews with a convenience sample of police officers of varying rank and position in Togliatti City in May 2002. There are three main police departments with regular contact with IDUs in Togliatti: Department for Illicit Drug Trafficking (OBNON) who are a "drugs squad" responsible for the control of trafficking of illegal drugs and primarily target large scale suppliers; the Community Security Patrol and the District Community Police Division who have direct and regular contact with IDUs through community patrol; and the Department for Matters relating to Minors. Policing departments with only occasional contact with IDUs were not included in the study.

A total of 27 police officers were interviewed of whom two were female. Participants were aged between 22 and 45 years. Interviewees represented the following police departments: District Community Police Division (n = 9); Community Security Patrol Unit (n = 11); Department for Illicit Drug Trafficking (n = 3); Department for Matters relating to Minors (n = 3); and Road Patrol Service (n = 1).

Data Collection and Analysis

Data collection was via loosely structured qualitative interviews. Interviews were undertaken by the authors (TR, LP, AS, GM) with one additional trained fieldworker. Interviews were confidential, lasted between 45 min and 1 h and took place at the interviewees' place of work. All interviews were tape recorded with informed consent, transcribed and translated from Russian into English. Interviews were conducted in Russian (n = 16) and in Russian via interpretation from English (n = 12). Interview conversation was framed by a topic guide, which was informed by a previous qualitative study.[22] The topic guide also informed the thematic coding of transcripts.

Ethics

All participants provided informed consent to participate, and no incentives were offered for participation. The study was undertaken with ethical approval granted from Riverside Research Ethics Committee in the UK and with the support of the Togliatti City Department of Health, Department of Internal Affairs and the City Narcological Services.

Findings

We present our findings in relation to the following themes: perceptions of the drug user; drug user surveillance and registration; carriage of needles and syringes; and policing and HIV prevention.

The Drug User and Surveillance

Conscious of evidence linking the "stigmatisation" of drug using populations with inequities in service access as well as elevated HIV risk,[38, 41, 47] it is worthy of note that we found it typical for drug users to be depicted in negative terms. Accounts often invoked notions of "citizenship," with distinctions drawn between "normal citizens" and drug users, who by virtue of having transgressed boundaries of normative citizenship were portrayed as having waived a right to be treated as normal. Drug users were described as having inherent criminal potential, warranting their ongoing surveillance, often resulting in temporary detainment: "Those in a state of narcotic inebriation already violate public order with their appearance. That's why they are detained" (Senior Inspector, Community Security Patrol).

The visible aspects of drug use were depicted by some as potential violations of "public order," and these pertained to signs of inebriation ("They can even be arrested for appearing in a state of intoxification"), made obvious "by their behaviour, their walk, by the look in their eyes." A number of Articles in the Administrative Violations Code of 1984 unrelated to drug use enabled police to conduct close surveillance of drug users, and these were described as Articles relating to "being intoxicated in a public place," "disorderly conduct" (including "swearing" or "disobeying a police officer"), and an Article relating to a person's appearance being "offensive to human dignity and public morality." The use of these Articles to conduct surveillance was justified largely for reasons of expedience. Articles relating to drug charges (such as Article 44: illegal acquisition and storage of narcotic drugs) were "complicated," required "paperwork," and "time," and might instead be "covered with a 'disorderly,'" often resulting in a "fine of 30–50 roubles":

> If he is walking around completely spaced out, with saliva running out of his mouth, then, I am sorry, but he's in a public place and should not disturb the public order. If he is not breaking the law, he can walk away. But most of the time, they are intoxicated [which justifies application of an administrative code] or carry drugs [which may justify arrest for possession]. (Chief Inspector, District Community Police Division)

The inherent criminal potential of drug users gave rationale for a pre-emptive approach to drug-related crime prevention. As one Senior Sergeant commented: "Not every thief is a drug user, but every drug user is a thief." Considerable efforts were placed upon street-level surveillance in which "we don't let anyone by," and where "we stop everyone" considered by "outward appearance" to be a drug user. The approach was said to "keep them [drug users] under surveillance, insofar as staff numbers allow." Such a strong emphasis upon surveillance was underpinned in some units by a quasi-formal system of performance indicators, such as a "points system where the more you catch the better" or being "obliged to discover one drug den a month." Targets set for offence reports were said to be invariably met ("They give a number like 20 for some month and everyone meets the quota for 20 reports"). Some rationalised that drug users were particularly at risk: "They are the easiest people to arrest. They never go and complain. And it is always possible to find them and write a report" (Chief Inspector, District Community Police Division).

Drug users were described as having most crime potential when in withdrawal, in which case "they start robbing all and sundry" and are "capable of committing any offence." Interviewees thus served to protect normal citizens from such transgressions:

> How does crime begin? They inject themselves, off they go, and on the next day they start getting withdrawal symptoms, but they're got no money. They start robbing all and sundry. There goes a woman with a gold chain, and they rip it off. What will she do to them? She won't do anything. It's us that have to run around and look for them. Normal people don't rip chains off people. (Sergeant, Community Patrol Service)

Drug users in withdrawal were said to become "aggressive," "dangerous," "unpredictable," "capable of anything," and may even "kill a person." With rationality overcome ("He no longer thinks of anything, and can do anything that comes to his mind"), the protection of community safety through pre-emptive detection was paramount:

A drug addict is capable of anything when they need a fix. God forbid, of course, but they would slit anybody's throat in a doorway for money. So we try to put them away as quickly as possible, so that they should not bother anyone. There are lots of instances of this! (Warrant officer, Community Patrol Service)

A fear of the violent drug user was also linked with the need for a firm policing approach. There were ambiguities as to what this constituted, with some accounts emphasising the need for, and acceptability of, "tough talk," if not a little "kicking" and "shoving," and the necessity to "grab them, drag them out and take them away" when "they put up a fight":

Well, pushing them [drug users] around and saying they are stupid. Is that really rude? That's alright. It would be rude if they [the police] beat up the drug addicts. But if they brought them in, kicked, shoved them round a couple of times, that is alright. (Patrol policeman, District Community Police Division)

Violence displayed towards drug users was not only described as an unavoidable feature of street surveillance, but by some as a means of displaying commonly held negative beliefs about drug users:

This [violence] is how they [the police] show their dislike of drug addicts. How many times have they had to cope with what addicts do? Drug addicts are scum. Bad people. And they steal. Drug users have committed most past crimes, and robberies are always down to them. (Chief Inspector, District Community Security Patrol)

Taken together, surveillance procedures were premised on the foundation that they enabled protection of the community from the potential crimes of the drug user, both from the person exhibiting signs of use and most importantly, the person exhibiting signs of withdrawal:

An addict is always unpredictable. Who knows what he will do—steal a car or rape somebody, or something else. That is why he must be barred from the community, at least until he has recovered from narcotic inebriation. [What do you mean "barred"?] Detained for 24 to 48 h until the high has passed. (Officer, Community Patrol Service)

We detain drug users when they are in the state of withdrawal. We have to detain them in that state because if we don't they will commit crime.

Drug users commit 88% of all crime. They steal, they rob ... (Senior Officer, Community Patrol Service)

Registration as a Stratagem of Surveillance

A key stratagem of surveillance, often made easier by the discovery of a syringe (see below), was the official registration of a person as an addict: "They'll be put on the register if they are not on it." As was commented:

We detain those who possess drugs or have some related information. We can also detain addicts even if they do not have drugs on them in order to register them. We keep their records in our books. (Junior officer, OBNON [Drug Squad])

Such official registration has potentially serious negative consequences for drug users associated with loss of employment and social stigma,[48] but gives rationale for "preventive work" and ongoing surveillance:

I can just approach a person and say: "Who are you? Could I see your ID?" Suppose he shows some ID. "Well, Mr Ivan Ivanovich Petrov." I make an inquiry in our information centre. And then I get the answer: "Yes, he is registered with us as a drug user." Then I say: "Well, let's search you." (Chief inspector, District Community Police Division)

We were told that surveillance is "what the register is for" and that registration endorses police "rights" to surveillance at the same time as waiving drug users certain rights of citizenship:

Our status allows us to check and search them [drug users]. If we have information that in certain flats drugs are being used, we put it on our books as a place of concentration for drug users. Once the flat is registered with us, we have rights to come there and search everyone. That means we have this right. (Senior Inspector, Community Security Unit)

All the addicts have to be listed. When we are dealing with them, you know that this person is an addict. You already know what sort of attitude to have. ["Attitude"? In what sense?] You can't trust an addict. You must always relate to him with a note of distrust. (Junior Officer, OBNON [Drugs Squad])

Such ongoing surveillance, and the experience of stop and search, has been described by drug users in the city as relentless.[22] However, police accounts emphasised that their suspicions that an individual they target is a drug user are usually correct:

I will stop them for a little chat if they have drugs [or] their behaviour is a slightly inadequate. That is how I know they did something illegal ... They get nervous, start twitching. They try to hide something. All these signs indicate that they have drugs. In 80–90% of cases I'm usually right. (Divisional Police Inspector, District Community Police Division)

It is important to note that we also found exceptions to the general depiction of drug users as potential criminals in need of close surveillance. Here an alternative view emerged in which drug use was depicted as an illness and drug users as citizens in need of help. In this minority view, drug users were envisaged as "quite normal people," as being "drug addicts who work, who don't steal and who don't rob anyone," and who "would not harm anyone":

In my opinion drug use is an illness. That's why you shouldn't put him behind bars, but should give him medical treatment. Before, there were Detoxification Medical Units. Alcoholics were held there. He isn't a criminal! He bought the drug for himself and uses it for himself. He doesn't see it. He has to have medical treatment. But that's just my opinion. (Senior inspector, Department for Matters relating to Minors)

Carriage of Needles and Syringes

We found there to be ambiguity in police accounts as to whether drug users should fear detention or arrest associated with carrying needles and syringes. This ambiguity centred on distinctions drawn between clean and previously used syringes, and between principle and practice. Accounts emphasised that in theory carrying a clean syringe was "not an offence," that "there is nothing we can prove if the syringe is cleaned" and that "we would be breaching their rights if we tried to use it as evidence." A clean syringe should therefore not be grounds for fear of arrest or detention among drug users:

They don't get caught with clean ones. What could happen to them because of that? But if they've already used drugs, then yes. (Sergeant, Community Security Patrol)

I don't know what they're afraid of. If the syringe is empty then it is empty, and that means there is no drug in it, doesn't it? What is there to be afraid of with an empty syringe? However, if there is solution in it then they should be afraid, because there is no difference between there being traces of heroin [in a previously used syringe] and solution currently in the syringe. (Inspector of training, Community Security Patrol)

However, in practice possession of a syringe, including if clean, was said to justifiably arouse suspicion of drug use, and thus also police interest:

> Let's say I saw a clean syringe. And let's assume this person is not registered with us. Of course, everything depends on his explanation why he carries it. If he says that he has medical treatment and looks normal, I am not going to humiliate him. Stopping this person already means that something about him drew my attention. For example, I do not carry a syringe. (District inspector, District Community Police Division)

A clean syringe was said to signal suspicion (especially "if he's on the register" of addicts) for which possible detention might follow subject to evidence, and by some was described as constituting "direct evidence" of injecting, thus permitting further investigation. The following extract provides an instance of where distinctions become blurred between a clean syringe constituting no offence in theory but signalling "suspicion" or "evidence" justifying police intervention in practice:

> Of course! If he is detained where there is usually a gathering of addicts, then he is a suspect right away. That's why they are afraid, because they can spend the night in the police station. [Why, if they have clean syringes?] I'm saying that they are under suspicion. If he is caught where there is a drug den that means that he has most likely come into contact with drugs somewhere ... [In other words, you feel that there is truth in what the addicts have told us?] Well, of course. They know themselves, that this is direct evidence of them injecting. (Officer, Community Security Patrol)

There was consensus that a drug user discovered with a previously used syringe had a justified fear of detention or arrest. At the time of the study, the Russian Criminal Code did not distinguish between smaller amounts of possession in that any amount of street heroin or liquid opiate up to 0.005 g was interpretable as a "large amount" potentially resulting in imprisonment. As a consequence, even "traces" of heroin in syringes might constitute possession: "As long as we can trace even a tiny bit of drug in it, it will be confiscated"; "We are talking milligrams"; "A little smear would be enough to be a criminal offence." When stopping a person with a previously used syringe, it was said that they would be detained if there was "reason or some sort of suspicion," while the syringe would be analysed for its contents:

> If it's not clear what was in there [a previously used syringe], you need to do an analysis and prove that there was a narcotic in it. A loaded syringe is also analysed. A person is brought to a station, in an order established by law, with witnesses, the syringe is confiscated from him, then it is

sealed and sent for analysis. Everything else is determined by the expert in narcotic substances. (Senior Inspector, District Community Police Division)

While the possession of a clean syringe is not an offence, in practice it therefore offers justification that a person already stopped or searched can be reasonably suspected of drug use, which may in turn lead to detention and further investigation. This may lead to eventual arrest, or far more commonly, the application of an administrative code (see above) for which small fines are sometimes payable and official registration as an addict.

Policing and HIV Prevention

Most we interviewed were aware of the needle and syringe distribution project which operated in two of the three districts of Togliatti:

> There are points around the city where syringes are exchanged for them, they are given condoms, handed out leaflets about how to do all that right, how to look after your veins, to avoid infection or an abscess. There is that. The feelings about this are double sided. On one hand, it's very necessary. Perhaps, someone will think of their future. It's a big plus. But on the other side, it's a Russian problem: they change them [syringes] for the addicts, but old people have to buy them with their own money! I think that the government ought to solve this problem some how. (Chief Sergeant, Community Patrol Service)

Our findings indicate evidence of willingness among police officials to consider how police can best work in partnership with community-based HIV prevention initiatives, including syringe exchange:

> It [syringe exchange] decreases the risk of HIV infection. If it's an illness then we have to fight it somehow. If they use drugs, then let them at least use clean syringes. (Senior Inspector, Department for Matters relating to Minors)

Positive depictions of the role or potential of syringe exchange in HIV prevention were tempered by perhaps predictable concerns that syringe exchange might encourage, or be interpreted as endorsing, drug use:

> It's a double-edged sword. On one hand, it seems that we are intercepting the spread of HIV, on the other hand, that we approve: "Here are new syringes for you, inject, comrades." On one hand, there won't be HIV, but on the other, it's a push toward drug use. (Senior Divisional Inspector, Department for Matters relating to Minors)

Importantly, pharmacies and syringe exchanges were described as providing ideal opportunities for police surveillance (and potential arrest) of drug users:

Exactly! That's what I'm talking about! Places where they are issued syringes, chemists, that is the very best place for finding drug addicts. Aha! Here he comes! Great! ... They cast their net and wait. That happens a lot. (Warrant Officer, Community Patrol Service)

Pharmacies may present a more cost efficient point of surveillance than the street, especially important given the pressure placed upon some units in relation to offence targets, and the relative difficulties seeking formal registration of apartments as places of drug use ("To prove it's a drug den you have to catch the drug addict who must say that he has previously been in this den several times and used drugs there, and only when we have two such declarations can we hand the matter over"). Targeting pharmacies was a necessity:

We have people in pharmacies who pass on information to us about the people who buy syringes, because drug users are often involved in crime. The police are already searching for some of them. It is easier to trace them when they come to pharmacies rather than look for them on the street or in somebody's flat. (Divisional Police Inspector, Community Security Unit)

The potential tensions between opportunities afforded by undertaking police surveillance at pharmacies and syringe exchanges and this limiting the success of such interventions was recognised by some: "He knows that he will be noticed by us. He doesn't want that." As others commented:

Of course it is a good idea [for police to target pharmacies and syringe exchanges]. However, as far as I can see, drug users rarely go to syringe exchange centres. I guess they're afraid that police might arrest them there. (Patrol Policeman, Community Security Patrol)

Despite acknowledgement that drug users in the city have cited police presence at pharmacies and syringe exchanges as a deterrent to their use, it was proffered that police presence at pharmacies was for surveillance rather than arrest purposes: "We won't arrest anyone who is just going to the chemist. We detain people for drug possession, not for the fact that they are drug users. I may stop them for a chat, ask some questions, and then let them go." As another described of syringe exchanges:

We don't go to syringe exchange centres in order to stop and search people. We go there to talk to drug users. If the person is nice, they will tell us where and at what time drugs are sold. We go to syringe centres to get this information. We are not against people exchanging their syringes. However, we often have to work in chemists. (Patrol Policeman, Community Security Patrol)

Discussion

Policing strategy may undermine ease of access to needles and syringes among IDUs, including in Russia.[10, 13, 17, 18, 49] Yet there are few studies exploring relationships between policing and HIV prevention for IDUs from police officer perspectives.[45, 46] This was an exploratory qualitative study which served to identify inductively key emerging themes in participant accounts, and therefore generalisability beyond this particular sample and city location cannot be assumed. Findings indicate willingness among police officers to work collaboratively alongside syringe distribution interventions, though show such voiced support potentially undermined by everyday policing strategy and practice. Interview accounts described a mainly punitive approach to the policing of drug users, based on an ethos of intensive street-based surveillance and pre-emptive action as a means of drug-related crime prevention, thus potentially undermining the efficacy of other city interventions seeking to promote HIV risk reduction among IDUs.

There have been close historical links between law enforcement and treatment services in Russia, whereby the practice of exchanging drug user registration lists between police and drug treatment services was commonplace. Current evidence suggests police and drug treatment registers have close overlap.[35] Research suggests that a strong emphasis on the registration of persons seeking help for their drug use acts as a disincentive among IDUs to access drug treatment or pharmacies and syringe exchange projects for clean injecting equipment, as well as contributes to their marginalisation through loss of employment opportunity once certified an addict.[22, 48] Studies have found association between registration at drug treatment services and HIV or HCV infection,[36] arrest and syphilis,[50] and drug-related arrest and elevated odds of syringe sharing.[37]

Our findings capture a strong emphasis on street policing as a mechanism of pervasive surveillance in the lives of IDUs. First, accounts emphasised a depiction of drug users as potential criminals. In combination with a common belief that when in withdrawal drug users were "capable of committing any offence," this gave rationale for an ethos of intense surveillance wherein IDUs would be repeatedly stopped and searched as a means of "pre-empting" drug-related crime. Second, accounts emphasised the registration of individuals suspected or proven as drug users, including as a means of enabling ongoing surveillance. While provision exists for the notification and follow-up of drug users for intelligence purposes in other countries (for example, the UK), our data suggest an intense concentration of police effort on monitoring and surveillance of IDUs as a stratagem of public order control. Third, our findings are indicative of policing strategies intersecting with a common portrayal of the drug user as a source of risk. Most accounts (there were exceptions) contrasted the drug user as "other" in comparison to "normal citizens," and as beyond rights of citizenship. The rationale for intensive surveillance of IDUs was reinforced in some accounts in relation to a perceived risk of physical harm associated with street policing. In this respect, some portrayed drug users as potentially aggressive or violent, especially when in withdrawal, and this gave some rationale for accepting as permissible physical aggression (falling short of "beating up") when policing drug users. Other qualitative studies of police officer perspectives have found relationships between police officers and drug users to be shaped by "misinformation" concerning drug use as well as perceived occupational risk.[46]

Aside from the potential negative health effects of aggressive street policing,[9, 12, 17, 20, 21] the pervasive surveillance of IDUs arguably contributes to more generalised marginalisation and social suffering.[38, 51] Some have described this as a form of "oppression illness" or "structural violence."[52–54] This may be felt at both an individual and community level in terms of reduced self-esteem and weakened capacity for risk avoidance, including in relation to HIV.[39, 40, 53, 54]

Importantly, our data suggests that a strong emphasis upon surveillance and registration may undermine efforts to maximise IDUs' ease of access to needles and syringes. While accounts emphasised that the carriage of clean needles and syringes posed no theoretical risk in relation to detention or arrest, there was a more blurred picture of what happens in practice. Carriage of a syringe, including if clean or unused, was said by some to constitute sufficient suspicion that an individual may be a drug user, thus opening up opportunities for additional questioning and official registration as an addict. Carriage of previously used syringes was said to constitute potential evidence of possession, for which a prison sentence was a possibility. This clearly may contribute to reluctance among IDUs to carry previously used equipment or to return it to a syringe exchange, and may also contribute to drug use at the point of drug sale as well as to hiding or storing syringes for re-use at dealers' houses.[22] While it was posited that relaxations made in May 2004 to Article 228 of the Criminal Code concerning drugs possession—which in effect decriminalised possession of small amounts of narcotic and psychotropic drugs—may have had some effect,[33] these relaxations were again revised in February 2006, with 0.5 g and above of heroin deemed "large scale." Surveys in Togliatti subsequent to the May 2004 revisions to Article 228 give no indication that the prevalence of drug-related arrest has diminished (personal communication, L. Platt).

There is considerable evidence underscoring the public health rationale for discretionary community policing strategies which enable IDUs' access to needles and syringes without fear of arrest.[10, 13, 17, 18] Cautioning rather than detention or arrest is one example of discretion in public health oriented policing.[17] An emphasis on referral to drug treatment services as alternatives to custodial sentence[55] and shifts from vertical to consultative decision-making in policing strategy[56, 57] are other examples. But such shifts are difficult to implement without generalised tacit approval at the community level. Shifts in policing strategy towards more public health and consultative approaches involve structural changes, and it is important to recognise that these are relative to wider structural challenges associated with police and law enforcement reform in Russia, including in relation to corruption.[34] Policing and harm reduction strategies may be described as "two cultures passing in the night."[58] The strength of scientific evidence alone, and repeated calls for a shift towards public health oriented policing, is not necessarily sufficient to bring about lasting or structural change.[24]

Given recent evidence of shifts in legislation in Russia which some have argued open up opportunities for a more public health oriented approach,[33] it is timely to consider the feasibility of local HIV prevention partnerships between policing and health agencies. Examples elsewhere demonstrate the potential impact of police training and consultation in facilitating reappraisal of the balance between law enforcement and harm reduction interventions at the local level.[58, 59] Critically, this has involved change that is "bottom-up."[58] There is an urgent need to pilot police training and intervention partnerships in HIV prevention in Russia. This is especially the case in cities where there is a combination of voiced positive support for such initiatives among police and yet policing practices which serve to undermine rather than enable access to needles and syringes among IDUs.

Acknowledgements

We are grateful for the support of the UK Department for International Development for project funding support, and to the UK Department of Health for core funding to the Centre for Research on Drugs and Health Behaviour. We also thank Alexandra Kornienko for her assistance during fieldwork. We would also like to thank the Togliatti City Department of Internal Affairs, the Togliatti City Department of Health, the Togliatti Harm Reduction Project Coordination Group, and the following individuals: Elvira Zhukova; Veronica Petrova; Yuri Pevzner; Alexander Shakhov; and Adrian Renton.

REFERENCES

1. Blankenship KM, Bray SJ, Merson MH. Structural interventions in public health. *AIDS*. 2000;14(Suppl 1):S11–S21.

2. Blankenship KM, Friedman SR, Dworkin S, Mantell JE. Structural interventions: concepts, challenges and opportunities for research. *J. Urban Health*; 2006 (in press).

3. Rhodes T, Singer M, Bourgois P, Friedman SR, Strathdee SA. The social structural production of HIV risk among injecting drug users. *Soc Sci Med*. 2005;61:1026–1044.

4. Galea S, Ahern J, Vlahov D. Contexual determinants of drug use risk behaviour: a theoretic framework. *J Urban Health*. 2003;80:50–58.

5. Galea S, Nandi A, Vlahov D. The social epidemiology of drug use. *Epidemiol Rev*. 2004;26:36–52.

6. Barnett T, Whiteside A. HIV/AIDS and development: case studies and a conceptual framework. *Eur J Dev Res*. 1999;11:200–234.

7. Rhodes T, Simic M. Transition and the HIV risk environment. *Br Med J*. 2005;331:220–223.

8. Rhodes T, Ball A, Stimson GV, Kobyshcha Y, Fitch C, Pokrovsky V, et al. HIV infection in the newly independent states, eastern Europe: the social and economic context of epidemics. *Addiction*. 1999;94:1323–1336.

9. Kerr T, Small W, Wood E. The public health and social impacts of drug market enforcement: a review of the evidence. *Int J Drug Policy*. 2005;16:210–220.

10. Burris S, Blankenship KM, Donoghoe M, Sherman S, Vernick JS, Case P, Lazzarini Z, Koester S. Addressing the "risk environment" for injection drug users: the mysterious case of the missing cop. *Milbank Q*. 2004;82:125–156.

11. Des Jarlais D. Structural interventions to reduce HIV transmission among injecting drug users. *AIDS*. 2000;14(Suppl 1):S41–S46.

12. Friedman SR, Cooper HLF, Tempalski B, Keem M, Friedman R, Flom PL, Des Jarlais DC. Relationships of deterrence and law enforcement to drug-related harms among drug injectors in U.S. metropolitan areas. *AIDS*. 2006;20:93–99.

13. Koester S. Copping, running and paraphernalia laws: contextual variables and needle risk behaviour among injection drug users in Denver. *Human Organ*. 1994;53:287–295.

14. Bluthenthal RN, Kral AH, Lorvick J, Watters J. Collateral damage in the war on drugs: HIV risk behaviors among injection drug users. *Int J Drug Policy*. 1999;10:25–38.

15. Taussig JA, Weinstein B, Burris S, Jones ST. Syringe laws and pharmacy regulations are structural constraints on HIV prevention in the U.S. *AIDS*. 2000;14(Suppl 1):S47–S51.

16. Fitzgerald J, Dovey K, Dietze P, Rumbold G. Health outcomes and quasi-supervised settings for street injecting drug use. *Int J Drug Policy*. 1994;15:247–257.

17. Maher L, Dixon D. Policing and public health. Law enforcement and harm minimization in a street-level drug market. *Br J Criminol*. 1999;49:488–508.

18. Aitken C, Moore D, Higgs P, Kelsall J, Kerger M. The impact of a police crackdown on a street drug scene: evidence from the street. *Int J Drug Policy*. 2002;13:193–202.

19. Small W, Kerr T, Charette J, Schechter M, Spittal P. Impacts of intensified police activity on injection drug users: evidence from an ethnographic investigation. *Int J Drug Policy*. 2006;17:85–95.

20. Bluthenthal RN, Kral AH, Lorvick J, Watters JK. Impact of law enforcement on syringe exchange programes: a look at Oakland and San Francisco. *Med Anthropol*. 1997;18:61–83.

21. Davis CS, Burris S, Kraut-Becher J, Lynch KG, Metzger D. Effects of an intensive street-level police intervention on syringe exchange program use in Philadelphia. *Am J Public Health*. 2005;95:233–235.

22. Rhodes T, Mikhailova L, Sarang A, Lowndes CM, Rylkov A, Khutorskoy M, et al. Situational Factors influencing drug injecting, risk reduction and syringe exchange practices in Togliatti City, Russian Federation. *Soc Sci Med*. 2003;57:39–54.

23. Wood E, Kerr T, Small W, Jones J, Schechter MT, Tyndall MW. The impact of police presence on access to needle exchange programs. *J Acquir Immune Defic Syndr*. 2003;34:116–118.

24. Fitzgerald J. Policing as public health menace in the policy struggles over public injecting. *Int J Drug Policy*. 2005;16:203–206.

25. Best D, Strang J, Beswick T, Gossop M. Assessment of a concentrated high-profile police operation: no discernable impact on drug availability price or purity. *Br J Criminol*. 2001;41:738–745.

26. Bastos FI, Strathdee S. Evaluating effectiveness of syringe exchange programmes. *Soc Sci Med*. 2000;51:1771–1782.

27. Rhodes T, Lowndes CM, Judd A, Mikhailova L, Sarang A, Rylkov A, et al. Explosive spread and high prevalence of HIV infection among injecting drug users in Togliatti City, Russia. *AIDS*. 2002;16:F25–F31.

28. Rhodes T, Sarang A, Bobrik A, Bobkov E, Platt L. HIV transmission and HIV prevention associated with injecting drug use in the Russian Federation. *Int J Drug Policy*. 2004;15:39–54.

29. Rhodes T, Platt L, Maximova S, Koshkina E, Latshevskaya N, Hickman M, Renton A, Bobrova N, McDonald T, Parry JV. Prevalence of HIV, hepatitis C and syphilis among injecting drug users in Russia: a multi-city study. *Addiction*. 2006;101:252–266.

30. Des Jarlais DC, Grund JP, Zadoretzky C, Milliken J, Friedman P, Titus S, et al. HIV risk behaviour among participants of syringe exchange programmes in central/eastern Europe and Russia. *Int J Drug Policy*. 2002;13:165–174.

31. Polobinskaya SV. *Russian Legislation and the Prevention of HIV among Intravenous Drug Users*. (Information booklet), Moscow: Open Society Institute; 2002.

32. Butler WE. *HIV/AIDS and Drug Misuse in Russia: Harm Reduction Programmes and the Russian Legal System*. London: International Family Health; 2003.

33. Burris S. Harm reduction: what's a lawyer to do? *Int J Drug Policy*. 2006;17:47–50.

34. Human Rights Watch (2004) *Lessons Not Learned: Human Rights Abuses and HIV/AIDS in the Russian Federation*, Human Rights Watch, 16:5(D).

35. Platt L, Hickman M, Rhodes T, Mikhailova L, Vlasov A, Tilling K, et al. The prevalence of injecting drug use in a Russian city: implications for harm reduction and coverage. *Addiction*. 2004;99:1430–1438.

36. Rhodes T, Platt L, Judd A, Mikhailova L, Sarang A, Wallis N, Alpatova T, Hickman M, Parry JV. Hepatitis C virus infection, HIV co-infection, and associated risk among injecting drug users in Togliatti, Russia. *Int J STD AIDS*. 2005b;16:749–754.

37. Rhodes T, Judd A, Mikhailova L, Sarang A, Khutorskoy M, Platt L, et al. Injecting equipment sharing among injecting drug users in Togliatti city, Russian Federation. *J Acquir Immune Defic Syndr*. 2004;35:293–300.

38. Bourgois P, Lettiere M, Quesada J. Social misery and the sanctions of substance use: confronting HIV risk among homeless heroin addicts in San Francisco. *Soc Probl*. 1997;44:155–173.

39. Bourgois P. U.S. inner-city apartheid: the contours of structural and interpersonal violence. In: Scheper-Hughes N, Bourgois P, eds. *Violence in War and Peace: An Anthology*. Oxford: Blackwell; 2003:297–303.

40. Cooper H, Moore L, Gruskin S, Krieger N. Characterising perceived police violence: implications for public health. *Am J Public Health*. 2004:94:1109–1118.

41. Iguchi MY, London JA, Forge NG, Hickman L, Fain T, Riehman KS. Elements of well-being affected by criminalizing the drug user. *Public Health Reports*. 2002;117(Suppl 1):S146–S150.

42. Roberts DE. The social and moral cost of mass incarceration in African American communities. *Stanford Law Rev*. 2004;56:1271–1305.

43. Singer M. AIDS and the health crisis of the U.S. urban poor: the perspective of critical medical anthropology. *Soc Sci Med*. 1994;39:931–948.

44. Parker RG, Easton D, Klein CH. Structural barriers and facilitators in HIV prevention: a review of international evidence. *AIDS*. 2000;14(Suppl 1):S22–S32.

45. Beyer L, Crofts N, Reid G. Drug offending and criminal justice responses: practitioners' perspectives. *Int J Drug Policy*, 2002;13:203–211.

46. Beletsky L, Macalino GE, Burris S. Attitudes of police officers towards syringe access, occupational needle-sticks, and drug use: a qualitative study of one city police department in the United States. *Int J Drug Policy*. 2005;16:267–274.

47. Parker R, Aggleton P. HIV and AIDS-related stigma and discrimination: a conceptual framework and implications for action. *Soc Sci Med*. 2003;57:13–24.

48. Bobrova N, Rhodes T, Power R, Alcorn R, Neifeld E, Kraskiukov N, Latyshevskaia N, Maksimova S. Barriers to accessing drug treatment in Russia: a qualitative study among drug injectors in two cities. *Drug Alcohol Depend*. 2006;82(Suppl 1):57–64.

49. Mokieno M, Mokienko I. Harm reduction programme in Sakhalin, Russia. *Twelfth International Conference on the Reduction of Drug Related Harm*, New Delhi, India; 2001.

50. Platt L, Rhodes T, Judd A, Koshkina E, Maximova S, Latishevskaya N, et al. Syphilis among injecting drug users in three cities in Russia: the effect of sex work. *Am J Public Health*; 2006 (in press).

51. Kleinman A, Das V, Lock M eds. *Social Suffering*. Berkeley: University of California Press; 1997.

52. Singer M, Toledo E. *Oppression Illness: Critical Theory and Intervention with Women at Risk for AIDS*. Washington, District of Columbia, American Anthropology Association; 1995.

53. Pederson D. Political violence, ethnic conflict, and contemporary wars: broad implications for health and social well-bring. *Soc Sci Med*. 2002;55:175–190.

54. Farmer P, Connors M, Simmons J. *Women, Poverty and AIDS: Sex, Drugs and Structural Violence*. Monroe, Maine: Common Courage; 1996.

55. Hough M. Drug user treatment within a criminal justice context. *Subst Use Misuse*. 2002;37:985–996.

56. Smith BW, Novak KJ, Frank J, Travis LF. Multi-jurisdictional drug task forces: an analysis of impacts. *J Crim Justice*. 2000;28:543–556.

57. Midford R, Acres J, Lenton S, Loxley W, Boots K. Cops, drugs and the community: establishing consultative harm reduction structures in two Western Australian locations. *Int J Drug Policy*. 2002;13:181–188.

58. Small W. Two cultures passing in the night. *Int J Drug Policy*. 2006;16:221–222.

59. Hammett TM, Bartlett NA, Chen Y, Ngu D, Cuong D, Dinh, Phuong N, Minh, et al. Law enforcement influences on HIV prevention for injection drug users: observations from a cross-border project in China and Vietnam. *Int J Drug Policy*. 2005;16:235–245.

---

*Tim Rhodes** and **Lucy Platt** are with the Centre for Research on Drugs and Health Behavior, Department of Public Health and Policy, London School of Hygiene and Tropical Medicine, UK.

Anya Sarang works advocating for the rights of drug users and PLHA with the Russian Harm Reduction Network in Moscow, Russia.

Alexander Vlasov is with the Department of Internal Affairs in the city of Togliatti, Russia.

Larissa Mikhailova works with the Togliatti City Narcological Services in Russia.

Geoff Monaghan is with the UN Office on Drugs and Crime, Regional Office for Russia and Belarus, Moscow, Russia.

T. Rhodes, L. Platt, A. Sarang, A. Vlasov, L. Mikhailova, G. Monaghan, "Street Policing, Injecting Drug Use and Harm Reduction in a Russian City: A Qualitative Study of Police Perspectives," *J. of Urban Health, Bulleting of the New York Academy of Medicine*, Vol. 83. No. 5, 2006

Used by permission.

DISCUSSION QUESTIONS

1. The article illustrates the numerous prejudices Togliatti's police have toward drug users. Is there a link between these prejudices and drug users' increased risks of HIV and AIDS in the city?

2. The article provides us with a number of statements from Togliatti police that speak to the breadth of stigma and prejudice towards drug users in. From where do you think these prejudices originate? Do they reflect reality? Do you think that the police use this high level of stigma to support their perceived need for firm policing and "allowable" violence towards drug users?

3. What is the impact of excessive policing on public health in the city?

4. Do you think that the registration of drug users and the increased police surveillance it entails results in discrimination against people living with HIV and AIDS?

5. Togliatti's police view drug users as potential criminals. What strategies might be used to change this perception?

PART 4:
Civil Society Taking Action Against HIV and Related Stigma

Civil society has driven the response to HIV and advocated for evidence-based interventions since the beginning of the epidemic. International, national, and grassroots organizations often have insights into the issues facing their communities, and are effective partners in designing and implementing prevention strategies to address these matters. Civil society actors actively promoted the rights of people living with HIV and AIDS, and advocated for universal access to treatment at the international level through coordinated participation in the preparation of the UN Declaration of Commitment on HIV/AIDS (2001) and the subsequent Political Declaration on HIV/AIDS (2006). While governments often failed to face and appropriately respond to the realities of the HIV epidemic, civil society actors hold them responsible to their national and international commitments.

Civil society offers powerful ways of combating HIV stigma and discrimination. Often those living with HIV and AIDS already belong to traditionally marginalized populations (e.g, injection drug users, men who have sex with men, sex workers) and so mutual support groups, set up by members and peers within a community, are often most successful in providing services and in challenging stigma.

Civil society also has been successful in forging innovative partnerships with governments and UN agencies in combating the HIV epidemic. As a strong voice for the affected community, civil society actors—from grassroots organizations to national NGOs—have been effective in talking openly about the challenges of HIV- and AIDS-related stigma, and often bringing cases of discrimination to the attention of the relevant authorities, thus helping victims of discrimination seek legal redress.

While the civil society in the countries of Central and Eastern Europe and Central Asia is still young, its active involvement in HIV prevention efforts in the region has been crucial in putting HIV and AIDS on the agendas of the national and regional policy makers.

In "Russia's Blossoming Civil Society Holds the Key to HIV," Hannah Brown describes how individuals affected by HIV and AIDS formed their own self-support groups, and addressed the government's rules that contribute to negative public attitudes toward people living with HIV/AIDS and further exacerbate stigmatization of the disease. The author believes that while addressing the poor public health structure is the government's responsibility, Russia's newly strengthened civil society must ensure that the government urgently addresses healthcare issues and changes policies that contribute to the further stigmatization.

In her speech at the international conference Health Security in Central Asia: Drug Use, HIV and AIDS, Joanne Csete, then director of the HIV/AIDS and Human Rights Program at Human Rights Watch, challenged the conference audience to think about human rights abuses related to HIV and AIDS as interconnected and overlapping. If prevention efforts are to succeed in Central Asia, civil society, NGOs, human rights activists, and especially those with HIV or at high risk of HIV infection must be empowered to advocate for effective prevention strategies and work together to address issues of stigma and discrimination.

Russia's Blossoming Civil Society Holds the Key to HIV

*by Hannah Brown**

Russia's leaders are facing an HIV epidemic that experts believe could become a national disaster. But ignorance and ingrained prejudices among the general population hinder efforts at control. Is Russia's nascent civil society strong enough to meet the challenge?

"I'm going to give up on Monday", promises Vadim with a wry smile, before listing heroin, cannabis, and hunka—a home-made opiate common in the west Siberian city of Tomsk, where Vadim lives—among the drugs he has been hooked on since 1993. "But it's not so easy to stop. Even if you don't feel a physical dependence".

As a young male drug user, Vadim, 29, could be the epitome of Russia's HIV epidemic. But he is not infected-at least not yet. After contracting hepatitis from sharing needles a few years ago, he has been a meticulous visitor to Tomsk's needle-exchange centre, housed in an anonymous dust-caked building on the city's outskirts. "There's no place to get clean needles other than here", he says.

The centre keeps tabs on its visitors, and operates under the watchful, if distant, eye of the authorities, but Vadim is worried enough about contracting HIV make sure his regular visits include blood tests. "My wife doesn't use drugs, so I have to be tested regularly to protect her", he explains.

Vadim blames his addiction on the turmoil that followed the Soviet collapse at the beginning of the 1990s, when the social institutions that had kept children like him on the straight and narrow imploded. "Teachers didn't want to teach", he explains. "There was no information about drugs, and it was fashionable". So, with time on his hands, and cheap drugs in plentiful supply, Vadim, like millions of his compatriots, succumbed to the lure of illegal intoxication.

This post-Soviet drug-use explosion paved the way for an HIV epidemic labelled by the Global Fund to Fight AIDS, Tuberculosis, and Malaria as the fastest spreading in the world. Although the virus was initially introduced to

Russia through sexual transmission, it was the thousands of drug users sharing needles that propelled it forward. By the end of 1995, there had only been seven cases out of a total of 1062 in which transmission was attributed to drug use. But over the next 10 years, unsafe injecting accounted for a massive 76% of the 342,000 official cases. UNAIDS believes the actual numbers could be twice as high.

CRISIS POINT

For international onlookers, Russia's HIV epidemic is now at a crucial stage. Rates of new infections seem to be levelling off, but scientists fear this development is not, as it might seem, a sign that control efforts are starting to work. Rather, the slowdown may indicate that the virus is leaving the confines of high-risk groups—drug users, commercial sex workers, and men who have sex with men—and is slowly seeping into the general population. The drop in new cases can be explained by the difference in efficiency of transmission routes: for drug users sharing needles, the chance of passing on HIV is close to 100%; for heterosexual partners, one of whom is infected, the probability of transmission can be as low as 1%.

Until this year, however, President Putin had seemed largely oblivious to the concerns of scientists and international AIDS organisations about Russia's burgeoning HIV crisis. A federal anti-AIDS law guaranteeing free medical care and social support for HIV-positive people was passed without any spending recommendations or action points. Prevention and treatment efforts were persistently starved of funds. And the lack of federal support for the country's hundred or so AIDS centres—part of a Soviet-designed nationwide network isolated from the rest of the healthcare system—left them with no option other than to look to international health agencies and western nongovernmental organisations (NGOs) for help.

Fortunately, aid has come, most notably from the Global Fund, now the country's largest external HIV/AIDS donor. The knock-on effects of this commitment seem also to have pushed HIV up the domestic agenda, evinced by this year's 20-fold federal funding increase, last month's pledge to fully reimburse the Global Fund for its grants, and Putin's powerful rhetoric on HIV/AIDS during Russia's first stint in the G8 chair.

But there has been a high price paid for the president's procrastination on

HIV, in the form of continuing ignorance about the virus among the general population. Sociological studies suggest that risky behaviours are getting more, not less, common in Russia, because people do not understand enough about AIDS. It is this situation that Russia's nascent civil society is now working hard to change.

UNCIVIL SOCIETY

As more of a managed democracy than a free one, the formation of activist groups to articulate the priorities of the populous and fight for individual rights in Russia has been slow and sporadic. But one beneficial side-effect of the country's reliance on external aid to combat HIV is that the international attention has helped strengthen the country's civic institutions—an essential component of successful anti-HIV efforts in all parts of the world.

These reenergised organisations do, however, have their work cut out. According to Alexey Bobrik, head of the GLOBUS project, a consortium of national and international NGOs which runs HIV prevention and treatment projects in 10 Russian regions, the general attitude towards HIV in Russia "is still one of denial and widespread stigmatisation, even in health facilities".

He says dental care and operations are routinely denied to HIV-positive people because of their infection status. And, he adds, the government requirement that infected individuals receive medical care only at AIDS centres essentially amounts to a public branding of HIV-positive people that perpetuates their marginalisation.

Richard Feachem, Executive Director of the Global Fund, has said of Russia's misconceptions about HIV that "denial of that degree puts Russia behind China and India, both of which have overcome the issue".

Part of the problem is that next to the heavy tolls wrought by Russia's daunting population-wide health burdens, which include very high rates of heart disease, alcoholism, and tuberculosis, the number of HIV cases is tiny. It simply isn't a serious health problem yet, Bobrik explains. "Many people in Russia don't believe it is a big social problem because of the low number of deaths and the fact that they are confined to groups such as drug addicts and other marginalised populations", he says. These beliefs are not only a problem for educating people at risk, however. They also prevent people already infected from seeking help.

In the southern city of Saratov, on the banks of the Volga river, the clean modern lines of the only AIDS clinic stand in stark contrast to the shabby wooden houses slumped along the neighbouring mud-track streets. Elena, a nurse at the centre, took up her job in 1999 after finding out she was HIV-positive. She now runs a peer-support group for people who come to the clinic for testing or treatment. "They all say it is so nice just to be normal people. We are always reminded about our disease, so it is a relief to have the opportunity to meet and discuss not as patients but as people", she says.

Luba Potemina, Elena's boss and head physician of the Saratov centre, says one of their main tasks is to "make sure that HIV-positive people don't feel any different from people with diabetes or vascular disease". Infected individuals are not separated from non-infected patients in hospital or maternity wards, which helps decrease discrimination outside the centre's walls, she says.

But the real battleground is in the community, among people too fearful of stigmatisation to seek the necessary treatment. Vitaly, a nervy young man who got engaged to Elena after they met at the AIDS centre, says many people "are afraid that their confidentiality will be breached, or that someone will see them", so they do not attend support meetings.

His experiences of being discriminated against in health centres and at school—he was only allowed to finish studying for the last 2 years on condition that he stayed at home-convinced him that people with HIV need somewhere to meet that is less public than the AIDS centre to get support. He is appreciative of the work of the AIDS centre, but believes the focus of local NGOs on raising awareness among young uninfected people means people actually living with the virus are ignored, which therefore perpetuates their marginalisation.

Vitaly has now set up his own NGO to help address what he perceives as a significant care gap. "When I was diagnosed, I was just told and that was it. But when people come to us, they feel like someone cares—and that's what's important", he says.

PREVENTION WORKS

The task of eliminating ingrained prejudices taken on by Russia's new clutch of NGOs is a daunting one, but a pleasant surprise has emerged from the country's recent experiences. What these dedicated groups have shown is how effective small well-run programmes can be, if given sufficient funds and a bit of attention.

Bobrik's GLOBUS project, named for the abbreviation of the Russian translation of Global Efforts Against HIV/AIDS in Russia—and of which Vadim's local needle-exchange centre in the Siberian city of Tomsk is part— is one of the most successful, despite only getting off the ground at the beginning of last year.

In just over 12 months, the GLOBUS project's activities, funded by the Global Fund, have already helped push down antiretroviral drug prices; improve access to prevention and treatment services; and have helped change national AIDS policy, through the lobbying efforts of the organisations it supports. In fact, according to Urban Weber, the Global Fund's Eastern Europe and Central Asia team leader, the region of Eastern Europe and Central Asia, of which Russia is part, "has produced some of the best results of any grants awarded by the Global Fund".

Bobrik attributes much of his consortium's success to the professionalism of NGOs in turning their hands to activities they had little previous experience of, including large-scale procurement, delivery of equipment, and the organisation of a large number of HIV/AIDS treatment programmes. But Weber believes the reason for the region's spectacular success is simpler. Russia combines four key ingredients: infrastructure, NGOs, government support, and cash. "That's the magic formula", he says.

But just as stigma and discrimination mark the lives of infected individuals, Bobrik says his organisation has encountered numerous problems caused by social resistance to expanding the scope of HIV-prevention activities, particularly those focused on drug use and raising awareness among homosexual men.

In April this year, one GLOBUS site was the subject of a series of attacks sanctioned by the Russian Orthodox Church, during which NGOs were accused of "destroying the moral grounds of society" and even of perpetuating paedophilia. However, Bobrik says such extreme outbursts are not his prime concern since the incident merely served to strengthen and unify the message from "all reasonable peoples—including the government and the academy of medical sciences". A bigger fear, he says, is the law.

After 2 years of subtle indications that drug-use laws were changing to make it easier to prosecute dealers, while protecting users by helping them to kick their habits, the State Drug Control Committee last year decided to re-tighten controls. Bobrik believes this decision will have a negative effect on HIV-prevention efforts by forcing addicts to boycott HIV-information centres because of fear of arrest.

But his greatest worry at the moment is that this move signals a more wide-ranging crackdown—a new Russian "war on drugs"—which could see the end of the legal protection currently extended to harm-reduction sites, such as needle-exchange centres, and put paid to hopes of a reversal in the government's currently strict prohibition of substitution treatment, used to help wean drug users off their habit. Without freedom to use substitution therapy when appropriate, international authorities agree that other harm-reduction strategies are next to useless.

PATCHY PROGRESS

For all their promise, these first forays into civil-society-led HIV prevention in Russia are necessarily small-scale, which means the good results they generate are inevitably isolated, and many regions still have no access to services at all.

For example, a specific criticism of the GLOBUS project in the west-Siberian oblast of Tomsk is that it has focused solely on the urban capital, which excludes many of the region's residents who are at the highest risk. In the frosty northern oil town of Strezhevoy, which borders the neighbouring high-HIV region of Tyumen, HIV transmission is much higher than in the student-dense capital because of the migration of HIV-positive individuals across the oblast border, and the concentration of heroin dealers bringing drugs into the town to help oil-revenue-rich workers offload their extra cash. HIV-positive people who have moved to get work are particularly vulnerable because oil companies inevitably prefer to hire new staff members rather than taking care of current ones. And with the recent politically messy break-up of oil-giant Yukos, widespread unemployment has added to Siberia's woes.

SYSTEM FAILURE

What Russia needs now to help its small-scale successes become sustainable improvements is for its reborn civil-society movement to make a lot more fuss about one issue common to all regions across Russia's great expanse: the fundamental barrier to uniformly good HIV-prevention and control posed by the decaying, fragmented health system.

Since the tight reins of central Soviet control have been loosened, Russia's 89 oblasts have been more or less allowed to go their separate ways when it comes to health. This means there is little uniformity between regions, and huge variations in quality and extent of care. Underfunding, however, is an affliction most regions can claim, and lack of money has led to appalling perversions of the concept of free emergency medical care—even for the HIV treatment promised by law. "In the early and mid-1990s it became routine for hospitals to require patients to provide their own food, linens, bandages, and even essential medications", recalls Bobrik.

What's more, even within regions different segments of the health system have little interaction. Care for people with HIV is the sole responsibility of a network of AIDS centres created under the Soviet system at the end of the 1980s and kept separate from the rest of the health system.

This vertical strategy worked fairly well at the epidemic's early stages, when case numbers were small and confined to high-risk groups. Over time, however, the restrictive structure has led to a gulf of misunderstanding about HIV/AIDS between the specialists in AIDS centres and doctors who work in the general health system. Even now, doctors and nurses in non-specialist health facilities are shockingly ignorant of basic facts about the disease.

Now that the epidemic is on a much larger scale, the inflexibility of the system is causing serious troubles. New treatment targets mean thousands of patients have to be treated very quickly all over the country. But the health systems' bias towards expensive tertiary centres and specialist care means there are neither the funds nor the capacity to cope.

Valery Chernyavskiy, a Russian doctor who now works for the Global Fund, believes the roots of these problems lie with the high degree of specialisation in medicine and the corresponding neglect Russia has shown to the discipline of primary care. But, he warns, resolving this misalignment will not come easily because of the vested interests that specialists have in their work. "The Russian system continues to miss the point", he says. "It has to look to the rest of the world."

The most obvious result of this sad state of affairs is the continued segregation of HIV-positive people through their necessary life-long ties to stigmatising AIDS centres. But the scarcity of local health providers with the capability to support HIV prevention and treatment presents practical problems, too, by hindering proper surveillance and detection of cases. "We need the health system to accurately identify people who are infected, to offer counselling and so on", explains Bobrik. At the moment, it doesn't do so.

Chernyavskiy believes these problems can all be traced back to deficiencies in local democracy—which, like civil society in Russia, is uncommonly weak. "Primary care is not only about GPs in surgeries, but it includes nurses and community involvement at a local level too", he explains.

So, if Russia's newly strengthened social mobilisation movement can turn its attention to health care in general, then system-transforming change should, at last, become a feasible goal to achieve.

---

*Hannah Brown works with the Lancet Group. She currently runs the features section, called World Report, and writes weekly editorials.

Reprinted from *The Lancet*, vol. 368, Brown, H., "Russia's blossoming civil society holds the key to HIV," pp. 437–440, ©2006, with permission from Elsevier.

DISCUSSION QUESTIONS

1. The article describes a harm reduction project in Tomsk that permits drug users to exchange dirty needles and syringes for clean ones and receive referrals to medical care. How would projects like that affect the stigma associated with HIV and AIDS? Do you think that the fact that the staff keeps track of visitors and that the project operates under the eye of local authorities has any impact on HIV and AIDS prevention in this community?

2. Sharing contaminated injection paraphernalia is among the easiest ways of transmitting HIV. How can this knowledge empower AIDS activists in their efforts to reduce the stigma?

3. The article mentions a Russian federal anti-AIDS law that guarantees free medical care and social support for people living with HIV and AIDS. However, the law was passed without any funding provision or action points. Do you think that such a law is effective? What do you think can be done to make laws more effective in tackling issues surrounding the HIV and AIDS epidemic?

4. What role can civil society play in HIV and AIDS prevention and in tackling the stigma associated with HIV and AIDS? Are there NGOs in your country/community working on this issue? What opportunities do young people in your community/country have to participate in HIV and AIDS prevention programs?

Facing Down the Ugly Politics of HIV/AIDS: What is the Role for Human Rights Groups and Other NGOs?

*by Joanne Csete**

It is a challenge to me to know how to structure a discussion of AIDS-related human rights abuses in the world when they are so many, so varied and so interconnected. I don't know if it helps to list the categories of abuse that human rights groups and AIDS NGOs have been contacting us about and that we ourselves with many NGO collaborators are trying to document and address. These overlap a great deal; they are not as discrete as this listing will make them seem. As I list these, you may wish to think about how relevant they are to the situation in your countries. They are:

- Discrimination and abuse faced by traditional "high-risk groups" (injection drug users, sex workers, men who have sex with men, migrant workers, etc.)

- Subordinate status of women and girls (rendering them unable to control the terms of their sexual lives, often combined with laws and polices forcing their economic dependence on their husbands or other men that keeps them in marriages they might otherwise leave)

- Sexual violence and coercion, including sexual violence as a weapon of war (which we have investigated in the Congo war)

- A horrific range of abuses against prisoners

- Discrimination on the grounds of HIV status (including many instances of legal discrimination embodied in national law)

- Immigration law and practice that limits people's entry into countries if they are HIV-positive (for which there is no public health justification)

- Criminalization of HIV transmission and other criminal law issues

- Compulsory testing and a wide variety of confidentiality and right to privacy issues

- Censorship and other violations of the right to information and free expression, including crackdowns against AIDS educators

- A wide range of violations of the rights of orphans and other children affected by AIDS

- Access to treatment and care

Those of you in the audience who are students of human rights will know that that last one on access to treatment would fall into the category of economic and social rights rather than the civil and political rights that make up the rest of the list. We should note, though, that access to treatment is related in important and direct ways to people's ability to realize their civil and political rights, including through reduction of the discrimination associated with overt illness.

How Has This Wide Range of Violations Been Allowed to Persist?

Human rights violations thrive for many reasons, but I think in the end the most important ones are political in a strict sense. In this case, the politics of HIV/AIDS has many ugly aspects. It is, first, a politics of denial—the very nature of the virus and its epidemiological course give politicians and policy-makers a window of denial that they readily take advantage of. A window, most sadly, that sets the epidemic up for the enormous mortality that becomes so hard to put the brakes on, especially in the absence of access to antiretroviral treatment. It is a politics of cowardice as most politicians in the world are not courageous about diving into any area in which the day-to-day struggles involve working side by side with gay men, drug users, sex workers, prisoners and others affected by AIDS. The politics of HIV/AIDS is also a politics of elitism and racism. As I suggested earlier, one of the main reasons the global AIDS epidemic took so long to find a place on the global stage and still does not have priority in global resource allocation is that it was brushed away as an "African problem". Moreover, in the world outside Africa, it is, in my experience, hard to find a policy-maker who readily embraces the idea that there are lessons to be learned from Africa. And within Africa and Asia, in spite of decades of dense and earnest rhetoric on the benefits of participation and participatory approaches, it is equally difficult to find policies or programs that take their real cue from the experiences of uneducated and poor and socially marginalized people.

As we all know too well, the politics of HIV/AIDS is a politics of moral judgementalism, in that the apparently growing political influence of religious fundamentalists of all kinds has unspeakably terrible consequences for HIV/AIDS. The power of religious extremists, once again, has hardened support for sodomy laws, has galvanized support for cruelly repressive drug laws, and has gone to great lengths to keep women and girls in subordinate roles. The influence of religious fundamentalists in the US, for example, is making it more and more difficult to bring basic information on HIV transmission to young people as a federal government heavily influenced by these fundamentalists is pushing comprehensive sex education out of the classroom in favor of "abstinence only until marriage" programs. These programs explicitly fail to inform young people about the effectiveness of condoms in preventing HIV transmission and focus on sexual abstinence as the only solution to HIV/AIDS.

How Do We Begin to Address Such a Wide Range of Abuses?

It is useful, first of all, to recognize that in the history of the HIV/AIDS epidemic, the successes in combating the disease (too few certainly) have largely been driven by civil society. NGOs, especially groups of people with AIDS and those who face high risk of HIV transmission, have tended to be far ahead of governments in advancing the policies and programs that have resulted in palpable reductions in transmission or in better access to treatment and care. This is a difficult message for Central Asia where civil society was for so long not allowed to flourish and there is a lot of catching up to do.

Human rights organization[s] have built and continue to build a record of achievement in the re[g]ion, and HIV/AIDS and harm reduction groups are growing in some countries in numbers and capacity. But these need to come together—that is, human rights groups on the one hand and HIV/AIDS and harm reduction on the other. The human rights movement, including my own organization, has been slow to come to HIV/AIDS issues with its full research capacity and advocacy voice. HIV/AIDS groups use the language of human rights but often need help exploiting most effectively the tools and mechanisms of human rights. I am happy that Human Rights Watch and the Open Society Institute are in discussion about how this kind of collaboration might be facilitated in Eastern Europe and Central Asia.

But that's the civil society side of the picture, and in the end not much will happen unless government and civil society are open to some degree of interaction. I was happy to hear in Dr. Kirichenko's interesting presentation earlier that this interaction is beginning on HIV/AIDS issues in Kyrgyzstan. In Kazakhstan, things are also happening. We spoke with one government AIDS center director over tea in the home of the director of a group representing men who have sex with men, for example. I have worked on HIV/AIDS in a lot of countries, and there are plenty of places where this still couldn't happen. Discussing the perils and potentials of civil society-state interaction in this area is beyond the scope both of my competence and of this talk, but I would like to suggest a few areas where collaboration will be very useful in the continuing struggle against AIDS in the region.

Review of laws and policies in light of the exigencies of combating HIV/AIDS is a crucial area that will be most effective if NGOs are involved. Kazakhstan is to be congratulated for initiating this kind of process, and many countries will be following that experience closely. The issues are quite clear, and the U.N. Guidelines on HIV/AIDS and Human Rights as well as the Legislators Handbook that goes with them and a number of other resources are available to use in such a process. A number of legal reform exercises that we have followed have resulted in useful changes to the law that have improved the environment for fighting AIDS. Our time in Kazakhstan was a reminder of how important it is to devote attention and resources not only to revising the law but also to implementation and follow-up. I am reminded of the observation of one author from India that too often passing laws is like passing water— it all winds up down the drain. ... that is, if there is not enough attention to implementation. It was exciting to be in Kazakhstan when Dr. Erasylova announced the ground-breaking change in the policy of mandatory HIV testing of all persons in detention in the country, which, as Marie Struthers mentioned earlier, would effectively eliminate the segregation of HIV-positive persons in the prison system. One doesn't expect a policy like this to be implemented overnight, but we hope the resources will be there to see this policy through to full implementation, especially in the pre-trial detention system. This is something that will also certainly be watched worldwide.

Another area crucial to HIV prevention that I think is an important one for government-NGO collaboration is the design and implementation of information campaigns and educational curricula on HIV/AIDS. How often do we see messages that include dark images of drug users and sex workers that are so demonizing that all they are missing is horns and a tail? We have to be careful that information and education campaigns don't feed stigma, that somehow the idea of the dignity and rights of everyone comes through. I believe this is best achieved by including persons at high risk in the process of designing information programs. Often the first step governments try to take, with the best of intentions, in "reforming" the image of the drug user is to encourage people to think of drug users as people with an illness, people who are sick. A high-level police officer in Kazakhstan explained to us that this idea of drug users as sick people is central to the "humanization" of drug policy in the country and that police are being trained to regard drug users as sick. This is certainly an important step forward from thinking of drug users only as criminals, but, at the risk of stating the obvious, I would note that labeling drug users as "sick" is not necessarily conducive to reducing discrimination against them and may constitute replacing one kind of discrimination with another, perhaps more benign. (This is especially the case if services are not provided that correspond to the idea that drug users have an illness that needs to be treated.) Again, it would be nice to see campaigns that not only do not criminalize people at high risk of HIV transmission but promote the idea that drug users have rights and deserve respect. This is not easy, but it's possible.

Another hard policy discussion that I think would benefit from inclusion of NGOs is the matter of antiretroviral treatment. As Marie noted, we found that in Kazakhstan the idea is widely held that drug users are not deserving of antiretroviral medicines. In an epidemic where 80 to 90 percent of persons with HIV/AIDS are injecting drug users, one would have to look hard for a more self-defeating policy. We know that this discussion will intensify throughout the region as more affordable antiretroviral drugs become available, as most people expect will happen. There is not adequate time in this talk to review the extensive body of research literature indicating that compliance with antiretroviral and other treatment protocols among active injecting drug users is as good as that of other people. But I hope that it will be possible to enter this discussion with the knowledge that banning antiretroviral medicines from drug users, aside from bring questionable from a public health point of view, is discrimination, pure and simple.

A particular action that I would also mention has to do with ratification of key human rights instruments. The part of international human rights law that deals with due process, fair and prompt trials, protection from arbitrary arrest and such crucial matters as the right to information and free expression is called the International Covenant on Civil and Political Rights. When a country rat- ifies this instrument, it becomes party to a treaty and sends a strong message of some level of commitment to these ideals. In Central Asia, every country but one has ratified this treaty, and we encourage our colleagues in Kazakhstan to join their neighbors as parties to this important law. It is tempting to think that ratification of such treaties doesn't mean much in practical terms, but in other parts of the world, it has been seen that even just the process of debating rati- fication in parliament, especially where NGOs are included, is important to opening the minds of policy-makers to think about protections of the rights that are so closely related to a state's ability to fight HIV/AIDS.

One final area I would mention where NGOs and governments may useful- ly work together in combating AIDS is the matter of understanding the real extent of the epidemic in a country—getting the numbers. I look forward to the day when I can hear a presentation on the epidemiology of HIV/AIDS in Central Asia where someone says "here are the official numbers of persons liv- ing with HIV/AIDS and they represent the real situation" rather than "here are the official numbers—multiply by ten" or "multiply by six". It is true that groups at high risk and people with AIDS can find surveys threatening, but the expe- rience of many countries has shown that if these persons are approached respectfully, they can be important allies in helping to accomplish good surveil- lance of HIV prevalence. It is in everyone's interest to know the real extent of the epidemic—obviously an essential matter for program planning and evalua- tion and for dealing with donors—and communities of persons at risk need this information as much as governments do. Repressive approaches to surveillance are as counterproductive as in any other domain of HIV/AIDS; working in col- laboration with persons living with the disease and persons at high risk can yield good results. Kazakhstan is beginning to do this, and others will be inter- ested in that experience.

I hope it will be possible to find many examples from Central Asia in the coming years of ways in which governments and NGOs, including human rights NGOs—if not always hand in hand, at least in discussion with each other—will find ways to confront and change the worst aspects of the politics of HIV/AIDS.

---

*Joanne Csete is currently the executive director with the Canadian HIV/AIDS Legal Network. Previously, she was director of the HIV/AIDS and human rights program at Human Rights

Watch in New York, where she oversaw research and advocacy on a wide range of human rights violations related to the AIDS epidemic.

As part of the latter role, in 2002 Joanne Csete delivered the above speech at the international conference Health Security in Central Asia: Drug Use, HIV and AIDS. The conference took place on October 14, 2002 in Dushanbe, Tajikistan.

Csete, Joanne, "Facing Down the Ugly Politics of HIV/AIDS: What Role for Human Rights Groups and other NGOs," Eurasianet, http//:www.eurasianet.org.

Used by permission.

DISCUSSION QUESTIONS

1. J. Csete notes that civil society actors have been driving the response to the HIV epidemic globally, and in Central Asia in particular. How do you think NGOs can improve the situation with regard to HIV- and AIDS-related rights abuses, such as sexual violence and coercion, and breach of confidentiality? How can we use the human rights framework to address these abuses?

2. The author suggests that the politics of moral judgmentalism negatively impacts the epidemic. Do you think these politics affect HIV- and AIDS-related stigma and discrimination? If yes, how do you think AIDS activists should tackle these politics? If no, then is it helpful for activists to protest the politics of moral judgmentalism?

3. Are civil society actions alone enough to reverse the epidemic? Are there any other key actors who need to be involved in prevention efforts?

4. Is government supportive of civil society prevention efforts in your community/country?

PART 5:
Background Reading

United Nations Declaration of Commitment on HIV/AIDS

"Global Crisis—Global Action"

1. We, Heads of State and Government and Representatives of States and Governments, assembled at the United Nations, from 25 to 27 June 2001, for the twenty-sixth special session of the General Assembly convened in accordance with resolution 55/13, as a matter of urgency, to review and address the problem of HIV/AIDS in all its aspects as well as to secure a global commitment to enhancing coordination and intensification of national, regional and international efforts to combat it in a comprehensive manner;

2. Deeply concerned that the global HIV/AIDS epidemic, through its devastating scale and impact, constitutes a global emergency and one of the most formidable challenges to human life and dignity, as well as to the effective enjoyment of human rights, which undermines social and economic development throughout the world and affects all levels of society—national, community, family and individual;

3. Noting with profound concern, that by the end of the year 2000, 36.1 million people worldwide were living with HIV/AIDS, 90 per cent in developing countries and 75 per cent in sub-Saharan Africa;

4. Noting with grave concern that all people, rich and poor, without distinction of age, gender or race are affected by the HIV/AIDS epidemic, further noting that people in developing countries are the most affected and that women, young adults and children, in particular girls, are the most vulnerable;

5. Concerned also that the continuing spread of HIV/AIDS will constitute a serious obstacle to the realization of the global development goals we adopted at the Millennium Summit;

6. Recalling and reaffirming our previous commitments on HIV/AIDS made through:

- The United Nations Millennium Declaration of 8 September 2000;[1]

- The political declaration and further actions and initiatives to implement the commitments made at the World Summit for Social Development of 1 July 2000;[2]

- The political declaration[3] and further action and initiatives to implement the Beijing Declaration and Platform for Action,[4] of 10 June 2000;

- Key actions for the further implementation of the Programme of Action of the International Conference on Population and Development of 2 July 1999;[5]

- The regional call for action to fight HIV/AIDS in Asia and the Pacific of 25 April 2001;

- The Abuja Declaration and Framework for Action for the Fight Against HIV/AIDS, Tuberculosis and other Related Infectious Diseases in Africa, 27 April 2001;

- The Declaration of the Ibero-America Summit of Heads of State of November 2000 in Panama;

- The Caribbean Partnership Against HIV/AIDS, 14 February, 2001;

- The European Union Programme for Action: Accelerated action on HIV/ AIDS, malaria and tuberculosis in the context of poverty reduction of 4 May 2001;

- The Baltic Sea Declaration on HIV/AIDS Prevention of 4 May 2000;

- The Central Asian Declaration on HIV/AIDS of 18 May 2001;

7. Convinced of the need to have an urgent, coordinated and sustained response to the HIV/AIDS epidemic, which will build on the experience and lessons learned over the past 20 years;

8. Noting with grave concern that Africa, in particular sub-Saharan Africa, is currently the worst affected region where HIV/AIDS is considered as a state of emergency, which threatens development, social cohesion, political stability, food security and life expectancy and imposes a devastating economic burden and that the dramatic situation on the continent needs urgent and exceptional national, regional and international action;

9. Welcoming the commitments of African Heads of State or Government, at the Abuja Special Summit in April 2001, particularly their pledge to set a target of allocating at least 15 per cent of their annual national budgets for the improvement of the health sector to help address the HIV/AIDS epidemic; and recognizing that action to reach this target, by those countries whose resources are limited, will need to be complemented by increased international assistance;

10. Recognizing also that other regions are seriously affected and confront similar threats, particularly the Caribbean region, with the second highest rate of HIV infection after sub-Saharan Africa, the Asia-Pacific region where 7.5

million people are already living with HIV/AIDS, the Latin America region with 1.5 million people living with HIV/AIDS, and the Central and Eastern European region with very rapidly rising infection rates; and that the potential exists for a rapid escalation of the epidemic and its impact throughout the world if no specific measures are taken;

11. Recognizing that poverty, underdevelopment and illiteracy are among the principal contributing factors to the spread of HIV/AIDS and noting with grave concern that HIV/AIDS is compounding poverty and is now reversing or impeding development in many countries and should therefore be addressed in an integrated manner;

12. Noting that armed conflicts and natural disasters also exacerbate the spread of the epidemic;

13. Noting further that stigma, silence, discrimination, and denial, as well as lack of confidentiality, undermine prevention, care and treatment efforts and increase the impact of the epidemic on individuals, families, communities and nations and must also be addressed;

14. Stressing that gender equality and the empowerment of women are fundamental elements in the reduction of the vulnerability of women and girls to HIV/AIDS;

15. Recognizing that access to medication in the context of pandemics such as HIV/AIDS is one of the fundamental elements to achieve progressively the full realization of the right of everyone to the enjoyment of the highest attainable standard of physical and mental health;

16. Recognizing that the full realization of human rights and fundamental freedoms for all is an essential element in a global response to the HIV/AIDS pandemic, including in the areas of prevention, care, support and treatment, and that it reduces vulnerability to HIV/AIDS and prevents stigma and related discrimination against people living with or at risk of HIV/AIDS;

17. Acknowledging that prevention of HIV infection must be the mainstay of the national, regional and international response to the epidemic; and that prevention, care, support and treatment for those infected and affected by HIV/AIDS are mutually reinforcing elements of an effective response and must be integrated in a comprehensive approach to combat the epidemic;

18. Recognizing the need to achieve the prevention goals set out in this Declaration in order to stop the spread of the epidemic and acknowledging that all countries must continue to emphasize widespread and effective prevention,

including awareness-raising campaigns through education, nutrition, information and health-care services;

19. Recognizing that care, support and treatment can contribute to effective prevention through increased acceptance of voluntary and confidential counselling and testing, and by keeping people living with HIV/AIDS and vulnerable groups in close contact with health-care systems and facilitating their access to information, counselling and preventive supplies;

20. Emphasizing the important role of cultural, family, ethical and religious factors in the prevention of the epidemic, and in treatment, care and support, taking into account the particularities of each country as well as the importance of respecting all human rights and fundamental freedoms;

21. Noting with concern that some negative economic, social, cultural, political, financial and legal factors are hampering awareness, education, prevention, care, treatment and support efforts;

22. Noting the importance of establishing and strengthening human resources and national health and social infrastructures as imperatives for the effective delivery of prevention, treatment, care and support services;

23. Recognizing that effective prevention, care and treatment strategies will require behavioural changes and increased availability of and non-discriminatory access to, *inter alia*, vaccines, condoms, microbicides, lubricants, sterile injecting equipment, drugs including anti-retroviral therapy, diagnostics and related technologies as well as increased research and development;

24. Recognizing also that the cost availability and affordability of drugs and related technology are significant factors to be reviewed and addressed in all aspects and that there is a need to reduce the cost of these drugs and technologies in close collaboration with the private sector and pharmaceutical companies;

25. Acknowledging that the lack of affordable pharmaceuticals and of feasible supply structures and health systems continue to hinder an effective response to HIV/AIDS in many countries, especially for the poorest people and recalling efforts to make drugs available at low prices for those in need;

26. Welcoming the efforts of countries to promote innovation and the development of domestic industries consistent with international law in order to increase access to medicines to protect the health of their populations; and noting that the impact of international trade agreements on access to or local manufacturing of, essential drugs and on the development of new drugs needs to be further evaluated;

27. Welcoming the progress made in some countries to contain the epidemic, particularly through: strong political commitment and leadership at the highest levels, including community leadership; effective use of available resources and traditional medicines; successful prevention, care, support and treatment strategies; education and information initiatives; working in partnership with communities, civil society, people living with HIV/AIDS and vulnerable groups; and the active promotion and protection of human rights; and recognizing the importance of sharing and building on our collective and diverse experiences, through regional and international cooperation including North/South, South/South cooperation and triangular cooperation;

28. Acknowledging that resources devoted to combating the epidemic both at the national and international levels are not commensurate with the magnitude of the problem;

29. Recognizing the fundamental importance of strengthening national, regional and subregional capacities to address and effectively combat HIV/AIDS and that this will require increased and sustained human, financial and technical resources through strengthened national action and cooperation and increased regional, subregional and international cooperation;

30. Recognizing that external debt and debt-servicing problems have substantially constrained the capacity of many developing countries, as well as countries with economies in transition, to finance the fight against HIV/AIDS;

31. Affirming the key role played by the family in prevention, care, support and treatment of persons affected and infected by HIV/AIDS, bearing in mind that in different cultural, social and political systems various forms of the family exist;

32. Affirming that beyond the key role played by communities, strong partnerships among Governments, the United Nations system, intergovernmental organizations, people living with HIV/AIDS and vulnerable groups, medical, scientific and educational institutions, non-governmental organizations, the business sector including generic and research-based pharmaceutical companies, trade unions, media, parliamentarians, foundations, community organizations, faith-based organizations and traditional leaders are important;

33. Acknowledging the particular role and significant contribution of people living with HIV/AIDS, young people and civil society actors in addressing the problem of HIV/AIDS in all its aspects and recognizing that their full involvement and participation in design, planning, implementation and evaluation of

programmes is crucial to the development of effective responses to the HIV/AIDS epidemic;

34. Further acknowledging the efforts of international humanitarian organizations combating the epidemic, including among others the volunteers of the International Federation of Red Cross and Red Crescent Societies in the most affected areas all over the world;

35. Commending the leadership role on HIV/AIDS policy and coordination in the United Nations system of the UNAIDS Programme Coordinating Board; noting its endorsement in December 2000 of the Global Strategy Framework for HIV/AIDS, which could assist, as appropriate, Member States and relevant civil society actors in the development of HIV/AIDS strategies, taking into account the particular context of the epidemic in different parts of the world;

36. Solemnly declare our commitment to address the HIV/AIDS crisis by taking action as follows, taking into account the diverse situations and circumstances in different regions and countries throughout the world;

LEADERSHIP

Strong leadership at all levels of society is essential for an effective response to the epidemic

Leadership by Governments in combating HIV/AIDS is essential and their efforts should be complemented by the full and active participation of civil society, the business community and the private sector

Leadership involves personal commitment and concrete actions

At the National Level

37. By 2003, ensure the development and implementation of multisectoral national strategies and financing plans for combating HIV/AIDS that: address the epidemic in forthright terms; confront stigma, silence and denial; address gender and age-based dimensions of the epidemic; eliminate discrimination and marginalization; involve partnerships with civil society and the business sector and the full participation of people living with HIV/AIDS, those in vulnerable

groups and people mostly at risk, particularly women and young people; are resourced to the extent possible from national budgets without excluding other sources, *inter alia* international cooperation; fully promote and protect all human rights and fundamental freedoms, including the right to the highest attainable standard of physical and mental health; integrate a gender perspective; and address risk, vulnerability, prevention, care, treatment and support and reduction of the impact of the epidemic; and strengthen health, education and legal system capacity;

38. By 2003, integrate HIV/AIDS prevention, care, treatment and support and impact mitigation priorities into the mainstream of development planning, including in poverty eradication strategies, national budget allocations and sectoral development plans;

At the Regional and Subregional Level

39. Urge and support regional organizations and partners to: be actively involved in addressing the crisis; intensify regional, subregional and interregional cooperation and coordination; and develop regional strategies and responses in support of expanded country level efforts;

40. Support all regional and subregional initiatives on HIV/AIDS including: the International Partnership against AIDS in Africa (IPAA) and the ECA-African Development Forum Consensus and Plan of Action: Leadership to Overcome HIV/AIDS; the Abuja Declaration and Framework for Action for the Fight Against HIV/AIDS, Tuberculosis and Other Diseases; the CARICOM Pan-Caribbean Partnership Against HIV/AIDS; the ESCAP Regional Call for Action to Fight HIV/AIDS in Asia and the Pacific; the Baltic Sea Initiative and Action Plan; the Horizontal Technical Cooperation Group on HIV/AIDS in Latin America and the Caribbean; the European Union Programme for Action: Accelerated Action on HIV/AIDS, Malaria and Tuberculosis in the context of poverty reduction;

41. Encourage the development of regional approaches and plans to address HIV/AIDS;

42. Encourage and support local and national organizations to expand and strengthen regional partnerships, coalitions and networks;

43. Encourage the United Nations Economic and Social Council to request the regional commissions within their respective mandates and resources to support national efforts in their respective regions in combating HIV/AIDS;

At the Global Level

44. Support greater action and coordination by all relevant United Nations system organizations, including their full participation in the development and implementation of a regularly updated United Nations strategic plan for HIV/AIDS, guided by the principles contained in this Declaration;

45. Support greater cooperation between relevant United Nations system organizations and international organizations combating HIV/AIDS;

46. Foster stronger collaboration and the development of innovative partnerships between the public and private sectors and by 2003, establish and strengthen mechanisms that involve the private sector and civil society partners and people living with HIV/AIDS and vulnerable groups in the fight against HIV/AIDS;

PREVENTION

Prevention must be the mainstay of our response

47. By 2003, establish time-bound national targets to achieve the internationally agreed global prevention goal to reduce by 2005 HIV prevalence among young men and women aged 15 to 24 in the most affected countries by 25 per cent and by 25 per cent globally by 2010, and to intensify efforts to achieve these targets as well as to challenge gender stereotypes and attitudes, and gender inequalities in relation to HIV/AIDS, encouraging the active involvement of men and boys;

48. By 2003, establish national prevention targets, recognizing and addressing factors leading to the spread of the epidemic and increasing people's vulnerability, to reduce HIV incidence for those identifiable groups, within particular local contexts, which currently have high or increasing rates of HIV infection, or which available public health information indicates are at the highest risk for new infection;

49. By 2005, strengthen the response to HIV/AIDS in the world of work by establishing and implementing prevention and care programmes in public, private and informal work sectors and take measures to provide a supportive workplace environment for people living with HIV/AIDS;

50. By 2005, develop and begin to implement national, regional and international strategies that facilitate access to HIV/AIDS prevention programmes

for migrants and mobile workers, including the provision of information on health and social services;

51. By 2003, implement universal precautions in health-care settings to prevent transmission of HIV infection;

52. By 2005, ensure: that a wide range of prevention programmes which take account of local circumstances, ethics and cultural values, is available in all countries, particularly the most affected countries, including information, education and communication, in languages most understood by communities and respectful of cultures, aimed at reducing risk-taking behaviour and encouraging responsible sexual behaviour, including abstinence and fidelity; expanded access to essential commodities, including male and female condoms and sterile injecting equipment; harm reduction efforts related to drug use; expanded access to voluntary and confidential counselling and testing; safe blood supplies; and early and effective treatment of sexually transmittable infections;

53. By 2005, ensure that at least 90 per cent, and by 2010 at least 95 per cent of young men and women aged 15 to 24 have access to the information, education, including peer education and youth-specific HIV education, and services necessary to develop the life skills required to reduce their vulnerability to HIV infection; in full partnership with youth, parents, families, educators and health-care providers;

54. By 2005, reduce the proportion of infants infected with HIV by 20 per cent, and by 50 per cent by 2010, by: ensuring that 80 per cent of pregnant women accessing antenatal care have information, counselling and other HIV prevention services available to them, increasing the availability of and by providing access for HIV-infected women and babies to effective treatment to reduce mother-to-child transmission of HIV, as well as through effective interventions for HIV-infected women, including voluntary and confidential counselling and testing, access to treatment, especially anti-retroviral therapy and, where appropriate, breast milk substitutes and the provision of a continuum of care;

CARE, SUPPORT AND TREATMENT

Care, support and treatment are fundamental elements of an effective response

55. By 2003, ensure that national strategies, supported by regional and international strategies, are developed in close collaboration with the international

community, including Governments and relevant intergovernmental organizations as well as with civil society and the business sector, to strengthen health care systems and address factors affecting the provision of HIV-related drugs, including anti-retroviral drugs, inter alia affordability and pricing, including differential pricing, and technical and health care systems capacity. Also, in an urgent manner make every effort to: provide progressively and in a sustainable manner, the highest attainable standard of treatment for HIV/AIDS, including the prevention and treatment of opportunistic infections, and effective use of quality-controlled anti-retroviral therapy in a careful and monitored manner to improve adherence and effectiveness and reduce the risk of developing resistance; to cooperate constructively in strengthening pharmaceutical policies and practices, including those applicable to generic drugs and intellectual property regimes, in order further to promote innovation and the development of domestic industries consistent with international law;

56. By 2005, develop and make significant progress in implementing comprehensive care strategies to: strengthen family and community-based care including that provided by the informal sector, and health care systems to provide and monitor treatment to people living with HIV/AIDS, including infected children, and to support individuals, households, families and communities affected by HIV/AIDS; improve the capacity and working conditions of health care personnel, and the effectiveness of supply systems, financing plans and referral mechanisms required to provide access to affordable medicines, including anti-retroviral drugs, diagnostics and related technologies, as well as quality medical, palliative and psycho-social care;

57. By 2003, ensure that national strategies are developed in order to provide psycho-social care for individuals, families, and communities affected by HIV/AIDS;

HIV/AIDS AND HUMAN RIGHTS

Realization of human rights and fundamental freedoms for all is essential to reduce vulnerability to HIV/AIDS

Respect for the rights of people living with HIV/AIDS drives an effective response

58. By 2003, enact, strengthen or enforce as appropriate legislation, regulations and other measures to eliminate all forms of discrimination against, and to ensure the full enjoyment of all human rights and fundamental freedoms by

people living with HIV/AIDS and members of vulnerable groups; in particular to ensure their access to, inter alia education, inheritance, employment, health care, social and health services, prevention, support, treatment, information and legal protection, while respecting their privacy and confidentiality; and develop strategies to combat stigma and social exclusion connected with the epidemic;

59. By 2005, bearing in mind the context and character of the epidemic and that globally women and girls are disproportionately affected by HIV/AIDS, develop and accelerate the implementation of national strategies that: promote the advancement of women and women's full enjoyment of all human rights; promote shared responsibility of men and women to ensure safe sex; empower women to have control over and decide freely and responsibly on matters related to their sexuality to increase their ability to protect themselves from HIV infection;

60. By 2005, implement measures to increase capacities of women and adolescent girls to protect themselves from the risk of HIV infection, principally through the provision of health care and health services, including sexual and reproductive health, and through prevention education that promotes gender equality within a culturally and gender sensitive framework;

61. By 2005, ensure development and accelerated implementation of national strategies for women's empowerment, promotion and protection of women's full enjoyment of all human rights and reduction of their vulnerability to HIV/AIDS through the elimination of all forms of discrimination, as well as all forms of violence against women and girls, including harmful traditional and customary practices, abuse, rape and other forms of sexual violence, battering and trafficking in women and girls;

REDUCING VULNERABILITY

The vulnerable must be given priority in the response

Empowering women is essential for reducing vulnerability

62. By 2003, in order to complement prevention programmes that address activities which place individuals at risk of HIV infection, such as risky and unsafe sexual behaviour and injecting drug use, have in place in all countries strategies, policies and programmes that identify and begin to address those factors that make individuals particularly vulnerable to HIV infection, including

underdevelopment, economic insecurity, poverty, lack of empowerment of women, lack of education, social exclusion, illiteracy, discrimination, lack of information and/or commodities for self-protection, all types of sexual exploitation of women, girls and boys, including for commercial reasons; such strategies, policies and programmes should address the gender dimension of the epidemic, specify the action that will be taken to address vulnerability and set targets for achievement;

63. By 2003, develop and/or strengthen strategies, policies and programmes, which recognize the importance of the family in reducing vulnerability, inter alia, in educating and guiding children and take account of cultural, religious and ethical factors, to reduce the vulnerability of children and young people by: ensuring access of both girls and boys to primary and secondary education, including on HIV/AIDS in curricula for adolescents; ensuring safe and secure environments, especially for young girls; expanding good quality youth-friendly information and sexual health education and counselling service; strengthening reproductive and sexual health programmes; and involving families and young people in planning, implementing and evaluating HIV/AIDS prevention and care programmes, to the extent possible;

64. By 2003, develop and/or strengthen national strategies, policies and programmes, supported by regional and international initiatives, as appropriate, through a participatory approach, to promote and protect the health of those identifiable groups which currently have high or increasing rates of HIV infection or which public health information indicates are at greatest risk of and most vulnerable to new infection as indicated by such factors as the local history of the epidemic, poverty, sexual practices, drug using behaviour, livelihood, institutional location, disrupted social structures and population movements forced or otherwise;

CHILDREN ORPHANED AND MADE VULNERABLE BY HIV/AIDS

Children orphaned and affected by HIV/AIDS need special assistance

65. By 2003, develop and by 2005 implement national policies and strategies to: build and strengthen governmental, family and community capacities to provide a supportive environment for orphans and girls and boys infected and affected by HIV/AIDS including by providing appropriate counselling and psycho-social support; ensuring their enrolment in school and access to shelter,

good nutrition, health and social services on an equal basis with other children; to protect orphans and vulnerable children from all forms of abuse, violence, exploitation, discrimination, trafficking and loss of inheritance;

66. Ensure non-discrimination and full and equal enjoyment of all human rights through the promotion of an active and visible policy of de-stigmatization of children orphaned and made vulnerable by HIV/AIDS;

67. Urge the international community, particularly donor countries, civil society, as well as the private sector to complement effectively national programmes to support programmes for children orphaned or made vulnerable by HIV/AIDS in affected regions, in countries at high risk and to direct special assistance to sub-Saharan Africa;

ALLEVIATING SOCIAL AND ECONOMIC IMPACT

To address HIV/AIDS is to invest in sustainable development

68. By 2003, evaluate the economic and social impact of the HIV/AIDS epidemic and develop multisectoral strategies to: address the impact at the individual, family, community and national levels; develop and accelerate the implementation of national poverty eradication strategies to address the impact of HIV/AIDS on household income, livelihoods, and access to basic social services, with special focus on individuals, families and communities severely affected by the epidemic; review the social and economic impact of HIV/AIDS at all levels of society especially on women and the elderly, particularly in their role as caregivers and in families affected by HIV/AIDS and address their special needs; adjust and adapt economic and social development policies, including social protection policies, to address the impact of HIV/AIDS on economic growth, provision of essential economic services, labour productivity, government revenues, and deficit-creating pressures on public resources;

69. By 2003, develop a national legal and policy framework that protects in the workplace the rights and dignity of persons living with and affected by HIV/AIDS and those at the greatest risk of HIV/AIDS in consultation with representatives of employers and workers, taking account of established international guidelines on HIV/AIDS in the workplace;

RESEARCH AND DEVELOPMENT

With no cure for HIV/AIDS yet found, further research and development is crucial

70. Increase investment and accelerate research on the development of HIV vaccines, while building national research capacity especially in developing countries, and especially for viral strains prevalent in highly affected regions; in addition, support and encourage increased national and international investment in HIV/AIDS-related research and development including biomedical, operations, social, cultural and behavioural research and in traditional medicine to: improve prevention and therapeutic approaches; accelerate access to prevention, care and treatment and care technologies for HIV/AIDS (and its associated opportunistic infections and malignancies and sexually transmitted diseases), including female controlled methods and microbicides, and in particular, appropriate, safe and affordable HIV vaccines and their delivery, and to diagnostics, tests, methods to prevent mother-to-child transmission; and improve our understanding of factors which influence the epidemic and actions which address it, *inter alia*, through increased funding and public/private partnerships; create a conducive environment for research and ensure that it is based on highest ethical standards;

71. Support and encourage the development of national and international research infrastructure, laboratory capacity, improved surveillance systems, data collection, processing and dissemination, and training of basic and clinical researchers, social scientists, health-care providers and technicians, with a focus on the countries most affected by HIV/AIDS, particularly developing countries and those countries experiencing or at risk of rapid expansion of the epidemic;

72. Develop and evaluate suitable approaches for monitoring treatment efficacy, toxicity, side effects, drug interactions, and drug resistance, develop methodologies to monitor the impact of treatment on HIV transmission and risk behaviours;

73. Strengthen international and regional cooperation in particular North/South, South/South and triangular cooperation, related to transfer of relevant technologies, suitable to the environment in prevention and care of HIV/AIDS, the exchange of experiences and best practices, researchers and research findings and strengthen the role of UNAIDS in this process. In this context, encourage that the end results of these cooperative research findings and technologies be owned by all parties to the research, reflecting their relevant contribution and dependent upon their providing legal protection to such

findings; and affirm that all such research should be free from bias;

74. By 2003, ensure that all research protocols for the investigation of HIV-related treatment including anti-retroviral therapies and vaccines based on international guidelines and best practices are evaluated by independent committees of ethics, in which persons living with HIV/AIDS and caregivers for anti-retroviral therapy participate;

HIV/AIDS IN CONFLICT AND DISASTER AFFECTED REGIONS

Conflicts and disasters contribute to the spread of HIV/AIDS

75. By 2003, develop and begin to implement national strategies that incorporate HIV/AIDS awareness, prevention, care and treatment elements into programmes or actions that respond to emergency situations, recognizing that populations destabilized by armed conflict, humanitarian emergencies and natural disasters, including refugees, internally displaced persons and in particular, women and children, are at increased risk of exposure to HIV infection; and, where appropriate, factor HIV/AIDS components into international assistance programmes;

76. Call on all United Nations agencies, regional and international organizations, as well as non-governmental organizations involved with the provision and delivery of international assistance to countries and regions affected by conflicts, humanitarian crises or natural disasters, to incorporate as a matter of urgency HIV/AIDS prevention, care and awareness elements into their plans and programmes and provide HIV/AIDS awareness and training to their personnel;

77. By 2003, have in place national strategies to address the spread of HIV among national uniformed services, where this is required, including armed forces and civil defence force and consider ways of using personnel from these services who are educated and trained in HIV/AIDS awareness and prevention to assist with HIV/AIDS awareness and prevention activities including participation in emergency, humanitarian, disaster relief and rehabilitation assistance;

78. By 2003, ensure the inclusion of HIV/AIDS awareness and training, including a gender component, into guidelines designed for use by defence personnel and other personnel involved in international peacekeeping operations while also continuing with ongoing education and prevention efforts, including pre-deployment orientation, for these personnel;

RESOURCES

The HIV/AIDS challenge cannot be met without new, additional and sustained resources

79. Ensure that the resources provided for the global response to address HIV/AIDS are substantial, sustained and geared towards achieving results;

80. By 2005, through a series of incremental steps, reach an overall target of annual expenditure on the epidemic of between US$7 billion and US$10 billion in low and middle-income countries and those countries experiencing or at risk of experiencing rapid expansion for prevention, care, treatment, support and mitigation of the impact of HIV/AIDS, and take measures to ensure that needed resources are made available, particularly from donor countries and also from national budgets, bearing in mind that resources of the most affected countries are seriously limited;

81. Call on the international community, where possible, to provide assistance for HIV/AIDS prevention, care and treatment in developing countries on a grant basis;

82. Increase and prioritize national budgetary allocations for HIV/AIDS programmes as required and ensure that adequate allocations are made by all ministries and other relevant stakeholders;

83. Urge the developed countries that have not done so to strive to meet the targets of 0.7 per cent of their gross national product for overall official development assistance and the targets of earmarking of 0.15 per cent to 0.20 per cent of gross national product as official development assistance for least developed countries as agreed, as soon as possible, taking into account the urgency and gravity of the HIV/AIDS epidemic;

84. Urge the international community to complement and supplement efforts of developing countries that commit increased national funds to fight the HIV/AIDS epidemic through increased international development assistance, particularly those countries most affected by HIV/AIDS, particularly in Africa, especially in sub-Saharan Africa, the Caribbean, countries at high risk of expansion of the HIV/AIDS epidemic and other affected regions whose resources to deal with the epidemic are seriously limited;

85. Integrate HIV/AIDS actions in development assistance programmes and poverty eradication strategies as appropriate and encourage the most effective and transparent use of all resources allocated;

86. Call on the international community and invite civil society and the pri-

vate sector to take appropriate measures to help alleviate the social and economic impact of HIV/AIDS in the most affected developing countries;

87. Without further delay implement the enhanced Heavily Indebted Poor Country (HIPC) Initiative and agree to cancel all bilateral official debts of HIPC countries as soon as possible, especially those most affected by HIV/AIDS, in return for their making demonstrable commitments to poverty eradication and urge the use of debt service savings to finance poverty eradication programmes, particularly for HIV/AIDS prevention, treatment, care and support and other infections;

88. Call for speedy and concerted action to address effectively the debt problems of least developed countries, low-income developing countries, and middle-income developing countries, particularly those affected by HIV/AIDS, in a comprehensive, equitable, development-oriented and durable way through various national and international measures designed to make their debt sustainable in the long term and thereby to improve their capacity to deal with the HIV/AIDS epidemic, including, as appropriate, existing orderly mechanisms for debt reduction, such as debt swaps for projects aimed at the prevention, care and treatment of HIV/AIDS;

89. Encourage increased investment in HIV/AIDS-related research, nationally, regionally and internationally, in particular for the development of sustainable and affordable prevention technologies, such as vaccines and microbicides, and encourage the proactive preparation of financial and logistic plans to facilitate rapid access to vaccines when they become available;

90. Support the establishment, on an urgent basis, of a global HIV/AIDS and health fund to finance an urgent and expanded response to the epidemic based on an integrated approach to prevention, care, support and treatment and to assist Governments inter alia in their efforts to combat HIV/AIDS with due priority to the most affected countries, notably in sub-Saharan Africa and the Caribbean and to those countries at high risk, mobilize contributions to the fund from public and private sources with a special appeal to donor countries, foundations, the business community including pharmaceutical companies, the private sector, philanthropists and wealthy individuals;

91. By 2002, launch a worldwide fund-raising campaign aimed at the general public as well as the private sector, conducted by UNAIDS with the support and collaboration of interested partners at all levels, to contribute to the global HIV/AIDS and health fund;

92. Direct increased funding to national, regional and subregional commissions and organizations to enable them to assist Governments at the national, subregional and regional level in their efforts to respond to the crisis;

93. Provide the UNAIDS co-sponsoring agencies and the UNAIDS secretariat with the resources needed to work with countries in support of the goals of this Declaration;

FOLLOW-UP

Maintaining the momentum and monitoring progress are essential

At the National Level

94. Conduct national periodic reviews involving the participation of civil society, particularly people living with HIV/AIDS, vulnerable groups and caregivers, of progress achieved in realizing these commitments and identify problems and obstacles to achieving progress and ensure wide dissemination of the results of these reviews;

95. Develop appropriate monitoring and evaluation mechanisms to assist with follow-up in measuring and assessing progress, develop appropriate monitoring and evaluation instruments, with adequate epidemiological data;

96. By 2003, establish or strengthen effective monitoring systems, where appropriate, for the promotion and protection of human rights of people living with HIV/AIDS;

At the Regional Level

97. Include HIV/AIDS and related public health concerns as appropriate on the agenda of regional meetings at the ministerial and Head of State and Government level;

98. Support data collection and processing to facilitate periodic reviews by regional commissions and/or regional organizations of progress in implementing regional strategies and addressing regional priorities and ensure wide dissemination of the results of these reviews;

99. Encourage the exchange between countries of information and experiences in implementing the measures and commitments contained in this Declaration, and in particular facilitate intensified South-South and triangular cooperation;

At the Global Level

100. Devote sufficient time and at least one full day of the annual General Assembly session to review and debate a report of the Secretary-General on progress achieved in realizing the commitments set out in this Declaration, with a view to identifying problems and constraints and making recommendations on action needed to make further progress;

101. Ensure that HIV/AIDS issues are included on the agenda of all appropriate United Nations conferences and meetings;

102. Support initiatives to convene conferences, seminars, workshops, training programmes and courses to follow up issues raised in this Declaration and in this regard encourage participation in and wide dissemination of the outcomes of: the forthcoming Dakar Conference on Access to Care for HIV Infection; the Sixth International Congress on AIDS in Asia and the Pacific; the XII International Conference on AIDS and Sexually Transmitted Infections in Africa; the XIV International Conference on AIDS, Barcelona; the X International Conference on People Living with HIV/AIDS, Port of Spain; the II Forum and III Conference of the Latin American and the Caribbean Horizontal Technical Cooperation on HIV/AIDS and Sexually Transmitted Infections, La Habana; the V International Conference on Home and Community Care for Persons Living with HIV/AIDS, Changmai, Thailand;

103. Explore, with a view to improving equity in access to essential drugs, the feasibility of developing and implementing, in collaboration with non-governmental organizations and other concerned partners, systems for voluntary monitoring and reporting of global drug prices;

We recognize and express our appreciation to those who have led the effort to raise awareness of the HIV/AIDS epidemic and to deal with its complex challenges;

We look forward to strong leadership by Governments, and concerted efforts with full and active participation of the United Nations, the entire multilateral system, civil society, the business community and private sector;

And finally, we call on all countries to take the necessary steps to implement this Declaration, in strengthened partnership and cooperation with other multilateral and bilateral partners and with civil society.

NOTES

1. See resolution 55/2.

2. Resolution S-24/2, annex, sects. I and III.

3. Resolution S-23/2, annex.

4. Resolution S-23/3, annex.

5. Resolution S-21/2, annex.

The UN Declaration of Commitment was adopted at the UN General Assembly Special Session on HIV/AIDS by Resolution A/Res/S-26/2 on August 2, 2001, www.un.org/ga/aids/docs/aress262.pdf.

United Nations General Assembly Political Declaration on HIV/AIDS

1. We, Heads of State and Government and representatives of States and Governments participating in the comprehensive review of the progress achieved in realizing the targets set out in the Declaration of Commitment on HIV/AIDS,[1] held on 31 May and 1 June 2006, and the High-Level Meeting, held on 2 June 2006;

2. Note with alarm that we are facing an unprecedented human catastrophe; that a quarter of a century into the pandemic, AIDS has inflicted immense suffering on countries and communities throughout the world; and that more than 65 million people have been infected with HIV, more than 25 million people have died of AIDS, 15 million children have been orphaned by AIDS and millions more made vulnerable, and 40 million people are currently living with HIV, more than 95 per cent of whom live in developing countries;

3. Recognize that HIV/AIDS constitutes a global emergency and poses one of the most formidable challenges to the development, progress and stability of our respective societies and the world at large, and requires an exceptional and comprehensive global response;

4. Acknowledge that national and international efforts have resulted in important progress since 2001 in the areas of funding, expanding access to HIV prevention, treatment, care and support and in mitigating the impact of AIDS, and in reducing HIV prevalence in a small but growing number of countries, and also acknowledge that many targets contained in the Declaration of Commitment on HIV/AIDS have not yet been met;

5. Commend the Secretariat and the Co-sponsors of the Joint United Nations Programme on HIV/AIDS for their leadership role on HIV/AIDS policy and coordination, and for the support they provide to countries through the Joint Programme;

6. Recognize the contribution of, and the role played by, various donors in combating HIV/AIDS, as well as the fact that one third of resources spent on HIV/AIDS responses in 2005 came from the domestic sources of low- and middle- income countries, and therefore emphasize the importance of enhanced

international cooperation and partnership in our responses to HIV/AIDS worldwide;

7. Remain deeply concerned, however, by the overall expansion and feminization of the pandemic and the fact that women now represent 50 per cent of people living with HIV worldwide and nearly 60 per cent of people living with HIV in Africa, and in this regard recognize that gender inequalities and all forms of violence against women and girls increase their vulnerability to HIV/AIDS;

8. Express grave concern that half of all new HIV infections occur among children and young people under the age of 25, and that there is a lack of information, skills and knowledge regarding HIV/AIDS among young people;

9. Remain gravely concerned that 2.3 million children are living with HIV/AIDS today, and recognize that the lack of paediatric drugs in many countries significantly hinders efforts to protect the health of children;

10. Reiterate with profound concern that the pandemic affects every region, that Africa, in particular sub-Saharan Africa, remains the worst-affected region, and that urgent and exceptional action is required at all levels to curb the devastating effects of this pandemic, and recognize the renewed commitment by African Governments and regional institutions to scale up their own HIV/AIDS responses;

11. Reaffirm that the full realization of all human rights and fundamental freedoms for all is an essential element in the global response to the HIV/AIDS pandemic, including in the areas of prevention, treatment, care and support, and recognize that addressing stigma and discrimination is also a critical element in combating the global HIV/AIDS pandemic;

12. Reaffirm also that access to medication in the context of pandemics, such as HIV/AIDS, is one of the fundamental elements to achieve progressively the full realization of the right of everyone to the enjoyment of the highest attainable standard of physical and mental health;

13. Recognize that in many parts of the world, the spread of HIV/AIDS is a cause and consequence of poverty, and that effectively combating HIV/AIDS is essential to the achievement of internationally agreed development goals and objectives, including the Millennium Development Goals;

14. Recognize also that we now have the means to reverse the global pandemic and to avert millions of needless deaths, and that to be effective, we must deliver an intensified, much more urgent and comprehensive response, in part-

nership with the United Nations system, intergovernmental organizations, people living with HIV and vulnerable groups, medical, scientific and educational institutions, non-governmental organizations, the business sector, including generic and research-based pharmaceutical companies, trade unions, the media, parliamentarians, foundations, community organizations, faith-based organizations and traditional leaders;

15. Recognize further that to mount a comprehensive response, we must overcome any legal, regulatory, trade and other barriers that block access to prevention, treatment, care and support; commit adequate resources; promote and protect all human rights and fundamental freedoms for all; promote gender equality and empowerment of women; promote and protect the rights of the girl child in order to reduce the vulnerability of the girl child to HIV/AIDS; strengthen health systems and support health workers; support greater involvement of people living with HIV; scale up the use of known effective and comprehensive prevention interventions; do everything necessary to ensure access to life-saving drugs and prevention tools; and develop with equal urgency better tools—drugs, diagnostics and prevention technologies, including vaccines and microbicides—for the future;

16. Convinced that without renewed political will, strong leadership and sustained commitment and concerted efforts on the part of all stakeholders at all levels, including people living with HIV, civil society and vulnerable groups, and without increased resources, the world will not succeed in bringing about the end of the pandemic;

17. Solemnly declare our commitment to address the HIV/AIDS crisis by taking action as follows, taking into account the diverse situations and circumstances in different regions and countries throughout the world;

Therefore, we:

18. Reaffirm our commitment to implement fully the Declaration of Commitment on HIV/AIDS, entitled "Global Crisis–Global Action", adopted by the General Assembly at its twenty-sixth special session, in 2001; and to achieve the internationally agreed development goals and objectives, including the Millennium Development Goals, in particular the goal to halt and begin to reverse the spread of HIV/AIDS, malaria and other major diseases, the agreements dealing with HIV/AIDS reached at all major United Nations conferences and summits, including the 2005 World Summit and its statement on treatment, and the goal of achieving universal access to reproductive health by 2015, as set out at the International Conference on Population and Development;

19. Recognize the importance, and encourage the implementation, of the recommendations of the inclusive, country-driven processes and regional consultations facilitated by the Secretariat and the Co-sponsors of the Joint United Nations Programme on HIV/AIDS for scaling up HIV prevention, treatment, care and support, and strongly recommend that this approach be continued;

20. Commit ourselves to pursuing all necessary efforts to scale up nationally driven, sustainable and comprehensive responses to achieve broad multisectoral coverage for prevention, treatment, care and support, with full and active participation of people living with HIV, vulnerable groups, most affected communities, civil society and the private sector, towards the goal of universal access to comprehensive prevention programmes, treatment, care and support by 2010;

21. Emphasize the need to strengthen policy and programme linkages and coordination between HIV/AIDS, sexual and reproductive health, national development plans and strategies, including poverty eradication strategies, and to address, where appropriate, the impact of HIV/AIDS on national development plans and strategies;

22. Reaffirm that the prevention of HIV infection must be the mainstay of national, regional and international responses to the pandemic, and therefore commit ourselves to intensifying efforts to ensure that a wide range of prevention programmes that take account of local circumstances, ethics and cultural values is available in all countries, particularly the most affected countries, including information, education and communication, in languages most understood by communities and respectful of cultures, aimed at reducing risk-taking behaviours and encouraging responsible sexual behaviour, including abstinence and fidelity; expanded access to essential commodities, including male and female condoms and sterile injecting equipment; harm-reduction efforts related to drug use; expanded access to voluntary and confidential counselling and testing; safe blood supplies; and early and effective treatment of sexually transmitted infections;

23. Reaffirm also that prevention, treatment, care and support for those infected and affected by HIV/AIDS are mutually reinforcing elements of an effective response and must be integrated in a comprehensive approach to combat the pandemic;

24. Commit ourselves to overcoming legal, regulatory or other barriers that block access to effective HIV prevention, treatment, care and support, medicines, commodities and services;

25. Pledge to promote, at the international, regional, national and local levels, access to HIV/AIDS education, information, voluntary counselling and testing and related services, with full protection of confidentiality and informed consent, and to promote a social and legal environment that is supportive of and safe for voluntary disclosure of HIV status;

26. Commit ourselves to addressing the rising rates of HIV infection among young people to ensure an HIV-free future generation through the implementation of comprehensive, evidence-based prevention strategies, responsible sexual behaviour, including the use of condoms, evidence- and skills-based, youth-specific HIV education, mass media interventions and the provision of youth-friendly health services;

27. Commit ourselves also to ensuring that pregnant women have access to antenatal care, information, counselling and other HIV services and to increasing the availability of and access to effective treatment to women living with HIV and infants in order to reduce mother-to-child transmission of HIV, as well as to ensuring effective interventions for women living with HIV, including voluntary and confidential counselling and testing, with informed consent, access to treatment, especially life-long antiretroviral therapy and, where appropriate, breast-milk substitutes and the provision of a continuum of care;

28. Resolve to integrate food and nutritional support, with the goal that all people at all times will have access to sufficient, safe and nutritious food to meet their dietary needs and food preferences, for an active and healthy life, as part of a comprehensive response to HIV/AIDS;

29. Commit ourselves to intensifying efforts to enact, strengthen or enforce, as appropriate, legislation, regulations and other measures to eliminate all forms of discrimination against and to ensure the full enjoyment of all human rights and fundamental freedoms by people living with HIV and members of vulnerable groups, in particular to ensure their access to, inter alia, education, inheritance, employment, health care, social and health services, prevention, support and treatment, information and legal protection, while respecting their privacy and confidentiality; and developing strategies to combat stigma and social exclusion connected with the epidemic;

30. Pledge to eliminate gender inequalities, gender-based abuse and violence; increase the capacity of women and adolescent girls to protect themselves from the risk of HIV infection, principally through the provision of health care and services, including, inter alia, sexual and reproductive health, and the provision of full access to comprehensive information and education;

ensure that women can exercise their right to have control over, and decide freely and responsibly on, matters related to their sexuality in order to increase their ability to protect themselves from HIV infection, including their sexual and reproductive health, free of coercion, discrimination and violence; and take all necessary measures to create an enabling environment for the empowerment of women and strengthen their economic independence; and in this context, reiterate the importance of the role of men and boys in achieving gender equality;

31. Commit ourselves to strengthening legal, policy, administrative and other measures for the promotion and protection of women's full enjoyment of all human rights and the reduction of their vulnerability to HIV/AIDS through the elimination of all forms of discrimination, as well as all types of sexual exploitation of women, girls and boys, including for commercial reasons, and all forms of violence against women and girls, including harmful traditional and customary practices, abuse, rape and other forms of sexual violence, battering and trafficking in women and girls;

32. Commit ourselves also to addressing as a priority the vulnerabilities faced by children affected by and living with HIV; providing support and rehabilitation to these children and their families, women and the elderly, particularly in their role as caregivers; promoting child-oriented HIV/AIDS policies and programmes and increased protection for children orphaned and affected by HIV/AIDS; ensuring access to treatment and intensifying efforts to develop new treatments for children; and building, where needed, and supporting the social security systems that protect them;

33. Emphasize the need for accelerated scale-up of collaborative activities on tuberculosis and HIV, in line with the Global Plan to Stop TB 2006–2015, and for investment in new drugs, diagnostics and vaccines that are appropriate for people with TB-HIV co-infection;

34. Commit ourselves to expanding to the greatest extent possible, supported by international cooperation and partnership, our capacity to deliver comprehensive HIV/AIDS programmes in ways that strengthen existing national health and social systems, including by integrating HIV/AIDS intervention into programmes for primary health care, mother and child health, sexual and reproductive health, tuberculosis, hepatitis C, sexually transmitted infections, nutrition, children affected, orphaned or made vulnerable by HIV/AIDS, as well as formal and informal education;

35. Undertake to reinforce, adopt and implement, where needed, national

plans and strategies, supported by international cooperation and partnership, to increase the capacity of human resources for health to meet the urgent need for the training and retention of a broad range of health workers, including community-based health workers; improve training and management and working conditions, including treatment for health workers; and effectively govern the recruitment, retention and deployment of new and existing health workers to mount a more effective HIV/AIDS response;

36. Commit ourselves, invite international financial institutions and the Global Fund to Fight AIDS, Tuberculosis and Malaria, according to its policy framework, and encourage other donors, to provide additional resources to low- and middle- income countries for the strengthening of HIV/AIDS programmes and health systems and for addressing human resources gaps, including the development of alternative and simplified service delivery models and the expansion of the community-level provision of HIV/AIDS prevention, treatment, care and support, as well as other health and social services;

37. Reiterate the need for Governments, United Nations agencies, regional and international organizations and non-governmental organizations involved with the provision and delivery of assistance to countries and regions affected by conflicts, humanitarian emergencies or natural disasters to incorporate HIV/AIDS prevention, care and treatment elements into their plans and programmes;

38. Pledge to provide the highest level of commitment to ensuring that costed, inclusive, sustainable, credible and evidence-based national HIV/AIDS plans are funded and implemented with transparency, accountability and effectiveness, in line with national priorities;

39. Commit ourselves to reducing the global HIV/AIDS resource gap through greater domestic and international funding to enable countries to have access to predictable and sustainable financial resources and ensuring that international funding is aligned with national HIV/AIDS plans and strategies; and in this regard welcome the increased resources that are being made available through bilateral and multilateral initiatives, as well as those that will become available as a result of the establishment of timetables by many developed countries to achieve the targets of 0.7 per cent of gross national product for official development assistance by 2015 and to reach at least 0.5 per cent of gross national product for official development assistance by 2010 as well as, pursuant to the Brussels Programme of Action for the Least Developed Countries for the Decade 2001–2010,[2] 0.15 per cent to 0.20 per cent for the

least developed countries no later than 2010, and urge those developed countries that have not yet done so to make concrete efforts in this regard in accordance with their commitments;

40. Recognize that the Joint United Nations Programme on HIV/AIDS has estimated that 20 to 23 billion United States dollars per annum is needed by 2010 to support rapidly scaled-up AIDS responses in low- and middle-income countries, and therefore commit ourselves to taking measures to ensure that new and additional resources are made available from donor countries and also from national budgets and other national sources;

41. Commit ourselves to supporting and strengthening existing financial mechanisms, including the Global Fund to Fight AIDS, Tuberculosis and Malaria, as well as relevant United Nations organizations, through the provision of funds in a sustained manner, while continuing to develop innovative sources of financing, as well as pursuing other efforts, aimed at generating additional funds;

42. Commit ourselves also to finding appropriate solutions to overcome barriers in pricing, tariffs and trade agreements, and to making improvements to legislation, regulatory policy, procurement and supply chain management in order to accelerate and intensify access to affordable and quality HIV/AIDS prevention products, diagnostics, medicines and treatment commodities;

43. Reaffirm that the World Trade Organization's Agreement on Trade-Related Aspects of Intellectual Property Rights[3] does not and should not prevent members from taking measures now and in the future to protect public health. Accordingly, while reiterating our commitment to the TRIPS Agreement, reaffirm that the Agreement can and should be interpreted and implemented in a manner supportive of the right to protect public health and, in particular, to promote access to medicines for all including the production of generic antiretroviral drugs and other essential drugs for AIDS-related infections. In this connection, we reaffirm the right to use, to the full, the provisions in the TRIPS Agreement, the Doha Declaration on the TRIPS Agreement and Public Health[4] and the World Trade Organization's General Council Decision of 2003[5] and amendments to Article 31, which provide flexibilities for this purpose;

44. Resolve to assist developing countries to enable them to employ the flexibilities outlined in the TRIPS Agreement, and to strengthen their capacities for this purpose;

45. Commit ourselves to intensifying investment in and efforts towards the research and development of new, safe and affordable HIV/AIDS-related medicines, products and technologies, such as vaccines, female-controlled methods and microbicides, paediatric antiretroviral formulations, including through such mechanisms as Advance Market Commitments, and to encouraging increased investment in HIV/AIDS-related research and development in traditional medicine;

46. Encourage pharmaceutical companies, donors, multilateral organizations and other partners to develop public-private partnerships in support of research and development and technology transfer, and in the comprehensive response to HIV/AIDS;

47. Encourage bilateral, regional and international efforts to promote bulk procurement, price negotiations and licensing to lower prices for HIV prevention products, diagnostics, medicines and treatment commodities, while recognizing that intellectual property protection is important for the development of new medicines and recognizing the concerns about its effects on prices;

48. Recognize the initiative by a group of countries, such as the International Drug Purchase Facility, based on innovative financing mechanisms that aim to provide further drug access at affordable prices to developing countries on a sustainable and predictable basis;

49. Commit ourselves to setting, in 2006, through inclusive, transparent processes, ambitious national targets, including interim targets for 2008 in accordance with the core indicators recommended by the Joint United Nations Programme on HIV/AIDS, that reflect the commitment of the present Declaration and the urgent need to scale up significantly towards the goal of universal access to comprehensive prevention programmes, treatment, care and support by 2010, and to setting up and maintaining sound and rigorous monitoring and evaluation frameworks within their HIV/AIDS strategies;

50. Call upon the Joint United Nations Programme on HIV/AIDS, including its Co-sponsors, to assist national efforts to coordinate the AIDS response, as elaborated in the "Three Ones" principles and in line with the recommendations of the Global Task Team on Improving AIDS Coordination among Multilateral Institutions and International Donors; assist national and regional efforts to monitor and report on efforts to achieve the targets set out above; and strengthen global coordination on HIV/AIDS, including through the thematic sessions of the Programme Coordinating Board;

51. Call upon Governments, national parliaments, donors, regional and sub-regional organizations, organizations of the United Nations system, the Global Fund to Fight AIDS, Tuberculosis and Malaria, civil society, people living with HIV, vulnerable groups, the private sector, communities most affected by HIV/AIDS and other stakeholders to work closely together to achieve the targets set out above, and to ensure accountability and transparency at all levels through participatory reviews of responses to HIV/AIDS;

52. Request the Secretary-General of the United Nations, with the support of the Joint United Nations Programme on HIV/AIDS, to include in his annual report to the General Assembly on the status of implementation of the Declaration of Commitment on HIV/AIDS, in accordance with General Assembly resolution S-26/2 of 27 June 2001, the progress achieved in realizing the commitments set out in the present Declaration;

53. Decide to undertake comprehensive reviews in 2008 and 2011, within the annual reviews of the General Assembly, of the progress achieved in realizing the Declaration of Commitment on HIV/AIDS, entitled "Global Crisis–Global Action," adopted by the General Assembly at its twenty-sixth special session, and the present Declaration.

NOTES

1. Resolution S-26/2 Annex.

2. A/CONF.191/13, chap. II.

3. See *Legal Instruments Embodying the Results of the Uruguay Round of Multilateral Trade Negotiations*, done at Marrakesh on 15 April 1994 (GATT secretariat publication, Sales No. GATT/1994-7).

4. See World Trade Organization, document WT/MIN(01)/DEC/2. Available at http://docsonline.wto.org.

5. See World Trade Organization, document WT/L/540 and Corr.1. Available at http://docsonline.wto.org.

The Political Declaration on HIV/AIDS was adopted by the United Nations General Assembly Resolution 60/262 on June 2, 2006. A/Res/60/262, UNAIDS, http://data.unaids.org/pub/Report/2006/20060615_HLM_PoliticalDeclaration_ARES60262_en.pdf.

This book is intended as a reference resource only, not as a medical manual. The information given here is designed to help you make informed decisions about your health. It is not intended as a substitute for any treatment that may have been prescribed by your doctor. If you suspect that you have a medical problem, we urge you to seek competent medical help.

Consult your physician prior to making any modifications to your diet and exercise program. Do not take yourself off of prescription medications without first consulting your physician.

The statements within this book have not been evaluated or approved by the FDA. This book has not been approved or endorsed by any cancer organization or any medical association.

Hallelujah Acres, Inc., 916 Cox Road, Gastonia, NC 28054
www.myHDiet.com

Printed in the United States of America

Cover designed by Dave Aldrich, *AldrichDesign.com*
Book layout by Westmoreland Printers, Inc. Shelby NC

ISBN 978-0-9914387-1-6
eISBN 978-0-9914387-0-9

www.UnravelTheMystery.com

Contents

Acknowledgement One

In 1976, Rev. George Malkmus was pastoring a successful church in upstate New York when he was told he had colon cancer. He had a protruding tumor the size of a baseball in his abdominal area. He had just witnessed his mother, who was a registered nurse, die from colon cancer after going the traditional medical route. He witnessed first-hand the terrible side effects his mother experienced as a result of the treatments. At the time, he felt the treatments had more to do with accelerating her death than the cancer did itself. When he was faced with the same type of cancer just a short time later he believed that there must be another way of dealing with this vicious disease.

A pastor friend explained to Rev. Malkmus that the body has the ability to heal itself if it is given the proper nourishment. Overnight, Rev. Malkmus changed his diet and within one year from making this diet change the tumor was gone as well as his arthritis, high blood pressure, and allergies. Even simple things like pimples and dandruff went away. It is now 2014 and Rev. Malkmus will turn 80 this year. He has never had an issue with cancer since his body healed itself nearly 40 years ago.

The program that Rev. Malkmus used is the basis for what we call the Hallelujah Diet Recovery Program today. Though it has been modified based on new findings from science and personal application, the basic principles are what many have used over the years to support their bodies while they battled cancer and other diseases. While it has taken science many years to catch up, Rev. Malkmus was sharing the message of hope and healing for the past 25 years.

Acknowledgement Two

There are many people who have assisted in getting this book to you. From the staff at Hallelujah Diet, Olin and Michael performing final reviews over the weekend, Alan, the graphic designer, to George and Rhonda Malkmus who pioneered this concept, to our children who have had to be patient with us this last year.

But there is one person who has been the most instrumental and has made all of the difference in getting this book to you; that man has been patiently praying for me, keeping me balanced, supporting my efforts and working by my side. He has been my editor, my publisher, my greatest critic and the most ardent supporter.

To my husband, Paul, who would balance so many details to get this book where it needed to be. Your sweet spirit throughout has been pivotal in keeping this book and me on track. Your exceptional guidance, direction and contributions are felt in every page of this book. I am deeply humbled by your attention towards me and the priority you gave to complete this book.

Finally, my most humble heart goes to my Creator. The One who embraced us as we buried our child from cancer. The One who placed the seed in my heart to reach out and speak the truth in love for all those confronting this disease. May He bless this work and all those who will read it, knowing that He is still the One who has control. No matter what anyone says, as long as you have breath, you have hope.

In Loving Memory

The process of writing this book was a bittersweet experience. Though it was my first book, the topic is near and dear to my heart. My husband, Paul and I are quite familiar with cancer. We know what chemotherapy treatments are and their horrible side effects. We know the sense of hope with the news of "remission" and the sense of despair each time we hear the phrase "it's back."

In life, you believe your children should outlive you. Unfortunately, that doesn't always happen. When our youngest was only 14 and just beginning his high school years, he was diagnosed with Hodgkins Lymphoma. He was introduced to this diet and lifestyle but chose a different direction. We cared for him as he went through the conventional methods and we rejoiced with him during the times of remission. It always seemed though, that the cancer came back around Christmas each time. Finally, when it was too late, he made an attempt at changing his diet and lifestyle.

About a month after he graduated from high school, Joshua Dean Malkmus went to be with the Lord and has been our guardian angel ever since.

We are one with those who have been in this battle against cancer. We truly see how difficult it is to not consider the conventional approaches when they are seen as absolutely the only chance and we are humbled by the incredible attention he received from the health care professionals.

As he was realizing that his time was near, he told his dad that he must have gotten this cancer for a reason and that he thought it might help people in some way. We believe that this book will help people and through their adopting this lifestyle, and subsequent victory, our son will live on. We love you Joshua!

Foreword by Neal Barnard, MD

This book presents vital information that can help you stay healthy—or help you regain health if it has slipped away. Of all the areas of health, perhaps the most important is tackling cancer.

Many of us live in fear of cancer. We view it as something that is completely out of our control. Thankfully, however, we have more control than we often think. As you read through this book, you will find an abundance of detailed information about the many toxins that can potentially play into cancer growth, and, more importantly, how to prevent exposure to these chemicals and environmental factors.

According to the National Cancer Institute, 80 percent of cancers are attributable to factors that have been identified and can potentially be controlled. Not only can we potentially prevent most cancers; those who already have cancer have the ability to improve their survival rates. Evidence is strongest for cancers of the breast, prostate, and colon, where the most research has been done, but many of the same principles apply to other numerous forms of cancer as well.

For example, it has become common knowledge that tobacco contains dangerous carcinogens. Thirty percent of cancers are caused by tobacco. And while lung cancer is the most obvious example, tobacco can also cause cancers of the mouth, throat, kidney, and bladder.

What most people don't know is how significantly diet affects cancer risk. By scientific estimates, at least one-third of annual cancer deaths in the United States are caused by dietary factors, and most likely the number is even higher than this. A review from the American Cancer Society on diet and cancer estimates that up to 80 percent of cancers of the large bowel, breast, and prostate are due to dietary factors—and studies indicate that the foods we eat have a substantial effect on other cancers as well.

The link between diet and cancer has been known—at least by some—for over a century. In January 1892, Scientific American printed the observation that "cancer is most frequent among those branches of the human race where carnivorous habits prevail." A decade later, the New York Times published an article entitled "Cancer Increasing among Meat Eaters," which described a seven-year epidemiological study showing that meat-eaters were at high cancer risk,

Increasing among Meat Eaters," which described a seven-year epidemiological study showing that meat-eaters were at high cancer risk, compared with those choosing other staples. Since then, numerous research studies have shown the same thing: Cancer is much more common in populations consuming diets heavy in animal-based foods and much less common in countries where diets consist primarily of grains, legumes, vegetables, and fruits.

But why does this happen? One reason is that foods affect the action of hormones in the body. In particular, dietary fat consumption drives the hormone production, which, in turn, promotes cancer cell growth in hormone-sensitive organs such as the breast and prostate. Major sources of unhealthy dietary fats in many people's diets are meat and dairy products. By cutting these out, we are reducing our chances of promoting cancer cell growth. Foods also affect the strength of the immune system. Fruits and vegetables contain a variety of vitamins, minerals, antioxidants, and phytochemicals to protect the body. In contrast, recent research shows that animal products contain potentially carcinogenic compounds that may contribute to increased cancer risk.

Furthermore, fiber, which has protective effects against cancer—namely colon cancer—is found exclusively in plant-based foods. Fiber greatly speeds the passage of food through the colon, which effectively removes carcinogens. Fiber also changes the type of bacteria that is present in our intestines, reducing the production of harmful carcinogenic acids. Plant-based foods are also completely cholesterol-free, which aids in keeping our bodies in a healthy state.

In our research studies at the Physicians Committee for Responsible Medicine, my colleagues and I have examined the effects of dietary interventions on a number of conditions. Whether we are looking to lower cholesterol or blood pressure levels, treat diabetes or migraines, or even simply trim waistlines, our studies have shown that a low-fat, vegan diet is a powerful way to promote health. The same goes for cancer—plant-based foods prevent and protect

Unraveling the Mystery is full of valuable information to help you do just that—prevent and protect against cancer.

We are surrounded everyday by forces we cannot control. Diet is not one of them. Follow the guidelines outlined in this book, and you will be on the road to a long, fulfilling, healthy future.

Unravel the mystery. Live a health-promoting lifestyle. Take this knowledge that Ann presents to you, and take control.

Neal Barnard, M.D., is a clinical researcher, author, and health advocate. He is the author of dozens of publications in scientific and medical journals as well as numerous nutrition books for lay readers. He is founder and president of Physicians Committee for Responsible Medicine (PCRM).

Foreword
By Francisco Contreras, MD

Ignorance is the stronghold of cancer. Fear is its fuel. For the majority of people, cancer is one big frightening mystery; and people think that it is genetics or bad luck that will determine whether a person will be diagnosed with a malignancy or not. That cannot be further from the truth. As a practicing integrative oncologist for thirty years, I am asked multiple times a week why more people are being diagnosed and dying from cancer every year. There is a cloud of confusion. This book thoroughly unravels cancer related issues in a way that provides clarity about what to do to prevent cancer or reverse it.

I have been honored to treat tens of thousands of people facing cancer over the last three decades and my patients have taught me more about cancer and beating it than the textbooks ever did. I have found that the three most important things you need to beat cancer, and all other diseases for that matter, are:

1. Knowledge
2. Faith
3. Healing Foods

Knowledge

Most people diagnosed with cancer are never told that the positive contribution of cytotoxic chemotherapy for advanced stage cancer is only two percent. Most patients are never informed by their oncologists that chemotherapy has been proved to be effective in less than five percent of all cancer types. Here is another fact people don't know: Only two percent of all women who have breast cancer have the BRCA1 or BRCA2 cancer gene. That means that genetics has nothing to do with ninety-eight percent of women diagnosed with breast cancer. The power to beat cancer comes by getting the correct information about the disease and treatment options.

Knowing that conventional treatment offers little hope for advanced stage cancer is a start. Then you need to acquire the information of natural therapies that can help. This book will give you a foundation of knowledge to understand everything that assaults our health and how to protect yourself from the attacks. It will provide information that will help you build a cancer free lifestyle.

Faith

The immune system is the most important defense against cancer. If the system is working perfectly, it is virtually impossible to get cancer. Researchers have mapped out the relationship between a person's thoughts and their immune system. From the moment of cognition, signals are sent to the hypothalamus, the pituitary glands and then the adrenal glands that release hormones into the bloodstream that will either boost or depress the immune system. Positive thoughts and emotions bolster the immune system. Negative thoughts and emotions break it down. Though much is known about the mind—body connection, science has been unable to explain what happens pre-cognition. Little is understood about the spirit and its impact on physical health. As a Christian oncologist, the Word of God speaks to me in an amazing way. When I read Proverbs 4:23, I take it literally. Your heart is the wellspring of life. If your spirit is healthy, living water will flow and stimulate your mind to have healing thoughts. Positive thoughts will improve the physical heart's function. If your spirit is conflicted, your wellspring will have stagnant water that will produce harmful thoughts. The physical heart will suffer. Please read this next line carefully and take note that it is an oncologist making this statement: Spiritual fortitude is the most powerful anti-cancer element at your disposal. Faith in God will overcome the fear of cancer. Prayer is not the last resort; it is the first line of defense.

Healing Foods

The human body is the pinnacle of God's creation. It is the only entity that was created in His image. Scripture states that your body was fearfully and wonderfully made (Psalm 139:14). Its divine design came complete with an instruction manual of the restorative fuel it requires. Everything God told us to eat has nutrients that boost the immune system, protect the DNA from mutation and provides energy while reducing inflammation. All of the foods that God told us not to eat depress the immune system, feed cancer cells and rob the body of energy while provoking inflammation and pain. Cancer prevention and reversal depends on what you feed your body. That is why the third section of this book is critical for you to embrace.

There is a clear ministerial calling on the Malkmus family and Ann has the spiritual gift of teaching. The wisdom contained in this book will change the quality of health and life you can experience as well as your generations to come. Read it, live it and add years of joy to your life and the call on it.

Francisco Contreras, MD is the director and chief of oncology at Oasis of Hope Hospital and the author of many books including 50 Critical Cancer Answers. www.oasisofhope.com

Introduction

What an incredible body!

Have you ever wondered just how the body really works? How does everything just . . . happen? The millions of processes that are running simultaneously without you ever having to give it a conscious thought.

- The heart beats effortlessly around 100,000 times, pumping 2,000 gallons of blood through 60,000 miles of blood vessels each and every day. No effort required, and you can't stop it by your thoughts no matter how hard you try.
- The lungs just automatically inflate and deflate bringing in 2,642 gallons of new oxygen into the body every day while expelling carbon dioxide. And it's doing this while continuing to pump blood.
- The skin feels, the eyes blink, the ears hear, the brain thinks, the kidneys and liver cleanse, the colon – well it does its thing – all without any effort.

So many bodily functions all taking place simultaneously in perfect harmony without any support or assistance needed by the person – You.

When you cut your finger the body immediately responds. Blood is rushed to the area to help cleanse the wound. Then the blood creates a scab that protects the area from the outside environment while the cells underneath begin the job of repairing. The body automatically starts to knit the skin back together knowing that it needs to fill in any gaps. As your cells multiply, nutrients and building blocks are carried to them through a blood supply that adapts to the particular size and shape of the wound. If blood vessels were destroyed, the growth of new blood vessels is spontaneously initiated to take their place, and they grow into the tissues within mere hours.

As the wound heals, the cell replication process is turned off. Your body's cells know exactly when to grow and exactly when to stop, and when it's all said and done, you're left with a near perfect replacement for the skin you previously lost.

So if this self-healing is inherent to the body then why do we develop cancer? There are approximately 37 trillion cells in an average adult body. About 300 million cells die and are replaced each minute – that's over 400 billion per day. As these cells are dying and being replaced there are from time to time cells that malfunction and become rogue. It is estimated that the average immune system eliminates cell mutations and their development into cancer over 10,000 times per day.

The amazing part is that this intelligence is automatically built within each of us. Just like our body automatically pumps blood and breathes, it heals while replacing cells that have outlived their purpose or could cause harm.

If all of these processes are going on behind the scene then what happens that allows cancer to develop? Are we focusing on what truly matters when we discuss "cure"? Or should we really be asking, "What is the cause?" Maybe the "cure" is more easily found in the "cause."

This book has been an interesting journey for me.

I learned first hand in the 1990's that my body could heal itself when I overcame Irritable Bowel Syndrome (IBS) and fibromyalgia. After my recovery I became a nutrition enthusiast. I couldn't get enough information. I studied everything I could get my eyes on. Eventually, I left my position as the Academic Dean of a college and ended up working for a company that teaches people how to use diet and lifestyle modifications to help their bodies heal.

While working for this company, I have seen some truly amazing things and I have had the privilege of working alongside many of the thought leaders in the functional medicine/alternative health movement. It's been amazing to learn how the body truly works and how nearly all sickness is caused by nutritional deficiency and toxicity. I've also had the privilege to work with people around the world learning their cultural lifestyles and helping them understand that by making simple (not always easy) changes that they too can find healing regardless of the disease or severity. The humbling part of this is, each year when we return to that part of the world, the testimonies that greet us are indeed remarkable and miraculous!

Over the last several years, two members of our family were diagnosed with cancer. One was our nephew, a 26 year-old veteran from the Iraq war. He had been diagnosed with colon cancer after his return from Iraq. He was married and had children. He followed the principles outlined in this book. It is now 6 years later and he is alive and cancer free today and has 5 beautiful children.

The other young man was diagnosed with Hodgkin's Lymphoma the end of his first year in high school and he was our son. He chose a different path, as he couldn't embrace the information in this book. He struggled to incorporate it into his life even after he came to live with us at the age of 15. His path included the conventional approach to treating cancer. This is when we saw first-hand the devastating effects of chemotherapy as his primary caregivers.

He was able to go into remission two different times. Each time the cancer returned, he chose the conventional approach. By the third time the cancer returned, the conventional approach no longer was effective. As we reflect on his lifestyle, his eating habits, his frame of mind and exercise routine, we realized that as a teenager it is hard to believe that this disease can take you. Blind faith in what appeared to be a convenient method of killing the cancer (just go to chemo once a week and get a few weeks off before you do it again) seemed easier than drinking a lot of carrot juices and eating a lot of unsalted, unsweetened vegetables. We lost our 18-year-old son to cancer on July 2, 2011. He had graduated from high school just 4 weeks earlier. He had chosen a college and had talked of marriage.

About this book

Have you ever thought you knew a lot about a subject only to discover later that you hardly knew anything of the topic? That's what happened to me in writing this book. I've understood for a long time the impact diet and lifestyle has on disease but it wasn't until I started compiling the scientific research for this book that I put so many pieces together as it related to health and sickness in general but to cancer specifically.

The more I have studied, the greater appreciation I've gained for our magnificent bodies. I knew they were self-healing and that toxicity and deficiency were the primary causes of sickness and disease, but I didn't realize the role that toxicity played in cancer specifically.

I was astonished by the amount of scientific studies that have been conducted and the associated research that is available directly linking certain substances to cancer.

The evidence is undeniable and overwhelming. Why this information isn't made more readily available is unconscionable. People need to know that so many of the things that they have put in and on their bodies for many years is actually responsible for the cancer they are experiencing today.

How does cancer develop?

The body's job is to keep everything working in harmony; a perfect balance. When something happens that threatens this balance the body quickly reacts to neutralize the situation and re-establish balance. As long as the cells have all of the resources that they need, the body is able to fend off the many threats it might be exposed to on a day-to-day basis – viruses, bacteria, bugs, stress, and even some toxic substances like cigarette smoke. But when cells are not being fed with adequate nutrition the immune system starts to become lethargic, losing its efficiency. The body cannot continue to remove toxins and repair the body simultaneously.

Because of this sluggish cell structure the body has a weakened immune system that isn't able to respond as quickly and effectively. Its power to protect and heal becomes compromised. As time goes on the body begins to fall further and further behind – too many stressors on the body without enough cell energy to continuously remove toxins and repair and rebuild healthy cells. This is when cancer begins to develop.

Cancer can take as long as 20 years to develop as the body gradually falls behind. Or, it could be triggered by a traumatic event that coupled with a weakened immune environment, is a breeding ground for cancer cells to develop. This event could be a divorce, loss of a loved one like a spouse or child, or it could be spawned by a move or loss of employment. In any of the above situations, the cells were in a weakened state allowing the disease to begin.

Once cancer has formed, the approach that tens of thousands have found successful includes flooding the cells with food that will make them strong and vibrant again while simultaneously identifying and removing those things that are causing additional stress – we call these toxins.

How do you give your cells the most energizing foods possible in a way that maximizes healthy new cell growth? This book goes into extensive detail on not just what to feed the cells but it also answers the why's and how's too. You'll learn the superfoods and supplements that will enhance and support the immune system if you choose chemotherapy that will significantly reduce or eliminate the devastating side effects.

Are you considering incorporating some alternative therapies? The options presented here have been specifically chosen so they won't cause harm to your body while working to attack the cancer cells and some of the methods will enhance your immune system.

Because toxin buildup plays such an important role in the formation of cancer a major section of this book identifies the toxins that may have contributed to a person's cancer. Documentation for the damage these toxins cause is provided with recommendations for how to reduce or eliminate exposure entirely. In some instances information is even provided that will assist in the safe removal of these toxins from the body.

The information in this book is presented in a way that will help you connect the dots ... what needs to change so the body will start healing itself of the cancer it is experiencing.

This book is for those who want to live. It is for those who are willing to place effort and faith in their own bodies. God gave everyone an incredible, self-healing body. We must not allow others to dissuade us of this extraordinary gift and fact.

As you read through this and observe the powerful testimonies of those who chose this approach, remember, you can do this too. Cancer isn't a death sentence. Your body has the power and the capability to be healthy – you just need to do your part and give it what it needs so it can do what it does best – heal itself.

I trust you will learn as much from reading this book as I have learned from the research that has gone into its creation. May your minds be open to the wonders that your body can create!

"Nothing great becomes great without overcoming great resistance."

What is Cancer?

Cancer is the second leading cause of death for Americans. The National Cancer Institute at the National Institution of Health estimates that there were 1,660,290 new cancer cases and 580,350 deaths from cancer within the United States in 2013. Among men, the top three cancer diagnoses are prostate cancer, lung cancer, and colorectal cancer. The leading types of cancer among women are breast cancer, lung cancer, and colorectal cancer. Cancer is a term used for diseases in which abnormal cells divide without control and are able to invade other tissues. Cancer cells can spread to other parts of the body through the blood and lymph systems.

According to the National Cancer Institute the nation is losing ground in many important areas that need attention:

- Incidence rates are rising for melanoma of the skin, non-Hodgkin lymphoma, childhood cancer, cancers of the kidney and renal pelvis, leukemia, thyroid, pancreas, liver and bile duct, testis, myeloma, and esophagus.
- Lung cancer incidence rates in women continue to rise.
- Death rates for cancer of the pancreas, liver, bile duct, and uterus are increasing.
- Initiation rates among 18-25 year olds have risen.
- More people are overweight and obese.
- Alcohol consumption has risen slightly since the mid 1990s. Fruit and vegetable intake is not increasing. Red meat and fat consumption are not decreasing.
- Cancer treatment spending continues to rise along with total health care spending.

Depending on the location in the body, normal healthy cells will typically divide; some, more often than others. A normal cell will divide an average of somewhere between 50 and 60 times during its lifetime. With each division, a cell runs the risk that its DNA will become damaged. The more times a cell divides the more chance of an injury. If the DNA is damaged, the injury is carried over to the newly formed cell. As this continues over time, if there has been no cellular repair, the genes that control the instructions on how much the cell should grow or divide will become damaged.

Each of the new, injured cells will no longer listen to the signals being sent out by the normal cells. The rogue cells gain so much strength that they no longer die. Cancer cells have been shown to divide thousands of times. They begin to produce and secrete a dangerous, poisonous substance to nearby tissues that only serve to accelerate and multiply the growth of these free radical cells.

Cancer cells have two characteristics in common:

1. They grow and divide uncontrollably
2. They have the ability to metastasize (spread)

Every living organism makes defective cells all the time. Human beings are no different. But the human body has numerous mechanisms in place to silence those free radicals so they cannot create too much damage and maintain control. Our cellular structure was designed to continue to produce antioxidant proteins and antioxidant enzymes that continuously fight those free radicals.

Through nutrients derived from food, these antioxidants will repair the damage done to the cells and continue this defensive process throughout our entire lives.

Another way of looking at this is known as "Immune-enhancement." If we continue to eat healthy foods, stay hydrated, keep our emotions and stress in check and ensure our bodies are not overfilled with toxins, the process of maintaining control over cancer cells is likely to be successful.

There are more than one hundred different varieties of cancer. Most types will be one of five broad categories:

1. Carcinoma - cancer that begins in the skin or in tissues that line or cover internal organs. There are a number of subtypes of carcinoma, including adenocarcinoma, basal cell carcinoma, squamous cell carcinoma, and transitional cell carcinoma.
2. Sarcoma - cancer that begins in bone, cartilage, fat, muscle, blood vessels, or other connective or supportive tissue.

3. Leukemia - cancer that starts in blood-forming tissue such as the bone marrow and causes large numbers of abnormal blood cells to be produced and enter the blood.
4. Lymphoma and myeloma - cancers that begin in the cells of the immune system.
5. Central nervous system cancers - cancers that begin in the tissues of the brain and spinal cord.

According to the American Cancer Society, 50% of all men and 33% of all women in the United States will develop some form of cancer at some point in their lives.

Some of the causes of cancer includes:

- Viruses
- Chemicals
- Inflammation
- Bacteria
- Fungus
- Foreign bodies
- Chronic infection
- Ionizing radiation

Other risk factors include:

- Growing older
- Tobacco
- Certain hormones
- Genetics
- Alcohol
- Poor diet
- Lack of physical activity
- Overweight

As we will discuss later, toxins abound in our lives. Internal and external toxins actually start accumulating upon conception. This continuous barrage of toxins through the years will wreak havoc on our filtering systems and inevitably weaken them and the entire body which will then allow the growth of yeast, bacteria, fungus and even a small virus that can create great difficulty for the body to recover.

Our diet, lifestyle and thought patterns are major factors to maintaining vibrant health. And the continuous consumption of inferior nutrition causes severe nutritional deficiencies that can lead to serious health problems.

These cancer statistics can be changed. Cancer doesn't need to be feared. This book will help guide you through the process of making wise decisions that will dramatically improve the odds of not getting cancer but of also beating this terrible disease if it does develop.

Section One

❧

Toxicity

A new video released in October, 2013 called The Human Experiment suggests that there are over 80,000 chemicals used legally in the United States and only 130 have been tested enough to be identified as hazardous to our health. As the incidences of cancer, and other immune suppressed issues continues to increase there is a definite validity in considering the role of toxins in this increase. Years ago, people could breathe clean air, drink pure water and eat vegetables that were raised in more pristine soil that was rich in nutrients and poor in pesticides, herbicides and other toxins. In this chapter we will discover some of the many chemicals, substances and environments that either contribute to or are a direct cause of many of the cancers that occur today.

Toxins are elements or substances that cause harm to an organism. Organisms that can be impacted include animal, plant or bacterium. Toxins not only can impact the whole of the organism but effects can be seen at the cellular level as well as in organs such as the liver.

Today, most people agree that smoking cigarettes is hazardous to the body. But, that hasn't always been the case. It wasn't until 1964 that the Surgeon General, Luther Terry, concluded that smoking is the direct cause of three diseases — lung cancer, heart disease and emphysema (now COPD). 40 years later the Surgeon General, Richard Carmona, released a report that for the first time linked conclusively smoking cigarettes and leukemia, cataracts, pneumonia and cancers of the cervix, bladder, kidney, pancreas and stomach. Although I don't blame them, my parents knew no better when they were both heavy smokers throughout all six of us children's young adult lives and before any of us were conceived. No one knows what effect that has had on each of us. As long ago as that was, it will not likely come up in any doctor's office questions if any of us were to develop a disease today.

How then can we feel confident that science today has caught up with the newest technologies of plastics, wireless, hybridized food, genetically modified organisms, and so on? Although there may not be studies that prove today, that the plastic containers we get our food in are dangerous, there may well be some in the next 10 years. Do we want to risk the constant exposure to something purely for convenience sake? The items we are using and eating that are still considered reasonably safe by most people (just like the cigarettes were not that long ago), may well end up as a potent carcinogen directly correlated with various diseases. Time will tell.

Admittedly, toxic substances abound in the world we live in today. From the radiation emitted through our cell phones, power lines and microwave ovens to the chemicals found in the foods many of us consume on a daily basis. Then there are the toxins that are generated from within the body that are being caused by the emotional and physical stress so many of us find ourselves burdened with each day. Toxins seem to be ever present and all around.

When we are sick, the body wants to heal. It desires to be healthy. But, in many instances the toxic load that has been placed on the body causes sickness and diseases like cancer. For healing to occur, we need to lighten this toxic load and help the body to detoxify — remove the toxins from the cells.

While it might be impossible to completely avoid all toxins, our goal is to help you understand the source of the toxins and the impact they may be having on your body. Once you realize the extent of these bombarding you all day, every day, and how it can impede on your endeavor to beat cancer, then your next goal should be to eliminate and remove as many of them as possible.

The Centers for Disease Control (CDC) conducts ongoing assessments of the levels of environmental chemicals in the U.S. population. This ongoing study utilizes lab samples from the individuals who are part of the National Health and Nutrition Examination Survey (NHANES). The NHANES samples from the years 1999-2000, 2001-2002, and 2003-2004 (each representing about 2,400 individuals) are used for the CDC's national reports. In the CDC Fourth National Report on Human Exposure to Environmental Chemicals, complete data from the above sample years were included. Each year additional chemicals are measured; the fourth report contains information on 75 previously untested compounds, for a total of 212 compounds measured. Table 1 on page 22 contains the list of chemicals found in the vast majority of individuals.

Sadly, as you continue to read into this chapter you will see that even fetuses are not exempt from growing in a contaminated environment. Although the information in the following pages may be alarming, it is meant to encourage awareness and lifestyle adjustment that will only serve to make the journey toward recovery easier.

Table 1. Common Chemicals

Acrylamides from fried foods	Cotinine	Trihalomethanes
Bisphenol	Chlorinated pesticides	Triclosan
Organophosphate pesticides	Pyrethroids	Heavy metals
Aromatic hydrocarbons	Polybrominated diphenyl ethers	Benzophenone from sunblock
Perfluorocarbons from non-stick coatings	A host of polychlorinated biphenyls and solvents	Mercury from seafood and dentistry
BPA from plastics	Teflon	Flame retardant

Chapter One: Air

"When you feel yourself to be in critical condition, you must treat yourself as gently as you would a sick friend."
—Julia Cameron

Oxygen may well be the most important nutrient we consume. Unlike many other nutrients it enters our bodies effortlessly. To be nourished with oxygen the only thing that the body needs to do is breathe. We rarely ask ourselves though what air is the healthiest? Are there chemicals and toxins in the air I'm breathing? What are the impacts on my health when I breathe in air that is contaminated?

There are literally thousands of ways that air can be contaminated. The following are some of the most prevalent and likeliest to cause significant health impairment and have even been associated with cancer.

1. Indoor Air Pollution

Most people spend the majority of their days inside buildings. Most of our modern structures are built to be as air tight as possible to ensure that the cold stays out during winter and the cool stays in during summer. While this air tight construction assists in maintaining more constant temperatures and reduces utility costs, the lack of quality, fresh air in the buildings has its share of consequences. Aerosol deodorant, bug repellent and killers, glues, solvents, paint, cleaning supplies, personal care products (perfumes and cologne) and even air fresheners all contain chemicals that are toxic to the body. These are examples of VOCs.

According to the EPA, Volatile Organic Compounds (VOCs) have been found at levels up to 10 times higher inside homes/buildings than outside. This was found regardless if the building was located in a rural or high-industrialized area. Eye and respiratory tract irritation, headaches, dizziness, vision disorders, and memory impairment are among the immediate symptoms that some people have experienced soon after exposure to some VOCs. Many organic compounds are known to cause cancer in animals; some are suspected of causing, or are known to cause cancer in humans.

VOCs are emitted by a wide array of products numbering in the thousands. Examples include: paints and lacquers, paint strippers, cleaning supplies, pesticides, building materials and furnishings, office equipment such as copiers and printers, correction fluids and carbonless copy paper, graphics and craft materials including glues and adhesives, permanent markers, and photographic solutions. Carpet emits VOCs, as do products that accompany carpet installation such as adhesives and padding.

As VOCs and other chemicals and substances are released into our homes and office buildings they are circulated throughout the building by the central heat and air conditioning systems. The lingering ill effects on our body and health continue well beyond the amount of time we are able to identify the existence of these compounds through smell.

Here are a few ways that exposure to many of these indoor air pollutants can be reduced:

- Increase the ventilation in the home. Leave a window open slightly.
- When having painting done in the building, use paint that is low in VOCs.
- When installing carpet select low VOC carpeting, solvents and pads.
- If at all possible, only use chemical based products (if they are necessary) outside and ensure that you are upwind from the spray so it is targeted away from you. Allow them to air out thoroughly before reintroducing them to the indoor environment.
- Replace chemical based home cleaning products with

ones that are chemical free. Water with a pH of 2.5 is effective at killing bacteria. 11.5 pH makes a great cleaning solvent.

• Consider purchasing an ozone-producing machine to assist in purifying the air.

2. Tobacco smoke

Francisco Contreras in his book, *Beating Cancer* states "Smoking is the single major cause of cancer deaths accounting for 30% of all deaths."

There are more than 4,000 chemicals in tobacco smoke, the smoke breathed in by smokers and nonsmokers. According to the American Heart Association, this exposure can cause cancer and heart and lung disease [1]. Of these 4,000 chemicals, 200 are known poisons and 43 are known to cause cancer.

3. Smog

Researchers at the University of California, Los Angeles School of Public Health have found that living near traffic pollution during pregnancy and the first year of life might increase the likelihood of developing childhood cancer. A pair of recently published European studies found that regularly breathing in air tainted with even low levels of air pollution raises your long-term risk of lung cancer:

A. One finding came from a review of data from nearly 313,000 people across nine European countries. The study was published online July 10 in The Lancet Oncology.

B. Short-term exposure to smog has also been linked to increased risk of hospitalization or death from heart failure, according to a study led by the University of Edinburgh that reviewed data from 12 countries worldwide, published the same day in The Lancet.

Living or working in environments with heavy traffic for any length of time can be considered detrimental to our health. Yet, uprooting isn't always an option. When faced with cancer, a person needs to evaluate the air they breathe and ensure that their body is only exposed to the purest air possible. Breathing only clean, non-toxic air is vital in creating an environment for healing.

4. Vehicle and factory emissions

In 2009, the Environmental Protection Agency released a landmark report estimating the concentrations of air pollutants across the United States. The report studied over 181 different air pollutants, 80 are thought to contribute to cancer in humans. For example, benzene is a toxin released from vehicle exhaust that may lead to cancer. Approximately 30% of the cancers caused by air pollution are due to vehicle exhaust; another 25% are due to local industrial activity.

Diesel Engine Exhaust

The following was taken from the American Cancer Society website: The International Agency for Research on Cancer (IARC) is part of the World Health Organization (WHO). Its major goal is to identify causes of cancer. IARC classifies diesel engine exhaust as "carcinogenic to humans," based on sufficient evidence that it is linked to an increased risk of lung cancer, as well as limited evidence linking it to an increased risk of bladder cancer.

- The National Toxicology Program (NTP) is formed from parts of several different US government agencies, including the National Institutes of Health (NIH), the Centers for Disease Control and Prevention (CDC), and the Food and Drug Administration (FDA). The NTP has classified exposure to diesel exhaust particulates as "reasonably anticipated to be a human carcinogen," based on limited evidence from studies in humans and supporting evidence from lab studies.
- The US Environmental Protection Agency (EPA) maintains the Integrated Risk Information System (IRIS), an electronic database that contains information on human health effects from exposure to various substances in the environment. The EPA classifies diesel exhaust as "likely to be carcinogenic to humans."
- The National Institute for Occupational Safety and Health (NIOSH) is part of the CDC that studies ex-

posures in the workplace. NIOSH has determined that
diesel exhaust is a "potential occupational carcinogen."

The evidence seems clear and thorough – vehicle exhaust, especially diesel exhaust poses significant danger to humans. While we can't choose which vehicle we get behind in traffic, we can turn on the inside air button in our car until we gain some distance between our vehicle and the one in front of us. Just having this knowledge will set you up to make different choices as they become apparent.

Chapter Two: Viruses and Infectious Organisms

"A sad soul can kill you quicker than a germ."
—John Steinbeck

Viruses, bacteria, infections and other strange but devastating phenomenon are infiltrating our lives more every day. Babies are born with ecoli in the fluid that surrounds them, small infants are getting urinary tract infections, babies are developing cancer before they leave the womb, children are dying of flesh eating amoeba, and the list goes on.

Why is this happening?

Worldwide, approximately 18% of cancers are related to infectious diseases [1]. This varies in different regions of the world from a high of 25% in Africa to less than 10% in parts of the developed world [1]. Viruses are usual infectious agents that cause cancer but bacteria and parasites may also have an effect.

A virus that can cause cancer is called an oncovirus. Some examples of these viruses include:

- Human papilloma virus which can cause cervical carcinoma
- Epstein-Barr virus which can cause B-cell lymph proliferative disease which can turn into nasopharyngeal carcinoma
- Karposi's sarcoma herpes virus which can turn into Kar-

posi's Sarcoma and some forms of lymphomas
- Hepatitis B and Hepatitis C viruses which can turn into Hepatocellular carcinoma
- Human T-cell leukemia virus-1 that can turn into T-cell leukemias [1]

Bacterial infections such as Helicobacter pylori can induce gastric cancer [2].

There are two parasitic infections that have been proven strongly associated with squamous cell carcinoma of the bladder and liver cancer [3].

Maintaining a strong immune system helps our bodies fend and fight off various parasites, bacteria, viruses, and infections that could weaken our bodies which may subsequently lead to cancer development. This must be a life-long process since the older a person grows, the weaker the immune system can become. Aging doesn't necessarily have to mean a weaker immune system, but it does mean that one must exert a more concerted effort in maintaining a higher level of immunity.

Chapter Three: Water

"Half the costs of illness are wasted on conditions that could be prevented."

—Dr. Joseph Pizzorno

Water may well be the second most important nutrient that we put in the body on a daily basis. Interesting note, according to H.H. Mitchell, Journal of Biological Chemistry 158:

- The brain and heart are composed of 73% water
- The lungs are about 83% water
- The skin contains 64% water
- The muscles and kidneys are 79% water
- The bones are 31% water

Of course the exact amount varies by an individual's age as well as other factors but the point is that we are comprised of mostly water.

Each day we expend a certain amount of our body's water reserve. Water is involved in hundreds of bodily functions. As we breathe we inhale oxygen and exhale carbon dioxide. With each exhale is a small amount of moisture which is evident when we breathe on a glass or mirror. The water within our body helps to regulate its temperature. It will sweat when too hot and create heat when too cold. Those actions will use more moisture. Water also helps to remove waste through our urine and feces.

Additionally, water acts as building material for every cell. It transports carbohydrates and proteins that our bodies need in the bloodstream. Water acts as a shock absorber for the brain, spinal cord

31

and fetus while lubricating joints and forming saliva.

Throughout all of these activities our bodies lose water that must be replaced. Just as the air we breathe needs to be pure so does the water that we consume so it can replenish what has been lost through normal everyday living.

Unfortunately, one of the greatest casualties to our nutrition has been in our water supply. Whether it is well water, municipal drinking supply or filtered water in a bottle, there seem to be very few if any, sources for pure, unadulterated drinking water.

My parents have lived in a small rural town in Wisconsin for over 60 years. I remember as I was growing up, many of our neighbors and community residents were diagnosed and died of cancer. The ages varied. Some were as young as 8 while others were in their 70's and 80's. What was interesting is that so many of the people who died from cancer in my neighborhood were in the prime of their lives – 40's 50's and 60's. Throughout the years since I have left home, my parents have continued to watch many of their friends and neighbors in this small town contract cancer.

What is causing so many of the people from this small community to succumb to some form of cancer? Is it the air they are breathing? Is it the water? How many other communities both large and small are finding their residents in similar situations? Once in a while the news will show a pocket in a state where there were an unusual number of people afflicted with some form of disease. It tends to be blamed on mining, or perhaps some other industry. There are likely many pockets in many states where, if the deaths were studied and tallied, a correlation to something else would likely be drawn.

Many studies have shown that this life-giving component (water) has become so terribly polluted that instead of cleansing, detoxifying, nourishing and satisfying the body it has become full of carcinogenic compounds contributing to, and perhaps may even be a direct cause of cancer.

Although there are numerous toxins in water, we will discuss the major ones if only to give an indication of the overall toxicity that exists in water today.

Chlorine, Bleach and Ammonia

Chlorine, a disinfectant, was first added to a community water system in 1908 in Chicago and was instrumental in eliminating many types of waterborne diseases, such as cholera and typhoid fever. Prior to chlorination, many major cities experienced death tolls of 1 in 1000 people from typhoid alone.

Chlorine has been used to disinfect municipal water for over 80 years and has had some positive effects on public health. In the 1970's, it was discovered that chlorine, when added to water, forms Trihalomethanes (chlorinated byproducts) by combining with certain naturally occurring organic matter. These are also known as disinfection byproducts (DBPs). The Environmental Protection agency reports that some people who drink water-containing Trihalomethanes over many years could experience a risk in certain types of cancers among other health concerns.

Researchers for the Division of Cancer Epidemiology & Genetics (DCEG), which is part of the National Cancer Institute performed a study of six cancer sites conducted in Iowa and found associations of rectal and bladder cancers with long-term (> 40 years) exposure to drinking water high in these unintentional byproducts.

A cancer control study conducted in Ontario Canada in 1996 demonstrated that the risk of bladder cancer increases 14 to 16% with exposure to chlorination by-products. The study indicates that these by-products represent a potentially "important" risk factor for bladder cancer [1][2].

In 1992, the American Journal of Public Health published a report that showed a 15% to 35% increase in certain types of cancer in people who consume chlorinated water. This report also stated that many of these effects were due not only to water consumption but showering in chlorinated water had a detrimental effect as well.

It seems that in the heroic attempt to purify municipal drinking water from deadly pathogens that the risk of long-term, life-threatening exposure to chlorine, bleach and ammonia has increased. Gastrointestinal, bladder and urinary tract health have been the areas of the body most affected by the chlorinated water.

Over The Counter and Prescription Medications

If you don't complete your cycle of antibiotics or other medications or if you find that your prescription or over the counter medication has expired, do you:

A. Flush the unused pills in the toilet?
B. Discard the unused pills and bottle in your trash can so
they can be moved to the mountain of other trash in
your local waste collection area?

The spectrum of medications is significant, including antibiotics (both human and veterinary), analgesics, anti-depressants, cholesterol-lowering and anti-hypertension drugs, anti-convulsants, acetaminophen, ibuprofen, and reproductive hormones. The list is endless. The average adult is now on 8 different prescription drugs.

People will more than likely either throw them away or drop them down the drain. In either case, these toxic substances end up in our soil and water supply. So what?

A recent five-month inquiry from the Associated Press into 62 major municipal water providers indicated that of the 28 who responded all had traces or greater detections of pharmaceutical ingredients as well as other toxins present in their municipal water supplies.

This Associated Press report indicated laboratory research that found even small amounts of pharmaceutical ingredients affected human embryonic kidney cells, human blood cells and human breast cancer cells. The cancer cells proliferated too quickly; the kidney cells grew too slowly; and the blood cells showed biological activity associated with inflammation. The report also indicated research showed that pharmaceutical drugs in waterways are damaging wildlife across the nation and around the globe. Notably, male fish are being feminized, creating egg yolk proteins, a process usually restricted to females [3].

A number of other studies found trace concentrations of pharmaceutical drugs in wastewater, various water sources and some drinking water. These investigations seemed to confirm that pharmaceutical drugs are present, albeit at trace concentrations, in many water sources.

Currently, EPA analysis of the available data indicates that there is a substantial margin of safety between the very low concentrations of pharmaceutical drugs that would be consumed in drinking water and the minimum therapeutic doses, which suggests a very low risk to human health. Based on this finding, the development of formal health-based guideline values for pharmaceutical drugs in the World

Health Organization's (WHO) Guidelines for drinking water quality is currently not considered to be necessary [4][5].

But, has anyone tested what long-term exposure of these low concentrations of pharmaceutical drugs in water can do to someone? What if they consume water with these components for thirty years? What if a small child consumes this low concentration? Will their minimal weight and rapidly producing cells be affected differently?

Water providers rarely disclose results of pharmaceutical screenings, unless pressed, the AP found. For example, the head of a group representing major California water suppliers said the public "doesn't know how to interpret the information" and might be unduly alarmed.

Drinking water isn't the only way that people are receiving lethal doses of toxins. The skin is the largest organ of the body covering about 3,000 square inches in the average adult and weighing about six pounds. This is nearly twice the weight of the average adult brain or liver. The skin receives about one third of the blood that circulates throughout the body.

An interesting method of getting "under the skin" is using a medical skin patch. These have become the new method of transferring drugs into the body. Medical skin patches have been designed to provide a specific dose of medicine through the skin into the blood stream. This is also called transdermal. There are patches for hormones, anti-depressant, ADHD, Ritalin, hypertension, motion sickness, B12, nitroglycerine, nicotine, contraception, lidocaine ... the list goes on. Then there are the creams that are rubbed onto the skin.

We've established that the skin acts as a receptor for the body allowing substances to enter the body and blood stream through its pores. Now what happens when warm or hot water is added to this equation? When we take a shower, a bath or sit in a hot tub the pores open even more, allowing the chlorine and other toxic chemicals in the water uninhibited access to our blood stream and ultimately our organs.

Furthermore, in a new study, researcher Julian Andelman, of the University of Pittsburg Graduate School of Public Health, the National Academy of Sciences has shown that volatile chemicals such as chloramine (a combination of water and ammonia) present in many municipal drinking water supplies are especially toxic to people when they are exposed to them while bathing or showering. He suggested that the major health threat posed by these water pollutants is far more likely to be from their inhalation as air pollutants in the home.

He says that in the past, this type of inhalation exposure to water pollutants has largely been ignored. But he found that hot showers can "expel" between 50 to 80% of the dissolved chemicals into the air. A hot bath reduces this exposure by 50%. One reason for this is that because water droplets distributed through the showerhead have a larger surface-to-volume ratio than water streaming into a bath, so the toxins can vaporize out [6].

Recent studies indicate that dermal (skin) and inhalation (breathing) exposures to what we discussed earlier, trihalomethanes (THM), a major component of DBP in treated water, can be significant. With collaborators in Spain, the DCEG evaluated disinfection by-products (DBP) in relation to bladder cancer risk in the Spanish Bladder Cancer Study, considering exposure via ingestion, showering/bathing, and swimming in pools. This was a large, interdisciplinary case-control study of bladder cancer (1,200 cases and 1,200 controls) in 18 hospitals from five different regions in Spain. The study indicates that dermal and inhalation exposures to THM exposure revealed an overall two-fold excess of bladder cancer among individuals with estimated household levels above 49 mg/L.

What this study revealed is that people who drank, showered, bathed and/or swam in chlorinated water were twice as likely to contract bladder cancer. This is just one study looking at one type of cancer. As research continues to unfold, what other direct associations will be uncovered linking the consumption of chlorinated water with cancer and other diseases?

The National Cancer Institute estimates cancer risks for people who consume chlorinated water to be 93% higher than for people who do not. The effects of drinking chlorinated water have been debated for decades. However, most experts now agree that there are significant risks related to consuming and inhaling chlorine and chlorinated byproducts.

With small pockets of communities all over the country and quite possibly around the world experiencing what could be mini-epidemics of various forms of cancer, multiple sclerosis, and other serious infirmities, it would be wise and prudent to take action in your own home to protect yourself and your loved ones from any contaminants that may be found in your water supply whether it is consumed or used in bathing.

Here are some ideas to help limit exposure and reduce the amount of toxic absorption through your water supply:

- Whole-house water filtration system. This not only protects the drinking water, but also removes the toxins from all water supplies throughout the house including bathroom sinks. (This is where people usually brush their teeth exposing the toxic chemicals to the receptors in the mouth.) We have one of these in our home.
- Individual shower filters. We take one of these with us when we travel overnight via car or air. Bring along a wrench and it's easy to change the showerhead in the hotel room. When we happen to forget this filter, our skin and body notice the difference in just a few days.
- Cold showers can reduce the vaporization of dissolved toxic chemicals by 50%.
- Shorter showers will reduce the exposure.
- To limit the spread of the released gases into the rest of the home, close the bathroom door while bathing and use an exhaust fan to move the toxins outdoors. Of course, this isn't necessary when using either a whole-house or shower filter system.

We've spent a lot of time discussing the toxic effects that chlorinated water has on the body but there is another reason it should be avoided. Since chlorine is a disinfectant, it cleans and disinfects the body removing beneficial compounds. Healthy bacteria in and on the body are beneficial and necessary for optimal body function. Putting chlorinated water on the body either while showering, bathing, or swimming kills these friendly bacteria that are vital in enhancing your immune system's ability to fight disease. Not only does it kill the bacteria but other nutrients are diminished like vitamin B12. Additionally, chlorinated water removes the healthy oils from the skin causing it to become dry and brittle.

Whether you are working to recover from cancer or another disease or just trying to stay healthy, avoid putting chlorinated/chemical laden water in your mouth, on your skin or in your lungs. Protect yourself!

In this section we focused on the chlorine, pharmaceutical drugs, disinfection byproducts (DBP) and other compounds. In future sections we'll be discussing fluoride as well as other chemicals from shampoos, skin lotions, cosmetics and deodorants that are washed off of our bodies through the bathing process then cycled into our water supply for consumption/absorption, yet another way of increasing our toxic load.

Chapter Four: Fluoride

"The... patient should be made to understand that he or she must take charge of his own life. Don't take your body to the doctor as if he were a repair shop."

—Quentin Regestein

With the abundance of advertisements, products, and dentists' recommendations of using fluoride, one would think that this country should have the most healthy teeth, gums and periodontal health.

Unfortunately, not only does our country still have terrible dental health, but this fluoride that has become falsely synonymous with better teeth health has actually been instrumental in degrading many facets of physical health. Sadly, there is evidence that the harmful effects of fluoride have been known by conventional medical and dental organizations for over half a century. For example, the Journal of the American Medical Association (JAMA) stated in their Sept. 18, 1943 issue that fluorides are general protoplasmic poisons that change the permeability of the cell membrane by certain enzymes. Also, an editorial published in the Journal of the American Dental Association on Oct. 1, 1944, stated: "Drinking water containing as little as 1.2 ppm fluoride will cause developmental disturbances. We cannot run the risk of producing such serious systemic disturbances. The potentialities for harm outweigh those for good."

A 1965 study indicated that there was clear evidence that cancer deaths were higher for cities with fluoridated water than for those that had no fluoridated water [1]. Today, nearly fifty years later, we would have difficulty finding a city that did not fluoridate the water.

So, why haven't we seen fluoride banned and not used so profusely all of these years later? Part of the problem is that it's an accumulative toxin that, over time, can lead to significant health problems but are not immediately linked to fluoride over-exposure.

The debate has been going on for many years. One book that seems to have excellent research to back up the dangers associated with fluoride is *Fluoride, The Aging Factor.* This book documents the cumulative effect of tissue damage by fluoride; commonly seen as aging (collagen damage), skin rashes and acne, gastrointestinal disorders, and many other conditions, including osteoporosis. Yiamouyannis, the author of the book, goes on to say that fluoride suppresses the immune system. Fluoride inhibits the movement of white blood cells by 70%, thereby decreasing their ability to reach their target. Yiamouyannis cites 15 references in his pamphlet, Lifesavers Guide to Fluoridation, that document immunosuppressive effects with as little as 10% of the amount of fluoride used in fluoridated water. Immune suppressing effects can look like anything from a cold that won't go away to increased risk of cancer and other infectious diseases [2].

The U.S. Center for Disease Control and the Safe Water Foundation reported that 30,000 to 50,000 excess deaths occur in the United States each year in areas in which the water contains only one ppm of fluoride. Another study performed in 1988 suggests that fluoride can increase the potency of carcinogens and increase tumor growth by as much as 25% [3]. Finally, a study done in the 1990's clearly suggests that since fluoride accumulates in the bone, there is good reason for the findings that young men had 50% more bone cancer in cities with fluoride.

In a 2005 paper entitled Fluoride – A Modern Toxic Waste, Lita Lee, Ph.D. writes: "Even though the EPA's recent studies don't seem to find a correlation between cancer and fluoridated water, it could be that they are not using the proper study materials. It is difficult to find connections using epidemiological studies that study studies and not individuals."

It is unwise to continue to believe the propaganda. It is better for our collective health if we incorporate some simple, easy steps to remove fluoride from our daily lives.

These are some proactive measures you can take:

1. Use toothpaste and mouthwash that contain no fluoride
2. Refuse the fluoride step when getting your teeth cleaned by a dental hygienist
3. Use a water filtration device that removes fluoride from your home water source
4. Reduce/eliminate drinking most forms of tea. Tea plants readily absorb fluoride from soil. As a result, tea drinks invariably contain high levels of fluoride. In the United States, brewed black tea averages about 3 to 4 parts ppm fluoride, while commercial iced tea drinks contain between 1 and 4 ppm [4]. Fluoride and bromide, having a similar structure as iodine, can competitively inhibit iodine absorption.

"The sad irony here is that the FDA, which does not regulate fluoride in drinking water, does regulate toothpaste and on the back of a tube of fluoridated toothpaste ... it must state that "if your child swallows more than the recommended amount, contact a poison control center."

The amount that they're talking about, the recommended amount, which is a pea-sized amount, is equivalent to one glass of water.

The FDA is not putting a label on the tap saying don't drink more than one glass of water. If you do, contact a poison center...

There is no question that fluoride – not an excessive amount – can cause serious harm."

—Paul Connett

Chapter Five: BPA

"A further sign of health is that we don't become undone by fear and trembling, but we take it as a message that it's time to stop struggling and look directly at what's threatening us. "
—Pema Chodron

How many times have you drank from a plastic bottle, stored your food in plastic, or purchased food in a styrofoam container? How about eating with a plastic fork or drinking from a plastic cup? And don't forget the plastic straw!

Bisphenol A (BPA) is an industrial chemical that has been used to make certain plastics and resins since the 1960's. BPA is found in polycarbonate plastics and epoxy resins. Polycarbonate plastics are often used in containers that store food and beverages, such as water bottles. They may also be used in other consumer goods. Epoxy resins are used to coat the inside of metal products, such as food cans, bottle tops and water supply lines. Some dental sealants and composites also may contain BPA.

BPA disrupts the endocrine system interfering with the production, secretion, transport, action, function and elimination of natural hormones. A body's own hormones can be imitated by BPA in a way that could be hazardous to health.

While safety levels have been set for BPA amounts many experts feel the health policies must be reviewed as recent studies are indicating there is truly reason for public safety concerns. What is more concerning is that with so many sources you can be exposed to BPA, how can any level really be set?

For most people the primary source of exposure to the chemical BPA is through diet. It can migrate into food from polycarbonate food and beverage containers or from food and beverage containers that contain or are lined with epoxy resin.

A study conducted by the Harvard School of Public Health found that participants who drank for a week from polycarbonate plastic bottles showed a two-thirds increase in BPA levels found in the participants urine [1]. In a similar study the Harvard School of Public Health found that those who ate one can of soup for five days straight had 1,221% more BPA in their urine than those who consumed home made soup for the same five days [2]. A CDC (Centers for Disease Control and Prevention) study found 95% of adult human urine samples and 93% of samples in children had bisphenol A [1].

Over 6 billion pounds per year of the estrogenic mimicker are used to manufacture polycarbonate plastic products. Numerous studies have clearly indicted BPA as a relatively strong estrogen receptor, disrupting endocrine especially in breast and other female hormonal areas as well as in prostate/testicle health.

While researching the link between BPA exposure and cancer many studies have confirmed that the bisphenol A introduced into the body can have a negative effect on our hormonal health:

- BPA may be linked to infertility in women. A study conducted by the Brigham and Women's Hospital identified the following effects on eggs that were exposed to BPA:
  – Percentage of eggs that matured decreased
  – Proportion that degenerated fell
  – Percentage of eggs that underwent spontaneous activation increased. (Spontaneous activation is an abnormal process in which an unfertilized egg acts as if it has been fertilized) [3].

Dr. Racowsky who, conducted the study says, "Our data show that BPA exposure can dramatically inhibit egg maturation and adds to a growing body of evidence about the impact of BPA on human health."

- BPA Linked To Erectile Dysfunction And Other Male Sexual Problems

– BPA-exposed workers had a significantly higher risk of sexual dysfunction compared to the unexposed workers.

– BPA-exposed workers had a nearly four-fold increased risk of reduced sexual desire and overall satisfaction with their sex life.

– They also had a greater than four-fold increased risk of erection difficulty, and more than seven-fold increased risk of ejaculation difficulty.

– There was a dose-response relationship between increased level of cumulative BPA exposure and higher risk of sexual dysfunction.

– Compared to unexposed workers, BPA-exposed workers reported significantly higher frequencies of reduced sexual function within one year of starting work in a BPA-exposed factory [4].

Some other studies you may find interesting:

- BPA linked to higher risk for obesity among young girls [5]
- Childhood Asthma Linked To BPA Exposure [6]
- Childhood Obesity Linked To BPA In Food Packaging [7]
- BPA In Rivers May Encourage Fish Species To Interbreed [8]
- BPA Exposure In Womb Linked To Behavior Problems In Young Girls [9]
- BPA Found In Canned Foods Aimed At Children [10]
- Switching To Fresh Foods Cuts Hormone Disruptors BPA and DEHP [11]
- 95% Of US Paper Money Tainted With BPA [12]
- BPA Now Linked To Poor Sperm [13]
- Dental Sealants Contain BPA Derivatives Which May Seep Into Children's Mouths [14]
- Study Suggests Sperm May Be Harmed By Exposure To BPA [15]
- Prenatal Exposure To Endocrine-Disrupting Chemicals

Linked To Breast Cancer [16]
- Law To Ban BPA In Children's Products Announced By US Senators [17]

The National Institutes of Health (NIH, NIDCR) and the United States Environmental Protection Agency convened an expert panel of scientists with experience in the field of environmental endocrine disruptors, particularly with knowledge and research on BPA. Five sub-panels were charged to review the published literature and previous reports in five specific areas and to compile a consensus report with recommendations. These were presented and discussed at an open forum entitled "Bisphenol A: An Expert Panel Examination of the Relevance of Ecological, In Vitro and Laboratory Animal Studies for Assessing Risks to Human Health" in Chapel Hill, NC on November 28-30, 2006 [18]. The preponderance of evidence suggests that BPA increases cancer susceptibility as a result of changes to DNA [19].

Important notes:
1. The risk of off-gassing from BPA is increased with exposure to sun and warm temperatures. We traveled to Nigeria for 2 months starting in November 2012. We saw pallets of bottled water sitting in the sun being exposed to warm temperatures. Interesting to note that many of the Nigerians who we counseled during our visit had hormone based cancers and infertility and erectile dysfunction were common complaints. It was obvious to us the direct correlation between the bottled water they were drinking and the poor health they were experiencing.
2. There is ample evidence that exposure to BPA creates imbalances within the body particularly to the endocrine system and hormone excretion.
3. There are many sources from which you can be exposed to BPA. Some of which you don't even know.

Every time you wrap your food in a sandwich bag, drink from a straw or use a plastic fork, you may be introducing a chemical to your body that will in time, create degradation to your endocrine system that will result in an imbalance in your hormones which can cause not only severe symptoms, but severe illness as well.

An easy, economical, "green" approach is to remove as much plastic and processed food from our daily life as possible. It is not difficult to store leftovers in glass containers. Nor would it be a problem to bring water in glass or stainless steel water bottles. There are even glass straws that can be purchased if one needs to drink from a straw. If you don't buy the microwave popcorn or the canned soups or the deli items, you will never have to eat from the chemically laden containers again. This is first and foremost best for your body and with the recycling of glass storage and cookware, it will help the environment as well.

Chapter Six: PFCs

"Sickness is the vengeance of nature for the
violation of her laws."
—Charles Simmons

There are numerous ways that we have introduced environmental chemicals into our bodies and the number of ways increase daily. For example, years ago, we would visit the Dry Cleaners maybe once every couple of months to clean special clothing. Now, people regularly drop off clothes two or three times a week. The chemicals they bring home in their laundry are so carcinogenic that even if they place the clothes outside for three days, the residual will still brush against their bodies. These chemicals are ingested through the skin requiring the filtration by the liver.

Perfluorinated Compounds (PFCs)

The chemicals in dry cleaning are called PFCs or perfluorinated compounds. These are a family of fluorine-containing chemicals with unique properties to make materials stain-and stick-resistant. Some PFCs are incredibly resistant to breakdown and are turning up in un-expected places around the world. Manufacturers have developed a host of chemicals in this family to repel oil and water from clothing, carpeting, furniture, and food packaging such as pizza boxes and paper food containers such as microwave popcorn and fast food wrappers. Fire-fighting foams have used them, as have dry cleaners, paints, roof treatments, and hardwood floor protectant.

PFCs are considered persistent organic pollutants (POPs) and resist chemical, biological, and photolytic degradation in the environment. These chemicals will biomagnify in the food chain and bioaccumulate in animal and human tissues.

There are many forms of PFCs, but the two most commonly found contaminants are:

- PFOA or perfluorooctanoic acid (PTFE) commercially known as Teflon™.
- PFOS or perfluorooctane sulfonate is a key ingredient in Scotch-guard, a fabric and carpeting stain repellent,

Exposure to PFC's occurs through our diet, from food wrapped or cooked in materials containing PFCs, and through the food chain and water pollution. Another route of exposure is inhalation of PFCs from clothing, home furnishings, carpeting, and other materials treated with PFCs to be stain and water-resistant.

Though there has not been much research on the effects of PFCs in humans, testing has shown that PFCs are present in both humans and wildlife. PFCs may be linked to:

- Thyroid dysfunction
- Preeclampsia
- Risk of high cholesterol
- Risk of cancer
- Liver dysfunction
- Immunotoxicity
- Endocrine disruption
- Developmental delays
- Fertility issues

Researchers are finding serious health concerns with PFCs, including increased risk of cancer. PFCs cause a range of other problems in laboratory animals, including liver and kidney damage, as well as reproductive problems. The time it would take to expel half of a dose of PFOAs, is estimated at more than 4 years. PFOSs half-life is estimated at more than 8 years. Exposure to PFOA or PFOS before birth has been linked with lower birth weight in both animal and human studies.

PFCs have been produced, used, and disposed of essentially without regulation for the last half-century. Rising levels of PFCs in the environment and increasing governmental pressure, however, have led to voluntary actions to reduce PFC production and use.

In 2002, 3M stopped using PFC's for its signature product, Scotch-guard®, because of concerns over release of PFOS and PFOA during manufacture and use. In early 2006, the EPA, Teflon™ manufacturer DuPont™, and seven other companies announced an agreement to reduce PFOA in emissions from manufacturing plants and in consumer products by 95% by the year 2010.

While some companies as outlined above are phasing out the use of PFOS and PFOA, the question is what chemical is replacing these substances? What are the long-term health risks that haven't been identified?

As dangerous as these persistent toxic chemicals are, it would be wise if the government didn't allow their use at all. There are certainly other components that can replace them without the deadly effects.

How can you reduce your exposure?

1. Avoid purchasing or, at a minimum, limit use of products that contain PFCs.
2. Beware of packaged foods. Stay away from greasy or oily packaged and fast foods, as the packages often contain grease repellent coatings. Examples include microwave popcorn bags, French fry boxes, and pizza boxes.
3. Avoid stain-resistance treatments. Choose furniture and carpets that aren't marketed as "stain-resistant," and don't apply finishing treatments such as Stainmaster® to these or other items. Where possible, choose alternatives to clothing that has been treated for water or stain resistance, such as outerwear and sportswear. Be wary of other products that may be treated including shoes, luggage, camping and sports equipment.
4. Check your personal-care products. Avoid personal-care products made with Teflon™ or containing ingredients that include the words "fluoro," "perfluoro," "PFOA," "perfluorooctanoic acid," or "PTFE." PFCs

can be found in dental floss and a variety of cosmetics, including nail polish, facial moisturizers, and eye make-up.

5. Avoid Teflon™ or non-stick cookware. If you choose to continue using non-stick cookware, be very careful not to let it heat to above 450ºF. Discard products if non-stick coatings show signs of deterioration [1].

At first glance, this information may appear unsettling and we may think we are doomed and have no recourse but to expect defeat when it comes to exposure to certain toxins. However, we actually do have more control than we are led to believe.

There are carpets, clothing, paints and cosmetics that are non-toxic. These may cost a little more and may take a little longer to find, but when it comes down to priorities, doesn't non-toxic make sense?

Chapter Seven: Radiation

"A man too busy to take care of his health is like a mechanic too busy to take care of his tools."
— Spanish Proverb

Our lives are dramatically different than they were 100 years ago. Today, babies are waking up next to video monitors, they chew on dad's cell phone and sit on mom's lap in front of the monitor or lap top watching mom type on the keyboard. Tablets like IPads are now used as babysitters. Teens and pre-teens have cell phones that they carry and use to communicate with their friends and families. They have computers and TVs in their bedrooms. As adults we put internet connectivity throughout our homes so we can connect all of these devices and even control them remotely – adjusting the temperature of the house, turning on/off lights or turning on the oven while driving home. We drive a hybrid car that takes us to the doctor where we have X-rays, mammograms or a CT scan.

Technology has certainly made our lives more convenient and productive but is there an impact on our health? Could it be that this technology that is providing so much pleasure as we listen to ITunes with our IPhones and our IPods might actually be one of the causes of the cancer so many people are experiencing today?

There are numerous studies that prove that living near a mobile phone station, or power lines can potentially increase cancer risk. But, with all of the electromagnetic devices that are currently in your home, have you created your very own mobile phone station or power line equivalent? Has convenience come with a cost?

Non-ionized radiation exposure

How many of the items below are in your home?
- Computers
- Cell phones
- Blue tooth devices
- Cordless phones
- Microwave ovens
- Digital baby monitors
- Fluorescent lights
- Wireless internet device (Wi-Fi)
- Routers
- Large screen televisions
- Any other types of wired and wireless electronic devices

These all generate electromagnetic fields (EMF) of varying strengths, which is a type of non-ionizing radiation, i.e. A type of low-frequency radiation. Radio waves, radar and radiation produced by electrical transmission are also examples of radiation sources that generate electromagnetic fields.

There have been numerous studies on the effects of the electromagnetic radiation emitted from these devices. All scientists agree that this radiation is dangerous at high levels, but it has been hoped that the low levels emitted from these household devices are safe. Many believe that when the body first experiences a new source of radiation, it reacts by strengthening its immune defenses, but then the immune system begins to weaken progressively the longer the exposure to the radiation continues.

The levels of radiation emitted from mobile and cordless phones on standby, and of Wi-Fi routers, digital baby monitors and Bluetooth are a fraction of those of a mobile or cordless phone in use on a call. But this does not mean they are safer.

The radiation exposure from wireless products is considered a "chronic" exposure, constantly at a low level rather than short burst of high power. There is evidence that this type of exposure might be more damaging in the long-term.

Even if the power level of one wireless router or computer is small, a home, school, or work environment may include many of these devices at once. Radiation exposure from a Wi-Fi system comes from the router and each of the computers. A cordless phone emits radiation from the base stations and the handsets. A mobile phone on standby, or worse, on a call, also adds to the radiation "load."

Most tests and studies only focus on one of these appliances at a time. And even then, the radiation has been questioned depending on the age of the person, the proximity of the device and the length of exposure. Few, if any, studies have been done on several devices that have now found their way into nearly everyone's home.

You will find numerous studies that easily provide the evidence needed to make informed decisions on how much electromagnetic frequency you will want to expose you and your family to on a daily basis, year after year.

Mobile Phones

A recent study, entitled Cellular Neoplastic Transformation Induced by 916 MHz Microwave Radiation was published in the Cellular and Molecular Neurobiology journal, confirms that the microwave radiation given off by a mobile phone is capable of transforming normal cells into cancerous ones. It found that after 5-8 weeks of exposure NIH/3T3 cells changed their form and rate of proliferation to a cancerous cell. These cells were also found to be tumor-forming when transplanted into mice [1]. (Prior to this study it was already noted that microwave radiation had been shown to alter brain molecules).

The World Health Organization now places mobile phone use in the same "carcinogenic hazard" category as lead, engine exhaust, and chloroform. The European Environment Agency has pushed for more studies, saying cell phones could be as big a public health risk as smoking, asbestos and leaded gasoline. There are currently 5.9 billion reported users of mobile phones. This number is growing rapidly making radiation exposure likely to be worldwide.

Unfortunately, inconsistent results have been published on potential risks for brain tumors tied to mobile phones because the studies used different methods that may not have lasted long enough to detect the increased risk of brain cancers, while others have chosen to group cell phones with cordless phones to create a different classification that deters people from seeing the true dangers. But even more recent analysis of these studies and their shortcomings from a number of authors find that brain tumor risks are significantly elevated for those who have used mobile phones for at least a decade.

High resolution computerized models based on human imaging data suggest that children are indeed more susceptible to the effects of EMF exposure at microwave frequencies [2][3]. Studies in Sweden indicate that those who begin using either cordless or mobile phones regularly before age 20 have greater than a fourfold increased risk of brain cancer [4]. No other environmental carcinogen has produced evidence of an increased risk in just one decade.

Brain cancer is the proverbial "tip of the iceberg"; the rest of the body is also showing effects other than cancers from cell phone radiation exposure.

The cell phone is as addictive as chocolate and it doesn't offer any antioxidant value at all! How many people are now using it to obtain their news, weather, e-mail, voicemail, internet searching, product purchases and map directions? Not to mention it is now a watch, a GPS, a camera, a radio and a compass. Many homes don't even have land line telephones anymore. If we don't take control over our addictive behaviors whether it is food, lack of exercise, or just using a radioactive device called a cell phone, our behaviors will surely dictate the future of our health.

Effects of Radiation on Children

Children are now being exposed to wireless products from a very early age and often throughout their developing childhood and teenage years. This should be considered experimental since no one has any idea of the cumulative effect of long-term exposure starting at such a young age. We know from the scientific studies relating to mobile phones that children are more vulnerable to this type of radiation, absorbing more radiation than adults through their thinner skulls [5]. Even the German and French governments have for years, advised against the use of wireless products like Wi-Fi and cordless phones at home.

The clearest evidence that this day-in day-out low-level exposure might be dangerous is from the studies of the health effects of both adults and children who live near mobile phone stations [6]. Several studies have shown significantly increased levels of cancers among

56

those living within a few hundred meters of a mobile phone station [7][8][9].

Even if they are not living near a mobile phone station, in a given day, at any one time, a child may be exposed to cumulative levels of radiation much higher than each product emits alone. The child may be exposed constantly at home and at school, even when asleep. This exposure generally starts when they are young and continues throughout the children's lives.

Mobile phones have only been used widely since the late 1990's so the early studies, mostly done in the early 2,000's, didn't involve long-term phone users. They were done when it was too early for the association to show up. However, even in 2008 the charity organization, Samantha Dickson Brain Tumor Trust, wrote "Brain tumors now account for more deaths among children and those under 40 than any other cancer." It will not be very long before the results become evident.

There is great evidence that is developing daily that consistent exposure to radiation, even if it is low frequency, will weaken the immune system making it easily susceptible to developing cancer. You can very easily reduce your exposure to more tolerant levels and still use some of the devices that have now become inseparable to your life.

Ways to more safely use your cell phone:
- Carry the cell phone or mobile device on your body as little as possible.
- Don't carry it on your hip or in your pocket other than to get it from point A to B.
- Lay it on the table or dashboard away from the body as much as possible.
- Use wired headphones instead of bluetooth ear devices.
- If using a bluetooth ear device, remove it from your ear when not in use.
- Consider turning off the Wi-Fi when sleeping.
- Sit farther away from TVs and other electronic devices.
- Place radiation guards, bio-chips, cell guards on computers, cell phones, etc. To reduce exposure. Research first and get the best available.
- Look for other ways to limit your exposure as much as

possible. Every little bit counts.

Microwave Ovens

Over 95% of American homes have microwave ovens used for meal preparation. Because microwave ovens are so convenient and energy efficient, as compared to conventional ovens, very few homes or restaurants are without them. In general, people believe that whatever a microwave does to foods cooked in it doesn't have any negative effect on either the food or them. Of course, if microwave ovens were really harmful, our government would never allow them on the market... would they? Regardless of what has been "officially" released concerning microwave ovens, we have personally stopped using ours based on the research from the past 30 years.

Ten Reasons Not to Use Your Microwave Oven

1. Continuous eating of food processed from a microwave oven may cause long-term, permanent, brain damage by "shorting out" electrical impulses in the brain (de-polarizing or de-magnetizing the brain tissue).
2. The human body cannot metabolize (break down) the unknown by-products created in microwaved food.
3. Male and female hormone production may shut down and/or become altered by continuous eating of microwaved foods.
4. The effects of microwaved food by-products are residual (long-term, permanent) within the human body.
5. Minerals, vitamins, and nutrients of all microwaved food is reduced or altered so that the body gets little or no benefit, or the body absorbs the altered compounds that cannot be broken down.
6. The minerals in vegetables are altered into cancerous free radicals when cooked in a microwave oven.
7. Microwaved foods may cause stomach and intestinal growths [tumors]. This may be a primary contributor to the rapidly increased rate of colon cancer in the

United States.

8. The prolonged eating of microwaved food may cause cancerous cells to increase in human blood.
9. Continual ingestion of microwaved food may cause immune system deficiencies through lymph gland and blood serum alterations.
10. Eating microwaved food may cause a loss of memory, concentration, emotional stability, and a decrease of intelligence.

Ionized radiation exposure from medical imaging machines

When X-rays or any ionizing radiation pass through the body they cause electrons to be ejected from atoms, leaving behind positive ions. These positive ions, or free radicals, can cause damage to DNA. DNA can also be damaged directly by radiation. If DNA is damaged there are three possible outcomes:

1. The cell dies (only occurs with very high doses).
2. The cell repairs itself perfectly (most common result).
3. The cell repairs itself with mistakes (rare).

The inaccurate repair of DNA is rare, but can cause a cell to act wild or grow into a cancer. Oftentimes it takes decades for cancer to be detected following radiation exposure.

Radiation from mammograms, bone density tests, computed tomography (CT) scans, PET scans, X-rays, and so forth will increase risks of developing cancer. While there are certainly concerns over low level tests like mammography and dental X-rays, many experts are extremely concerned about an explosion in the use of the higher radiation tests such as CT and nuclear imaging.

The radiation you get from X-ray, mammogram, CT and nuclear imaging is ionizing radiation – high-energy wavelengths or particles that penetrates tissues to reveal the body's internal organs and structures. Ionizing radiation can damage DNA, and although your cells repair most of the damage, they sometimes do the job imperfectly, leaving small areas of "misrepair." The result is DNA mutations that may contribute to cancer years down the road.

In 2006, about 62 million CT scans were performed in the United States, compared with just three million in 1980. There are good reasons for this trend. CT scanning and nuclear imaging have revolutionized diagnosis and treatment, almost eliminating the need for once-common exploratory surgeries and many other invasive and potentially risky procedures. The benefits of these tests, when they're appropriate, far outweigh any radiation-associated cancer risks, and the risk from a single CT scan or nuclear imaging test is quite small. However, in light of the 20-fold increase in the use of these tests, experts wonder if we are looking at future public health problems.

Some of this worry was fueled by the April 2010 release of the President's Cancer Panel report, "Reducing Environmental Cancer Risk: What We Can Do Now." Among other concerns, the report highlighted the rise in radiation exposure from medical imaging. The panel outlined ways to minimize radiation exposure from medical sources and recommended health care providers keep a running tally of the amount of radiation their patients receive from medical imaging.

It is clearly known that children and teens who receive high doses of radiation to treat lymphoma or other cancers are more likely to develop additional cancers later in life. But we have no clinical trials to guide our thinking about cancer risk from medical radiation in healthy adults. Most of what we know about the risks of ionizing radiation comes from long-term studies of people who survived the 1945 atomic bomb blasts at Hiroshima and Nagasaki. These studies show a slight but significantly increased risk of cancer in those exposed to the blasts, including a group of 25,000 Hiroshima survivors who received an amount of radiation that would be equal to two or three CT scans today.

The atomic blast isn't a perfect model for exposure to medical radiation, because the bomb released its radiation all at once, unlike today, where the doses from medical imaging are smaller and spread over time. Still, most experts believe that can be almost as harmful as getting an equivalent dose all at once.

Most of the increased exposure in the United States is due to CT scanning and nuclear imaging, which require larger radiation doses than traditional X-rays. A CT scan for example, delivers 70 times as much radiation as one chest X-ray.

In a 2009 study from Brigham and Women's Hospital in Boston, researchers estimated the potential risk of cancer from CT scans in 31,462 patients over 22 years. For the group as a whole, the increase in risk was slight – 0.7% above overall lifetime risk of cancer. In the United States the risk of developing cancer combined for men and women is around 42%. But for patients who had multiple CT scans, the increase in risk was higher, ranging from 2.7% to 12% (In this group, 33% had received more than five CT scans; 5% more than 22 scans; and 15 more than 38).

What Can You Do?

Here are several ways to keep your exposure to medical radiation as low as possible:

- Discuss any high-dose diagnostic imaging with your health care provider. If you need a CT or nuclear scan to treat or diagnose a medical condition, the benefits may outweigh the risks. Still, if your health care provider has ordered a CT, it's reasonable to ask what difference the result will make in how your condition is managed; for example, will it save you from an invasive procedure?
- Keep track of your radiation exposure. Not only should your health care provider and the image device makers indicate the radiation dose for each exposure, but you can keep track of your own PET scan, CT scan, and X-ray history. It may not be completely accurate because different machines deliver different amounts of radiation, and because the dose you absorb depends on your size, your weight, and the part of the body targeted by the X-ray. Note any radiation treatment for cancer. Include, any occupational radiation exposure. An example is if you work on an airline or travel extensively and use TSA imaging machines. Both you and your health care provider will get a decent estimate of your exposure.
- Consider a lower-dose radiation test. If your health care provider recommends a CT or nuclear medicine scan, ask if another technique would work, such as a lower-

dose X-ray or a test that uses no radiation such as ultrasound (which uses high-frequency sound waves) or MRI (which relies on magnetic energy). Neither ultrasound nor MRI appears to harm DNA or increase cancer risk. If you must have a CT scan and weigh less than 180 pounds you might be able to get the radiation dose reduced.

- Consider less-frequent testing. If you're getting regular CT scans for a chronic condition, ask your health care provider if it's possible to increase the time between scans. And if you feel the CT scans aren't helping, discuss whether you might take a different approach, such as lower-dose imaging or even observation without imaging.
- Don't seek out scans. Don't ask for a CT scan just because you want to feel assured that you've had a "thorough checkup." CT scans rarely produce important findings in people without relevant symptoms. And there's a chance the scan will find something incidental, spurring additional CT scans or X-rays that add to your radiation exposure.
- If possible, wear a thyroid guard and lead apron during dental X-rays. Also, ask whether you can receive a digital X-ray, which uses less radiation than film.
- Can you use an older test result? Let your health care practitioner know if you've received imaging at another office or hospital within the past 5 years. He may be able to re-examine the results and spare you another round of radiation.

It is important to note that each exposure to radiation compounds in our body increasing the risk of cancer. So even though a single source of exposure to radiation is unlikely to cause cancer by itself, the combined exposures add up to more damage than the sum of each individual one increasing our risk of cancer over time [10].

Children are at the greatest risk of developing cancer from radiation exposure. There are two theories why. First, rapidly dividing or growing cells are at a greater risk of damage from ionizing radiation.

Second, children have a long life ahead of them; therefore the chance of detecting a slow growing cancer is higher when compared to someone exposed later in life.

In general, women are at a slightly higher risk of developing cancer when compared to men exposed to the same dose of radiation. This is based again on the exposure data from survivors of atomic bombs, nuclear accidents and the early use of X-rays. As we learned earlier in the book, men and women also have different average risks from developing cancer.

Natural methods to remove ionizing radiation from the body:

- Iodine – one of the first diseases that can occur in people living near nuclear facilities that have faced nuclear fallout is thyroid cancer. Iodine can greatly help in preventing thyroid cancer. Before the thyroid gland can use iodine, it has to activate it to a nascent form so that it reacts and combines to form thyroid hormones. Nascent iodine can overcome barriers that prevent the uptake of iodine by the thyroid, such as competition from fluoride, bromide-containing molecules, or perchlorate. These are serious issues for thyroid health and have to be overcome by supplying enough iodine to compete with the other molecules. The thyroid can more easily take up nascent iodine than other forms of iodine. And since it is already activated, the necessary thyroid hormones can be readily made. It will help protect the thyroid from both hyper and hypothyroidism. It is available without prescription. It is more expensive than potassium iodide, but it is more absorbable and high doses of it can be given even to children. It may be useful to consult a health care practitioner on dosage.
- Spirulina – this is a superfood that is derived from blue green algae and it has many health benefits. Recent studies have indicated that spirulina is quite helpful in anti-radiation therapy and according to research that has been conducted with children in Chernobyl; spirulina can also help as a medication for radiation poisoning. It is known to protect bone marrow cells from

DNA damage [11]. It can assist in the prevention of diseases such as leukemia and help the body fight bacterial and viral infections. When taken orally, it can also help in removing barium from the body.

- Chlorella – a fresh water, single celled algae that contains the highest amount of chlorophyll in any known plant. Apart from having numerous benefits for the body, it is also known as one of the best methods of expelling radiation from the body. Chlorella, in particular, has the ability to neutralize radiation and remove toxins such as cadmium, dioxins, and PCB's from the body. Its ability to detoxify uranium, lead and copper has also made it very valuable, especially considering the toxins we are exposed to today.
- Reishi Mushrooms – they are known to strengthen the immune system and improve circulation. This mushroom has relevance today as it plays an important role in protection against ionizing radiation.
- Magnesium – this is an important mineral in removing heavy metals from the body that encourage radiation damage. Magnesium oil is a valuable way to introduce it to the body.
- Fulvic Acid – when it comes to getting rid of radiation from your body, fulvic acid is on the top of the list as it can break down heavy metals and toxins in the body and remove them from the body. Fulvic acid is a water-soluble organic substance that is found in surface water and it has some amazing benefits although scientists the world over are just learning of it. Fulvic acid is a humic acid that transforms the molecular structure of water and enhances the functions of water.
- Zeolites – minerals that are effective at binding and expelling heavy metals from the body.
- Vitamins A, C, and E – also known as the ACE vitamins, they offer proven antioxidant protection. High intake of these vitamins and other antioxidants protect airline pilots from radiation-induced chromosomal damage, an occupational hazard in those who work

at high altitudes [12]. In fact, ACE supplements have been proposed as "space foods" to protect astronauts from high radiation levels [13].

• Zinc and Manganese – vitally important for sustaining whole-body resistance to ionizing radiation.

• Melatonin – protects dividing cells and circulating blood cells from chromosomal injury by radiation [14][15].

• Licorice Extracts – block DNA damage and protect lipids from radiation-induced peroxidation [16].

• The Indian Gooseberry – increases survival time and reduces mortality of mice exposed to whole-body radiation [17].

Every exposure to radiation, whether it is ionized or non-ionized, and whether the level is high or low continues to place a burden on your body. These exposures are constantly happening throughout the day and into the night. It would seem that your body is always trying to recover from the barrage of radiation that keeps coming at it day after day, month after month, and year after year. At some point, the body gives up and breaks down setting the stage for cancer to develop.

Chapter Eight: Mold

"Sickness is felt, but health not at all."
—Thomas Fuller, M.D.

Mycotoxins are toxins produced by organisms of the fungi kingdom, commonly known as molds. If you eat grains or legumes like corn, barley, oats, wheat, rice, sorghum and peanuts, or grain-fed animal products, there is a good chance you are already being exposed because mold infestation and mycotoxin contamination affects as much as one-quarter of the global food and feed supply [1].

Evidence is mounting regarding the connection between mycotoxins (molds) and cancer. It seems that when mold is present, it will change how bodies use estrogen. A groundbreaking study published in the journal The Science of Total Environment in 2011 found that the estrogen-disrupting mycotoxin known as zearalenone (ZEA), produced by a microscopic fungus, was detectable in the urine of 78.5% of New Jersey girls sampled, and that these ZEA-positive girls, aged 9 and 10 years, "tended to be shorter and less likely to have reached the onset of breast development" [2]. Mycotoxin has also been found in eggs and dairy products, and even found in beer. The researchers were able to find an association between the young girls' urinary levels of ZEA and their intake of commonly contaminated sources such as beef and popcorn.

Interestingly, derivatives of ZEA mycotoxin have been patented as oral contraceptives. And, according to a recent article, ZEA has been widely used in the United States since 1969 to fatten cattle. Observations of premature puberty in girls demonstrates evidence that this practice can cause physical harm in humans. As a result, this practice has been banned by the European Union. There has since been other research that has confirmed the link between mycotoxins and premature puberty.

Surprisingly, the ZEA study in the young New Jersey girls was the first ever performed to evaluate this mycotoxin's potential estrogen-disrupting properties, and indicates just how great a need there is for further research on the topic, as far as public health is concerned. There are already over 40 mycotoxins of great enough concern to be subject to regulation by over 100 countries and yet, most of these have not been fully evaluated for their potential health risks [3].

Since research has already proven that the younger a girl is when she goes into puberty, her risk of developing hormone-based cancer increases as she ages, then, it would be logical to assume that our food supply has significantly increased our young girls' chances of developing cancer.

Other Toxic Molds

Experts suspect that toxic black mold can cause cancer, although there still needs to be more research. Some other toxic molds, like Aspergillus for example, definitely cause cancer though. The aflatoxin mycotoxins which Aspergillus produce are among the most powerful carcinogens. Ground nuts or peanuts are noted to be grown in aflatoxin. Alfalfa sprouts have the tendency to grow in aflatoxin as well.

As early as 1999, findings of a link between inhaled mycotoxins (such as aflatoxin) and cancer were reported by the National Institute for Occupational Safety and Health (NIOSH), their study noted: "Several studies have provided evidence for the association of cancer in humans with inhalation of aflatoxin contaminated dust, e.g., lung cancer or colon cancer...elevated risks for liver cancer and cancers of biliary tract". The NIOSH study further warned: "Diseases associated with inhalation of fungal spores include toxic pneumonitis, hypersensitivity pneumonitis, tremors, chronic fatigue syndrome, kidney failure, and cancer."

Anyone with compromised immune systems (in which cancer is one) would be wise to examine the area in which they live to ensure no mold is lurking in the basement or in the attic. They should also avoid any food item that has any potential of being grown in mold.

Chapter Nine: Heavy Metals

"The secret of health for both mind and body is not to mourn for the past, not to worry about the future, or not to anticipate troubles, but to live the present moment wisely and earnestly."
—Siddartha Guatama

New technology brings new pollutants. As lead was to paint 30 years ago, mercury is to amalgam fillings today. Mercury is just one of numerous heavy metal toxins that we are learning more about daily. It is of vital importance that people learn about heavy metals, how they have become insidiously toxic within our bodies, what we can do to prevent undue exposure and what effort we should be making to eliminate as much as we can from our bodies. Although we will not discuss every heavy metal in great detail, we will discuss the most prominent ones and their detrimental effects on the body.

Mercury

Mercury is the most toxic naturally occurring substance on the planet, yet, according to the EPA, there is currently over 1,000 tons of mercury from amalgam fillings in the mouths of Americans. Over 67 million Americans exceed the exposure of mercury vapors considered "safe" by the EPA because of amalgams in their teeth [1].

Dental amalgams can increase your risk of cancer in a variety of ways. Mercury is a known carcinogen (cancer-causing agent), and exposure to it can significantly impair your body's immune system, which is your primary defense against cancer, as well as many other diseases. Additionally, mercury exposure can cause increased production of free radicals. Free-radical damage to cellular DNA is a primary

69

cause of cancer. Once in the body, mercury can also block the enzymes necessary for the body's normal processes of detoxification. When these processes are impaired, toxins more easily spread through the body, where they can harm cellular DNA, setting the stage for cancer to develop [2].

Several other studies suggest that there is a link between accumulation of metals such as mercury, nickel and cadmium and the malignant growth and proliferation process of breast cancer [3]. A Canadian research team recently (2011) assessed breast cancer tissue biopsies and discovered a highly significant accumulation of heavy metals in the diseased breast tissues [4].

In 2001, the US National Health and Nutrition Examination surveyed 31,000 adults and found that the number of dental fillings correlated to the incidence of cancer, mental conditions, thyroid conditions, neurological issues (including MS), diseases of the respiratory system, and diseases of the eye. However, the United States, FDA and various Supreme Court justices determined that "the correlations do not sufficiently demonstrate causation." What this means is that statistical evidence showing mercury vapor emitting from amalgams does not have a direct causative effect on the various diseases that are being implicated, and correlation does NOT mean causation.

In 2003, the World Health Organization called for further studies to be done. In 2009, the FDA issued a new regulation placing dental amalgams into Class II (moderate risk) from Class I (low risk), allowing them to impose special controls and recommendations surrounding the use of amalgams.

The current ADA and FDA position is that amalgam is a safe restorative material. Silver fillings have been used for 150 years. Today, around 47% of all dentists still use amalgam fillings [5].

A person who has been recently diagnosed with cancer may want to first, consider going to a "biological dentist," one who has been trained to properly extract the mercury, having prepared the patient's body prior to extraction, and using methods to significantly reduce any further risk or complication to the body.

All the conventional and/or alternative methods used in the fight against cancer will be less effective while the mouth still has the toxic fillings in it and the vapors are still wreaking havoc on the body and all of its vital organs. More discussions on oral health pathology and cancer will be in a later section.

Arsenic

Exposure to arsenic is mainly through intake of food and drinking water, food being the most important source in most populations. Long-term exposure to arsenic in drinking water is mainly related to increased risk of skin cancer, but also some other cancers, as well as other skin lesions. Occupational exposure to arsenic, primarily by inhalation, is considered causally associated with lung cancer [6].

Since there are effective water filtration devices within a reasonable price range, there should be no reason to continue to expose yourself to many of these toxins.

Cadmium

A recent study published in the journal Cancer Research indicates that women whose diets contain higher levels of cadmium are at a greater risk of developing breast cancer. Cadmium is a heavy metal long known to be carcinogenic, and, it's also been identified as a metal that can bind to estrogen receptors, effectively mimicking the female hormone estrogen. The study found that among close to 56,000 women, those with the highest intakes of cadmium were 21% more likely to develop breast cancer [7].

Cadmium leaches into crops from fertilizers, or when rainfall or sewage sludge deposits it onto farmland. Potatoes and whole grains are a couple of the primary sources cadmium, but it's also present in air pollution from the burning of fossil fuel, and can therefore also be inhaled according to a report entitled, Breast Cancer and the Environment: A Life Course Approach by the Institute of Medicine (IOM) issued in December of last year, which discusses environmental impacts on breast cancer risk [8][9].

This study offers new evidence in a large human population that environmental chemicals that mimic the effects of the female hormone estrogen may contribute to women's risk of certain cancers, including endometrial and breast cancers. The finding came just three months after the IOM, a prestigious body of independent biomedical researchers, concluded that a host of other factors – most within a woman's power to control, such as obesity and hormone-replacement medication – were the most important sources of breast cancer risk.

The following metals have been identified as being capable of binding to cellular estrogen receptors and then mimicking the actions of physiological estrogens [10]:

Aluminum	Antimony	Arsenite	Barium
Cadmium	Chromium	Cobalt	Copper
Lead	Mercury	Nickel	Selenite
Tin	Vanadate		

The best way to determine your heavy metal load is with a 24-hour urine collection test. A holistic health care provider can assist you in assessing your heavy metal toxin load. Then, they will discuss with you methods of removal. There are oral and IV chelators as well as various types of chelating foods you can incorporate. It is a slow process removing heavy metals, but the long-term benefits are valuable.

How to Remove Heavy Metals from Your Body

Metals hide in the fat cells of the body. The more fat cells one has, the more chemicals they can harbor. Chelators bond to a toxic metal ion and form a stable complex that can be removed from the body.

1. The herb cilantro helps remove metals such as mercury, lead and aluminum from the body. Cilantro is a variation of parsley and is widely available in grocery stores. The seeds of the cilantro plant are commonly known as "coriander". Chop the cilantro finely and mix in soups and salads frequently to cleanse these metals from your body.
2. Malic acid (found in apples and apple cider vinegar) helps remove aluminum from the body.
3. Other natural chelators include vitamin C, sulphur-containing amino acids such as methionine and cysteine (grass-fed whey powder is a good source of these amino acids), yellow dock root, and chlorella.
4. Iodine chelates metals such as mercury, lead, cadmium and aluminum and halogens such as fluoride and bromide. Iodine also removes perchlorate (rocket

fuel) from the body. In the United States, perchlorate frequently contaminates drinking water, milk, and other foods. There are many health benefits from increased iodine intake. Consuming nascent iodine is optimal.

5. Increasing the amount of glutathione in your body will help remove heavy metals such as mercury, lead, and cadmium. (Isolated grass-fed whey protein dramatically increases glutathione)

6. Heavy metals and other toxins stored in the liver and gall bladder as "stones" can be eliminated from the colon when you do a liver and gall bladder cleanse.

7. Alpha Lipoic acid helps remove mercury from inside cells and the brain. The mercury is then carried to the liver where it is mixed with bile, and then goes into the intestinal tract.

8. Sulfur-rich foods can bind with mercury in the intestinal tract so that the body does not reabsorb it.

9. Algin is a non-digestible fiber from brown seaweeds such as kelp. Algin will bind with mercury in the digestive tract, and will also bind with cadmium and radioactive materials.

10. Other intestinal chelators include spirulina, chlorella, aloe, and bentonite clay.

Chapter Ten: Aluminum

"To insure good health: Eat lightly, breathe deeply, live moder-
ately, cultivate cheerfulness, and maintain an interest in life."
—William Londen

Aluminum is a widely recognized neurotoxin that inhibits more than 200 biologically important functions and causes various adverse effects in plants, animals, and humans. The relationship between aluminum exposure and neurodegenerative diseases, including Parkinson's, Multiple Sclerosis and Alzheimer's Disease has been established by extensive research and is reason enough to avoid aluminum exposure. Now research has confirmed the relationship between aluminum exposure and breast cancer.

Several recent studies have linked aluminum to breast cancer. A study published in the Journal of Inorganic Biochemistry in July 2013 found that breast cancer patients had significantly higher levels of aluminum in their nipple aspirate fluids when compared to a control group of healthy women without breast cancer. The study compared 19 breast cancer patients with 16 healthy women in a control group [1].

Another recent study published in the Journal of Inorganic Biochemistry found that aluminum can increase the spread of breast cancer cells. Because the metastasizing or spread of cancer is correlated with increased mortality, this finding is highly significant [2].

In a 2011 study, The Journal of Inorganic Biochemistry noted that the presence of aluminum in the human breast may alter the breast microenvironment causing disruption to iron metabolism, oxidative damage to cellular components, inflammatory responses and alterations to the mobility of cells [3].

New research published in the Journal of Applied Toxicology has revealed that long-term exposure of breast cells to aluminum results in increased cultured tumor cells and of cells on the way to malignant transformation. This study also found that even shorter exposure to aluminum results in a weakened cell state [4].

Another study published in 2003 by the European Journal of Cancer Prevention also found a correlation between earlier diagnosis of breast cancer and antiperspirant deodorant use [5]. This study also indicated "underarm shaving with antiperspirant deodorant" use may play a role in breast cancer.

While science is catching up to the dangers of aluminum and the connection between its presence in the body and various diseases, the natural health movement has espoused the dangers of aluminum for many years.

Aluminum is thought to be particularly poisonous to the nervous system with a range of symptoms that can include disturbed sleep, nervousness, emotional instability, memory loss, headaches, and impaired intellect. It can stop the body's ability to digest and make use of calcium and phosphorus. This prevents bone growth and reduces bone density. Aluminum can also cause conditions, which actually force calcium out of the bones. Either of these situations can bring on weakness and deformation in the bone structure with crippling effects. Aluminum toxicity can also result in aching muscles, speech problems, anemia, digestive problems, lowered liver function, colic and impaired kidney function [6].

Sources of aluminum:

In the kitchen: Pots/pans, cookware, aluminum foil, and utensils are all sources. Boiling water in aluminum pots produces toxic hydrooxides, boiling meat produces chlorides and frying foods in an aluminum pan increases nitrates. Aluminum teapots should be avoided because the tannic acid in the tea tends to allow aluminum to leak into the tea.

Food additives: The following food additives contain aluminum compounds: E173, E520, E521, E523 E541, E545, E554, E555 E556, E559. Aluminum is a common food additive found in foods such as processed cheeses, table salt, baking powder, pickles, bleached flour, self-rising flour, prepared dough (including frozen), cake mixes, pancake mixes, non-dairy creamers, vanilla powders and some donuts and waffles. Spices and food colorings contain aluminum compounds. Milk formulas for babies can contain up to four hundred times more aluminum than breast milk.

Medications: Antacids quite often contain aluminum trisilicate as does buffered aspirin. Antacids can contain 200 milligrams or more of elemental aluminum in a single tablet. Certain popular antacids contain aluminum hydroxide. It is present in popular over-the-counter and prescription medicines such as certain pain-killers, anti-diarrhea medicines and anti-hemorrhoid preparations. Many vaccines also contain aluminum.

Personal care items: Toothpastes, nasal sprays, anti-antiperspirants/deodorants, many body lotions and creams, most cosmetics, shampoos and conditioners, soaps, suntan lotions and lip balm are all possible sources of aluminum.

Other products containing aluminum: It can be found in dental amalgams, cigarette filters and pesticides. Some metal cleaners contain aluminum oxide.

After viewing this partial list, how many times have you ingested, consumed, slathered, or rubbed on aluminum or it's derivative today?

It is not difficult to eliminate many of the products that you are using every day. There are aluminum-free products that can easily replace these. Read the labels, spend a couple of extra dollars and protect yourself.

Chapter Eleven: Parabens

"Wisdom is to the mind what health is to the body."
—Francois De La Rochefoucauld

The market is saturated with products that will make you smell good, have smooth skin, have clean breath, not sweat, thicker looking hair, and so on. The way they are portrayed they are harmless and will make you feel and look better. The manufacturers are employing exceptional marketing skills but have refrained from revealing the true contents behind the magic: Parabens. These chemicals are in nearly every over-the-counter product and seem to have infiltrated our water sources and even food products!

The detrimental effects of parabens have not even begun to be felt yet, though this chemical in particular, will heavily influence the health of the next generation.

Parabens are chemicals with estrogen-mimicking properties, and excess estrogen is one of the hormonal links involved in the development of breast cancer. There are 6 types of parabens:

- Methyl paraben
- Propyl paraben
- Isobutyl paraben
- Ethyl paraben
- Butyl paraben
- E216

The list below is some of the primary sources of parabens. It's important to recognize that whatever you spread on your skin can be absorbed into your body and potentially cause serious damage over time, as this research demonstrates.

- Deodorants and antiperspirants
- Shampoos and conditioners
- Shaving gel
- Toothpaste
- Lotions and sunscreens
- Make-up and cosmetics
- Pharmaceutical drugs
- Food additives

Numerous studies have shown that parabens can affect your body much like the estrogens, which can lead to diminished muscle mass, extra fat storage, and male breast growth. Other studies have also linked parabens to breast cancer. The US Environmental Protection Agency (EPA) has linked methyl parabens in particular to metabolic, developmental, hormonal, and neurological disorders, as well as various cancers. There is also a highly disturbing find in one of the studies linking parabens with childhood diseases.

A new study published in the Journal of Applied Toxicology has raised some disturbing possibilities regarding the dangers of common hormone-mimicking preservatives, particularly parabens found in thousands of consumer products on the market today [1].

A recent study from the UK's University of Reading established that parabens in human breast tissue can proliferate into cancer cells. The researchers also found significant parabens concentrations within the breast tissue of 160 people who submitted tissue samples. They found that 27% of all the samples contained parabens concentrations that could potentially stimulate breast cancer growth because of their capability to disrupt estrogen production.

In this final highlighted study entitled "Parabens detection in different zones of the human breast: consideration of source and implications of findings," researchers discussed the role that parabens may have in breast cancer and childhood disease.

The report focused on the findings of The Genesis Breast Cancer Prevention Centre at the University Hospital of South Manchester NHS Foundation Trust published in March 2012, which discovered five paraben esters in human breast tissue samples collected from 40 mastectomies from women with primary breast cancer [2].

The report revealed three things:

1.   The ester form of parabens found within the breast tissue samples indicated exposure occurred through the skin, which may indicate skin care products, and underarm deodorants had a factor.
2.   The parabens residues were found at concentrations up to 1 million times higher than the estrogen (estradiol) levels naturally found in human breast tissue.
3.   Propylparaben was found in the highest concentration in the underarm area (axilla), where underarm deodorants are most used and breast cancer prevalence is at its highest.

While the World Health Organization considers the estrogenic properties of parabens to be a low toxicological risk because it is 10,000-100,000 less potent than estradiol (E2), the 1 million-fold higher levels found within breast tissue sampled clearly indicate the magnitude of exposure more than compensates for the lesser potency.

Also noted in the new study was a highly disturbing possibility: "For exposures in children, concern has already been raised that 'the estrogenic burden of parabens and their metabolites in blood may exceed the action of endogenous estradiol in childhood and the safety margin for propylparaben is very low when comparing worst-case exposure' (Boberg et al., 2010)."

In other words, synthetic hormones from chemicals like parabens may actually be eclipsing the activity of naturally produced hormones in our children. Given that 99.1% of the US population's urine samples (ages 6 or older) contain methylparaben, this issue has broad-ranging implications.

At this time European regulations allow for the use of parabens in cosmetics at up to 0.4% by volume. The limits in the US are much less restricted. According to the FDA's website "The Cosmetic Ingredient Review (CIR) reviewed the safety of methylparaben, propylparaben, and butylparaben in 1984 and concluded they were safe for use in cosmetic products at levels up to 25%. Typically parabens are used at levels ranging from 0.01 to 0.3%." What a difference in range from the European regulations in cosmetics verses the US standards! Parabens are also FDA-approved for use as food preservatives. A separate section is dedicated to parabens in the food industry.

There doesn't seem to be any consideration for the chronic low dose exposure and how it will affect people and children long term. And as I have stated elsewhere in this book, there just doesn't seem to be any thought when setting up regulations or performing these studies as to how these toxins will be amplified when combined with other chemical toxins.

This research does however point to an area that has cause for great concern: Commonly used chemicals and preservatives may be contributing in a certain segment of the population that is vulnerable due to their lower body weight and may be more susceptible to chemically-induced gene toxicity because their cells are naturally dividing more rapidly and because their detoxification systems are less developed. Who is this vulnerable group? Infants and children.

It is becoming increasingly clear that in order to protect ourselves and especially our offspring from avoidable chemical exposures this country needs to implement the precautionary principle in its toxicological risk assessments: if there is indication that a chemical could do harm (based on cell and animal studies), it should be treated as if it does do harm, and be regulated accordingly. Until then, we are effectively a living and breathing nation of guinea pigs.

Although we are only half way through the Toxins chapter, it is clearly evident that these toxins are having a serious detrimental impact not only on adults but will likely have an even greater deadly impact on our children and grandchildren. As you continue to read the rest of this section, imagine how the combined toxins may have an even more serious impact.

Chapter Twelve: Toxic Teeth

"The healthy, the strong individual, is the one who asks for help when he needs it. Whether he has an abscess on his knee or in his soul."

—Rona Barrett

One issue that can exert a significant negative influence on the immune system's ability to improve our health is oral pathology. Even with the best of diets, some people find that over time they succumb to cancer and ask the question – How could this happen?

There are three primary areas of concern: Mercury amalgam fillings or other metals in the mouth, cavitations – primarily from wisdom teeth extraction sites, and root canals.

Mercury

Mercury is a highly toxic heavy metal and has no place in the human body. Mercury fillings must be removed with caution and specific safety measures in place. Only a dentist well experienced in this area should do the removal of mercury. If removed improperly, the resulting mercury vapors can be extremely dangerous with devastating impact.

In describing the efficient absorption of mercury through the tissues of the cheeks and under the tongue into the blood stream, Hal Huggins, D.D.S states: "From the blood stream, mercury can travel to any cell in the body, where it can either disable or destroy the tissues. Mercury can also travel directly from the fillings into the lungs, into the blood stream and, as before described, every cell in the body becomes a valid target" [1]. According to Dr. Huggins, mercury may change forms in the body, from organic to inorganic with either form attacking different aspects of the cell membrane, DNA, or enzymes.

Cavitations

Wisdom teeth are normally extracted, leaving the periodontal ligament in the jawbone. The bone heals over, encapsulating the decaying ligament in a small hole in the bone. Pathogenic bacteria develop in a highly protected environment and continually intoxicate the body and stress the immunes system. Antibiotics cannot get into that protected area. The immune system may be under stress for decades before cancer or other illness will manifest.

To determine the frequency of cavitations, Dr Huggins reviewed the charts of over 100 clinic patients. Extraction sites of wisdom teeth (third molars) were found to have cavitations 88% of the time; second molars had a 70% incidence of cavitations; and, first molars an incidence of 85%! (Uninformed Consent, Huggins, Hal, D.D.S and Levy, Thomas, M.D. p. 212)

Once the extraction site healing at the top is complete, the oxygen-deprived (anaerobic) environment becomes host to highly toxic metabolic by-products. The native mouth bacteria normally resides in harmony in an oxygen-enriched environment but in the anaerobic environment of a cavitation site, the by-products become potentially deadly. "In fact, some of these toxins show anywhere from 100 to 1000 times the toxicity of botulism toxin on certain enzymes tested!" (Huggins, p 215)

Root Canals

According to George Mening, DDS, author of Root Canal Cover-Up a single root-canaled tooth will have an estimated 3 miles of micro-canals – an extremely wide area for bacterial growth. Once bacteria start to gain a foothold inside a devitalized tooth, antibiotics can't kill them because such drugs cannot penetrate into the affected tooth. This leaves the bacteria free to migrate down into other areas of the body where they can set the stage for a variety of crippling degenerative diseases, including cancer.

In an interview in July, 2013 with Patrick Timpone, Dr. Huggins states that "ALL cavitation sites and root canal teeth harbor pathogenic bacteria."To date, Dr. Huggins has identified 53 different bacteria in root canal teeth and 82 in cavitations! Different types of bacteria destroy different enzymes that impact different organs/tissues of the body [2]. With ongoing stress of the immune system, it is usually just a matter of time (maybe decades) before illness is manifest due to the inability of the immune system to keep the constant onslaught of bacteria under control.

Interestingly, independent researcher, Robert Dowling, PhD has discovered that oral pathology does not cross the body's mid-line. Left side oral pathology manifest in pathology in the left side of the body. "A man with prostate cancer, for example, has oral pathology in the front of the mouth. A woman with right breast cancer has right-side oral pathology. A man with right lung cancer has right-side oral pathology. There are no exceptions, . . ." (Am I Dead? . . . or do I just feel like it, Fred Hughes)

Most dentists are unaware of cavitations and are unable to detect them. Routine X-ray is not adequate to detect cavitations or toxicity of root canals. Thermal imaging of the face and digital panoramic X-ray can be most beneficial in detection of cavitations. If a cavitation is suspected, it is prudent to seek out a knowledgeable, holistic, mercury free dentist to help locate and repair it.

Root canal teeth are dead structures protruding from the jawbone. Over time, bacteria develop in the dead canals as they do in cavitations which will constantly stress the immune system. In his July 16, 2013 interview, Dr. Huggins states that 100% of root canal teeth contain pathogenic bacteria. With an immune system overstressed, it may be impossible for the body to heal itself of chronic diseases. Again, if a tooth with a root canal is suspect, it will need the attention of a knowledgeable and experienced holistic dentist.

My Story

Around 10 years ago I had a root canal done on the lower quadrant of the right side of my mouth. I went to a highly regarded root canal specialist who taught at a prestigious dental college in the area and after the procedure was over, I never thought of it again. About 5 years later I noticed two strange occurrences. First, I developed a lump on my right breast. Second I developed a small lump on my jaw line. I had been on a clean living food diet for several years by that time so I had no idea why these had developed. In 2010, I went to a biological dentist in Fairfax, VA and had all of the 14 plus mercury amalgam fillings removed from my teeth. He also found that one of those mercury fillings was placed over the root canal in the back corner of the right side of my mouth. As he was removing the root canal and the mercury filling, he found a cavitation that was filled with bacteria beside the root canal from a 30 year old wisdom tooth extraction. The two areas were side-by-side and the toxins from both had been filling my body daily for many years.

The lump on my jaw immediately disappeared. It took longer for the breast lump to reduce and then subsequently disappear. Not all breast lumps may disappear, however, to have a non-cancerous lump isn't too difficult to live with.

There is a book called *Saving Victoria's Breast* by Fred Hughes. Another excellent book that seems to confirm the connection between oral pathology and the rest of the body.

As we have met more and more people fighting this battle, we are witnessing certain similar threads. One of them is the oral pathology connection to cancer.

Chapter Thirteen: Emotional, Mental, Spiritual and Stress

"Health isn't about being "perfect" with food or exercise or herbs. Health is about balancing those things with your desires. It's about nourishing your spirit as well as your body."
—Golda Poretsky

Does Stress Feed Cancer?

A little stress can be good for us – it pushes us to move ahead and be innovate. But chronic stress can increase the risk of diseases such as depression, heart disease and even cancer. Many studies have shown that stress can promote cancer indirectly by weakening the immune system's anti-tumor defense or by encouraging new tumor-feeding blood vessels to form as evidenced by a study published in April, 2012 in The Journal of Clinical Investigation which shows that stress hormones, such as adrenalin, can directly support tumor growth and spread.

The study's lead author Anil Sood from The University of Texas M. D, Anderson Cancer Center in Houston suggests that stress can trigger cancer cells to break off from tumors and spread throughout the body (metastasizing). It is already known that a chemical process has already taken place in cancer cells preventing them from experiencing a timely death like normal healthy cells do. This was one of the first of its kind of studies to see how stress influenced tumor progression. Since stress influences so many normal physiological processes,

87

it would be be logical to assess this form of biological connection. After witnessing this phenomenon in vitro, on mice and finally in samples of human ovarian cancer, they concluded that people under a certain amount of stress, along with elevated stress hormone activity were associated with higher levels of a protein that allowed the cells to strengthen individually and create a faster disease progression [1][2].

In the same publication, The Journal of Clinical Investigation there is a commentary entitled Why Stress is Bad For Cancer Patients. In this paper, Hassan et al., looked closely at the growth of prostate cancer. Here are some highlights:

1. There are a growing number of studies that have uncovered major roles for chronic stress in cancer progression.
2. Adrenalin activation has been implicated as the key factor of these effects by modulating several growth factors in multiple cancers.
3. Chronic stress plays a significant role in cancer progression, and decreased cancer incidence is observed among patients who take beta blockers for the treatment of other diseases.
4. Cancer diagnosis and associated treatment can potentially elevate a patient's stress levels, whereas social support has been associated with increased patient survival.
5. Recent findings regarding the role of stress hormones in chemoresistance, metastasis, cancer relapse, and surgical recovery have moved the field forward, but the molecular mechanisms underlying these effects are still not fully understood [3].

Fortunately, the psychological stress/cancer-connection is now supported by ample scientific evidence. The Centers for Disease Control and Prevention (CDC) make this important statement on their web site: "Intensive and prolonged stress can lead to a variety of short - and long-term negative health effects. It can disrupt early brain development and compromise functioning of the nervous and immune systems. In addition, childhood stress can lead to health problems later in life including alcoholism, depression, eating disorders, heart disease, cancer, and other chronic diseases."

There is also substantial evidence from both healthy populations as well as individuals who have cancer linking psychological stress with reduced immune function highlighting natural killer (NK) cells, because of the role that they may play in malignant disease. In addition, distress or depression is also associated with two important processes for the development of cancer: poor repair of damaged DNA, and alterations in cell reproduction and growth.

There is also the possibility that psychological interventions may enhance immune function and survival among cancer patients and the results clearly merit further exploration, as does the evidence suggesting that social support (relationships) may be a key psychological element. These studies and others suggest that psychological or behavioral factors may influence the incidence or progression of cancer [4].

The following situations that can induce stress along with certain personality types have been known to be associated with people who have developed breast cancer:

A. The coping strategy used is denial or repression
B. Experiencing separation or loss
C. Several stressful experiences throughout life
D. Seeing life from a melancholy or hopeless point of view
E. Nurturing and trying to please others
F. One who avoids conflict

The theory is that the gene that is used to avoid conflict may be the same gene that has an increased susceptibility of cancer [5].

There are likely personality traits that if studied, would be identified in many cancers, not just breast cancer. But remember, many factors contribute to developing cancer. Some are obvious; others may need some investigative work to identify.

Finally, according to a well-known study published in The American Journal of Public Health in 1987, men and women suffering from the loss of a spouse have an increased risk of death – from not only heart attacks, but from cancer, accidents, suicide, and violence.

Even harboring negative thoughts and unforgiveness can weaken the immune system and ultimately be a contributor to cancer. Our son is a powerful testimony of one who desperately needed to forgive someone so he could experience the freedom. On our first visit to a toxicologist, one of the first questions the doctor asked was how Josh's relationship was with those in his life. We soon found out there was one who Joshua had strong negative feelings for and the doctor told him he must forgive, whether they ever had a relationship or not. He must forgive to allow his body to heal. After we learned of this, we made several attempts to work with him on this, but a young, quiet teenage boy may not have much ability to articulate or even come to terms with his own emotions. As time went on it was clearly evident he could not get beyond his feelings. It may be quite difficult to forgive, but it can be deadly to be unforgiving.

There is no way of dividing our spirit, mind or body. They all affect each other. Therefore, it is imperative that when a diagnosis of cancer is made, that we not only evaluate our eating habits and sleep patterns, but we must also evaluate our happiness and peace quotient. If we do not manage our stress properly, if we do not enjoy meaningful relationships, if we are not at peace with others and ourselves, then there is no way our bodies can fight this battle and recover.

"As a man thinks in his heart, so is he."
—Proverbs 23:7

Chapter Fourteen: Food Additives, Dyes, Preservatives and Parabens

"If you don't take care of this the most magnificent machine that you will ever be given...where are you going to live?"

—Karen Calabrese

When you walk down an aisle in the grocery store, you see row upon row of cans, jars, packages and boxes filled with food that you can conveniently open, heat and enjoy! This convenience factor not only costs a little more but when you eat the contents of the package you are getting much more than what the ingredients say you are. It has been estimated that there are more than 14,000 substances added to processed foods which include flavoring agents, food colors, preservatives and thickeners. The way that these are advertised would make you think the manufacturers are using them for safety and protection from spoiled or contaminated foods.

The truth is cooked or processed food has very little flavor, color or texture so additives are used to make them more appealing. For example, breads and bagels need to be large, fluffy and white so bulking agents and bleach are added. Most tomatoes, bananas, avocados and mangos are not ripe when they are harvested, cooled, stored and transported significant distances to where they will be marketed and consumed. Not long before they reach their destination, they are placed into specially constructed ripening rooms and brought to optimum ripening through the introduction of liquid ethanol, which activates the ethylene hormone in them to ripen at a uniform rate.

Another example is dried fruit. Sulfur dioxide is used as a preservative in dried fruit to prevent it from spoiling, and also to preserve the fruit's gorgeous and appetizingly bright color. That's why unsulfured fruits tend to look brownish or black. Sulfur dioxide is a gas that's created by burning coal or oil, which both contain sulfur. This gas smells similar to rotten eggs and though used as a food preservative, it's also used in products as disinfectant or bleaching agents.

Are these safe for us to consume? Wouldn't the FDA ensure this? Interestingly, the FDA has only 3,000 of the 14,000 substances in its database. Obviously there are many that no one has ever tested. Regarding those that have been tested, many of the 3,000 the FDA says are safe have only been tested with industry tests performed by the manufacturers. Those are the tests the FDA have been using to say these items are safe. Few, if any independent tests have been given any serious consideration by the FDA.

Dr. Russell Blaylock has found that of the independent studies that test the safety of additives most are based on animal trials. Although it is difficult to deduce whether the results of an animal study equate to human health, many of these studies show that some additives could be cancer causing. Many animal studies have been used to identify toxic levels in some of the other sections we just studied. It would be logical then, to presume that the results in the food additives studies should be taken seriously.

The great difficulty with connecting cancer as well as other neurotoxic diseases to food additives is that they may take many years to develop and the cause would not likely be tied to the real culprit any more. It appears this is a common thread we have been seeing regarding toxins potentially causing cancer in later years.

An area that we will discuss again later is that few food products contain only one of these substances. Tested individually it may appear to be below toxic levels, but there are typically multiple components of these substances in one food product, and no testing is ever done to test synergistic toxicity.

Although there are many food additives we will focus on the most common ones:

1. Nitrites and Nitrates

Although these two have differences, they both present dangers when ingested in food. Sodium nitrate/nitrite is used to preserve, color, and flavor meat products. Sodium nitrite is commonly added to bacon, ham, hot dogs, luncheon meats, smoked fish, and corned beef to stabilize the red color and add flavor. It prevents bacterial growth and rapid decaying of meat. Studies have linked eating it to various types of cancer. Under certain high-temperature cooking conditions such as grilling, it transforms into a reactive compound that has been shown to promote cancer. This preservative stimulates the formation of nitrosamines, which are highly carcinogenic (cancer causing).

In 2005, a study at the University of Hawaii, linked consumption of processed meats to a 67% increase in the risk of pancreatic cancer. Interestingly enough, the researchers in this case did not find that eating unprocessed meat at the same rate led to nearly the same risk [1]. What's the difference in the meats that contain similar amounts of saturated fat and cholesterol? The processed meats had four times the amount of sodium and 50% more sodium nitrite.

2. BHA and BHT

Butylated hydroxyanisole (BHP) and butylated hydrozytoluene (BHT) are antioxidants used to preserve common household foods by preventing them from oxidizing. Both keep fats and oils from going rancid and are found in cereals, chewing gum, potato chips, and vegetable oils, but there is concern that they may cause cancer. The structure of BHA and BHT will change during the process of preserving food, and may form a compound that reacts in the body. BHA and BHT are not stable or inert. They don't easily get expelled after entering the body. The research has suggested they have a major role in causing cancerous tumors in rats.

3. Propyl gallate

Used to prevent fats and oils from spoiling, propyl gallate is often used in conjunction with BHA and BHT. This additive is sometimes found in meat products, chicken soup base, potato sticks, ready-to-make soups, and chewing gum. Studies show that regular consumption of these products may cause colon and stomach cancer.

4. Monosodium glutamate

MSG was introduced into processed foods in 1948 and is an amino acid used as a flavor enhancer in soups, salad dressings, chips, frozen entrees, most restaurant food as well as hundreds of other processed foods. It is commonly associated with Asian foods and flavorings. Incredibly, even infant formulas and baby food contain this toxin, even though babies and infants, who are four times more sensitive than adults to the toxic effects of this chemical, are the most at risk. Animal studies link it to damaging nerve cells in the brains of infant mice. The dangers surrounding MSG are, perhaps, most concerning for new moms who are unable to breastfeed, and are looking for an alternative to the MSG – laden infant formulas on the market. MSG is now a part of almost everything you consume during the entire day.

Studies conducted on a number of rats showed that almost all of the rats displayed a damaged hypothalamus (an important part of the brain concerned with regulatory activities of the body) and neurons of the inner retinal layer with just one dose of MSG. It is also used to lab-induce obesity among rats. What makes it far more dangerous is the fact that humans are 3-5 times more sensitive to MSG than rats. Humans are more sensitive to glutamate than any other species.

Two other considerations as to why MSG is so dangerous are first; MSG is an excitotoxin, which means that it overexcites your cells to the point of damage, acting as a poison. The second part of the equation is that MSG can be literally hidden in food labels, under names like broth, casein, hydrolyzed, autolyzed, and more, making it extremely difficult to identify.

MSG is also a probable cause contributing to the obesity epidemic. Scientists have known that MSG causes obesity since the 1960's.

Common Hidden Names for MSG: (there are over 40 others):
- Gelatin
- Hydrolyzed Vegetable Protein (HVP)
- Yeast Extract
- Malted Barley
- Rice Syrup or Brown Rice Syrup
- Citric acid

Check out Appendix D for all of the other names it has.

Sadly, oncologists rarely advise people who are fighting cancer to avoid foods that have glutamate even though several studies show that many forms of cancer have glutamate receptors that will enhance tumor growth [2][3]. Unfortunately, not only will they increase the tumor growth but they will encourage the rapid spreading of the cancer. Dr. Russell Blaylock calls glutamate a "Cancer Fertilizer."

Since its introduction into food, the amount of MSG and other glutamate additives in processed food has doubled every ten years. The average American consumes huge amounts of glutamate every day. Obviously, the best approach is to avoid them. Plant-based diets have been shown to be protective of the excitotoxicity effects, but only when the toxins are greatly reduced in consumption.

5. *Food colorings*

You may think that all dangerous artificial food colorings were banned by the FDA long ago, but in fact only Red Dye No. 2 was banned by the FDA after some studies found that large doses could cause cancer in rats. There are still several food colorings on the market that are linked with cancer in animal testing [4]. Some specific dye colors promote tumor formation, in the right combination and under certain conditions. If you aren't confident that the color you are seeing in or on the food product is coming from natural sources, don't buy it.

Food dyes that are still on the market:
- Blue #1 and #2 are found in beverages, candy, baked goods and pet food, have been linked to cancer in mice. Blue #2 increased tumor incidence and death rate in exposed hamsters.
- Red #3 is used to dye cherries, fruit cocktail, candy, and baked goods, and has been shown to cause thyroid tumors in rats.
- Red #40 is contaminated with benzidine or other carcinogens. It increased tumor incidence and death rate in exposed hamsters.
- Green #2024 is added to candy and beverages, though rarely used, has been linked to bladder cancer. It increased tumor incidence and death rate in exposed hamsters.

- Yellow #5 is contaminated with benzidine or other carcinogens, damages DNA, and has been found to mimic estrogen [5].
- Yellow #6 is added to beverages, sausage, gelatin, baked goods, and candy and has been linked to tumors of the adrenal gland and kidney. It has been found to be contaminated with benzidine or other carcinogens and it has been found to mimic estrogen [6][7].

Foods that contain multiple dyes as well as other toxic additives, when combined, will often magnify the toxicity effect. Although most toxic substance studies rarely get that far in their research.

6. Olestra

Olestra, a synthetic fat known as the brand name Olean and found in some brands of potato chips, prevents fat from getting absorbed in the digestive system. This often leads to severe diarrhea, abdominal cramps, and gas.

More frightening, it is known to bind to fat soluble vitamins A, D, E and K, which protect the body from cancer and boost immunity. Binding of olestra to these vitamins in general, makes you much more prone to cancer.

7. Potassium bromate

Rare, but still legal in the U.S., and used as an oxidizing agent to increase volume in white flour, breads, and rolls. It is known to cause cancer in animals while even small amounts in bread can create a risk for humans.

It has also proven to be toxic to the kidneys both in man and animals. It has developed thyroid and kidney tumors among rats, when they were fed with bread using potassium bromate as the oxidizing agent.

California requires a cancer warning on the product label if potassium bromate is an ingredient.

8. Sulfites

Chemical compounds with anti-fungal and antibacterial properties that are used to preserve produce. Sulfites are a preservative used to prevent discoloration of food, bleach food starches, impede bacterial growth, and add stability to medication.

Sodium sulfite, sodium bisulfite, sodium metabisulfite, and sulfur dioxide are the most common names for sulfites, and the ones, which pose the greatest sulfite dangers. In 1986 the FDA banned sulfites as a preservative on fresh fruits and vegetables. Grapes, however, are exempt from this rule because grape farmers have a tradition of spraying grapes heavily with sulfites.

A lot of prescription and over-the-counter medications contain sulfites. Some products and produce containing sulfites include: Grapes, cornstarch, corn syrup, jarred peppers and olives, wine vinegar, wine, spinach (lower if organic) dried fruit, lemon juice concentrate, shredded coconut, dehydrated potatoes.

Also relatively high in sulfites: all jams and jellies, guacamole, horseradish, pickles, shrimp, scallops, crab and lobster, soy protein, processed cheeses and beer.

9. Parabens

Chemicals widely used in skin cosmetics, lotions and pharmaceuticals. There is only one study that was published in April 2013 and we believe it is the first of its kind testing various foods for paraben. Researchers from the New York State Department of Health and the Department of Environmental Health Sciences, along with the University of New York at Albany studied foods purchased from local markets and have determined that much of the U.S. food supply is contaminated with parabens. Although there are numerous studies linking parabens with breast cancer and specifically deodorant, there just was no way of understanding or explaining the high paraben levels in people using just skin products.

This study likely explains an increasing body of evidence showing that humans have much higher blood and urine concentrations of parabens than could be explained with the use of body lotions and cosmetics.

The researchers tested 267 samples of food collected from stores and markets around Albany New York. These included juices, soft drinks, alcoholic beverages, infant formula, dairy products such as milk, yogurt, cheese and ice cream, oils, fats, breads, flours, rice, pasta, corn, fruits, baked goods, meats, shellfish and seafood and many others.

Of all the foods, pancake syrup had the highest levels of methyl-parabens. Others that contained high levels of methyl-parabens included muffins, iced tea, pudding and turkey roast. The highest levels of propyl-parabens were found in turkey breasts, yogurt, turkey roast and apple pie. The highest levels of ethyl-parabens were found in red wine. The researchers found parabens in 98% of grain foods, 91% of fish and shellfish, 87% of dairy products, and 85% of fruit products.

Five different types of parabens were tested. These were:
• butyl-parabens
• benzyl-parabens
• propyl-parabens
• methyl- parabens
• ethyl-parabens

The researchers found that an astonishing 90% of the food samples tested contained "measurable" concentrations of parabens.

Dr. Kurunthachalam Kannan, primary author of the study stated: "This is the first study to report the occurrence of parabens in U.S. foods, and preserved foods. We have found them to be an important source of paraben exposure in people." The findings were a major surprise to many experts [8]. More recent studies have found paraben content among our waterways, soils and even house dust.

Since we have ample evidence of the dangers of all forms of parabens, it is wise to see that the foods we have been consuming have been compromising our health every time we eat them. If you are concerned with what to eat, stay reading, the best is yet to come!

"There are few chemicals that we as a people are exposed to that have as many far reaching physiological affects on living beings as Monosodium Glutamate does. MSG directly causes obesity, diabetes, triggers epilepsy, destroys eye tissues, is genotoxic in many organs and is the probable cause of ADHD and Autism. Considering that MSG's only reported role in food is that of 'flavor enhancer' is that use worth the risk of the myriad of physical ailments associated with it? Does the public really want to be tricked into eating more food and faster by a food additive?"

—John E. Erb

Chapter Fifteen: Pesticides

"We should resolve now that the health of this nation is a national concern; that financial barriers in the way of attaining health shall be removed; that the health of all it's citizens deserves the help of all the nation."
—Harry S. Truman

Recent studies have shown that there's a 600% greater risk of childhood leukemia when kids are exposed to pesticides. Products used to kill household pests and the ones that are spread on your lawn can affect your children and pets. (Source: School of Public Health, University of California, Berkeley; Environmental Health Investigations Branch, California Department of Health Services; Stamford University of Medicine)

But what about the pesticides that are on the foods we eat? If you have ever tried to grow fruits or vegetables you quickly realize the challenge you have of trying to save the valuable fruit of the plant from the insects, the blights or the fungus. Diseases are a major source of crop and plant damage that can be caused by a number of disease-causing organisms. Fungi are the number one cause of crop loss worldwide. Viruses, nematodes, and bacteria also cause diseases in plants. Fungicides, herbicides, and insecticides are all pesticides used in plant protection. We will just call them pesticides for the purposes of this section.

Through the many years that man has used the soil to grow crops, the hundreds of millions of pounds of pesticides that have gone into the soil have permeated into the water, into the root system of the plant and of course, into the fruits and vegetables themselves. Technology has improved so much that now, instead of spraying the pesticides on to the external parts of the plants, seed manufacturers have now been able to inject the seed with the pesticides so the seed becomes more resistant to weeds, fungus, bacteria, mold, insects, drought, etc. This is called genetically modifying the plant. A separate section has been chosen to discuss the health ramifications of this process.

Numerous studies have been found linking those who have consistent exposure to pesticides, herbicides, insecticides and fungicides are at significantly greater risk of developing lymphomas, breast cancers, aggressive prostate cancers and even their children have a greater risk of developing various cancers including brain cancers [1][2][3][4]. While agriculture has traditionally been tied to pesticide-related diseases, 19 of 30 frequently used lawn pesticides and 28 of 40 frequently used school and home pesticides are also linked to cancer.

The increase in male breast cancer, autism, childhood cancers and more may be caused from the increased amounts of pesticides in blood lines that weaken genes that produce weakened humans.

The report entitled Reducing Environmental Cancer Risk: What We Can Do Now indicates that you don't need constant exposure for damage to occur. It also suggests that the connection between pesticide use and cancer is not being taken seriously and the nation's cancer program needs to consider the carcinogenic effects of the thousands of pesticides that are found in our clothing, drinking water, foods and air daily.

Weakened immune systems, small children, elderly, all will have greater reactions to these pesticides and there doesn't seem to be enough effort or focus placed on the dangers these bring. An excellent website to illustrate the types of studies done on various forms of cancer is: www.beyondpesticides.org/health/cancer.php. This compilation of studies is not exhaustive but clearly suggests that enough people have taken this issue seriously to study certain pesticides and their effect on the body that can result in various types of cancer.

This section of the book is not intended to explain the dangers of the thousands of pesticides being used all over the world or the hundreds that are being used in this country. However, as you are attempting to recover from any type of cancer, be aware that you must choose foods, water and air that can be as pure as possible so as not to compromise your immune system any further.

The Environmental Working Group (EWG) has a website that establishes the best and worst list of vegetables and fruits associated with the amount of pesticides are used on them. Later, in the Nutrition section, you will see the two lists to assist you in purchasing the cleanest produce possible.

Two particular crops – United States grown summer squash and leafy greens, specifically kale and collards, did not meet traditional Dirty Dozen list criteria but were commonly contaminated with pesticides exceptionally toxic to the nervous system.

Though the Environmental Protection Agency has been encouraging restricting the uses of the most toxic pesticides, they are still detected on some foods. For example, green beans were on the most toxic list because they were often contaminated with two highly toxic organophosphates. Those pesticides are slowly being withdrawn from US agriculture. But leafy greens still show residues of several risky pesticides. That's why they are on the toxic list for 2013.

Tests in 2008 found that some United States grown summer squash – zucchini and yellow crookneck squash – contained residues of harmful pesticides that were phased out of agriculture in the 1970s and 1980s but that linger on some farm fields.

Genetically modified plants (GMO), are not often found in the fresh produce section of grocery stores. The genetically modified crops likely to be found in fresh produce aisles of American supermarkets are yellow crooked neck squash, zucchini, Hawaiian papaya and some varieties of sweet corn. Most Hawaiian papaya is a GMO. Only a small fraction of zucchini and sweet corn are GMO. Since U.S. law does not require labeling of GMO produce, EWG advises people who want to avoid it to purchase the organically grown versions [1].

Field corn, nearly all of which is produced with genetically modified seeds, is used to make tortillas, corn chips, corn syrup, animal feed and biofuels. Because it is not sold as a fresh vegetable, it is not included in EWG's Shopper's Guide to Pesticides in Produce. Nor is soy, another heavily GMO crop that makes its way into processed food.

To avoid the greatest number of pesticides, purchasing organic produce is the best option. No matter how many people question its benefits, the regulations surrounding the "organic" label dictate that no pesticides be used. You do have some safety measures in that.

You don't have to have the perfect, weed-free lawn in the neighborhood and you can find natural remedies to kill the ants in your kitchen instead of bringing in some toxic chemical. Awareness is the key. There are numerous methods to reduce your level of exposure. It is really up to you.

Chapter Sixteen: Genetically Modified Organisms (GMO)

"Very simply, we subsidize high-fructose corn syrup in this country, but not carrots. While the surgeon general is raising alarms over the epidemic of obesity, the president is signing farm bills designed to keep the river of cheap corn flowing, guaranteeing that the cheapest calories in the supermarket will continue to be the unhealthiest."

—Michael Pollan

The United States has allowed genetically modified foods to be incorporated into the American diet since around 1996. The Food and Drug Administration proclaimed in 1992 they had no information showing that GM foods were substantially different from conventionally grown foods. The FDA has labeled them "Generally Recognized as Safe," or GRAS. This status allows a product to be commercialized without any additional testing. According to US law, to be considered GRAS the substance must be the subject of a substantial amount of peer-reviewed published studies (or equivalent) and there must be overwhelming consensus among the scientific community that the product is safe. GM foods had neither. They were deemed safe to eat, and absolutely no safety studies were required.

Unfortunately, the rest of the story involves corruption and secret memos but this isn't the direction I wanted this story to go so suffice it to say, there were politics involved and as such, little or no tests were ever done when these seeds were introduced into the American diet despite actual FDA scientists who had repeatedly warned that GM

103

foods can create unpredictable, hard-to-detect side effects, including allergies, toxins, new diseases, and nutritional problems. They urged long-term safety studies, but were ignored.

Today, the corruption continues so the industry-backed testing that has trickled in is questionable and lacks efficacy to truly trust the results. And of course, any independent testing has been thoroughly criticized and ultimately downtrodden so as not to appear credible.

The process of genetic engineering itself involves inserting into the seed a gene or genes by either shooting genes from a "gene gun" into a plate of cells, or using bacteria to infect the cell with foreign DNA. Both create mutations in and around the insertion site and elsewhere [1][2], The "transformed" cell is then cloned into a plant through a process called tissue culture, which results in hundreds or thousands of mutations throughout the plant's gene structure. In the end, the GM plant's DNA can look quite different from its natural parent.

How do these foods affect our health?

- Soon after GM soy was introduced into the UK, allergies to it increased by 50% [3].
- Cooked GM soy has as much as 7 times the amount of a soy allergen as does cooked un-GMO soy [4].
- GM soy has a new protein allergen that is not in an un GMO soy plant [5].
- GM foods may make you allergic to non-GM foods.

A couple of interesting points are first, that in the five years immediately after GM soy was introduced, US peanut allergies doubled. It is known that a protein in natural soybeans cross-reacts with peanut allergies; therefore, soy may trigger reactions in some people who are allergic to peanuts. There has been a great surge in peanut allergies and it may be that people who consume soy grow an allergy toward peanuts [6]. Second, there has been a great surge in the number of gluten sensitivities since the inception of GMO foods. It is possible that scientists may find a correlation between the increase in these sensitivities and the ingesting of the new protein found in GMO soy or other GMO foods.

- GM soy also produced an unpredicted side effect in the pancreas of mice--the amount of digestive enzymes produced was dramatically reduced [7][8]. If a shortage of enzymes causes food proteins to breakdown more slowly, then they have more time to trigger allergic reactions. Thus, digestive problems from GM soy might promote allergies to a wide range of proteins, not just soy.
- Bt is a bacterium that was used as an insecticide and sprayed on crops for years. Then, it was genetically placed into the crop so the farmers would no longer need to spray. In the process, the levels became at least three thousand times more concentrated than the spray ever was, but the assumption was that since the spray was safe, so would the bacteria when it is placed in the gene. The results have so far indicated that this toxin is highly allergenic and the dangers of this are quite far-reaching. Several studies on people have found that the gene transfer effect involved severe allergic reactions in people who were in the fields where this crop was growing [9][10][11].

GM foods and liver problems
- Rats fed GM potatoes had smaller and partially atrophied livers [12].
- Rats fed GM corn, engineered to produce Bt-toxin, had liver lesions and other indications of toxicity [13].
- Rabbits fed GM soy showed altered enzyme production in their livers as well as higher metabolic activity [14].
- The livers of rats fed Roundup Ready canola were 12%–16% heavier, possibly due to liver disease or inflammation [15].
- Rats fed Roundup Ready soybeans also showed structural changes in their livers [16].
- GM crops have also been linked to reproductive problems, sterility, disease and death.

Since the research has been limited, but the increase of certain bacterial infections, immune-suppressive disorders, allergies and other phenomenon have been prevalent, is it a coincidence that the increases seem to have taken place not long after the introduction of these crops? It is quite obvious that further objective research is desperately needed. One would hope that as the illnesses continue to increase and their origins cannot be explained, further exploration can be made.

What crops and foods are genetically modified?

There are eight GM food crops. The five major varieties – soy, corn, canola, cotton, and sugar beets – have bacterial genes inserted, which allow the plants to survive extremely heavy doses of weed killer. Farmers use considerably more herbicides on these GM crops and so the food has higher herbicide residues. About 68% of GM crops are herbicide tolerant [17].

The second group of GM foods have a built-in pesticide. It is found in GM corn and cotton. A gene from the soil bacterium called Bt (for Bacillus thuringiensis) is inserted into the plant's DNA, where it secretes the insect-killing Bt-toxin in every cell. About 19% of GM crops produce their own pesticide. Another 13% produce a pesticide and are herbicide tolerant [18].

There is also Hawaiian papaya and a small amount of zucchini and yellow crookneck squash, which are genetically modified to resist a plant virus.

Chapter Seventeen: Alcohol

"Half the costs of illness are wasted on conditions that could be prevented."
—Dr. Joseph Pizzorno

There are several studies that discuss the value of resveratrol, a powerful antioxidant that is found in wine. While the antioxidant may be found in it, there are other factors to consider when determining if that drink is the best way to acquire the antioxidant.

There is evidence that indicates that the amount of alcohol consumed over time, not the type of alcoholic beverage, seems to be the most important factor in raising cancer risk. Most evidence suggests that it is the ethanol itself that is responsible for the increased risk, not other things in the drink. However, the exact way in which alcohol affects cancer risk isn't completely understood. In fact, there may be several different ways in which it raises risk, and this may depend on the type of cancer.

- We do know that alcohol depletes zinc, magnesium, B-complex vitamins especially folate by lowering the body's ability to absorb folate from foods. This problem can be compounded in heavy drinkers, who often do not get enough nutrients such as folate in their diet. Low folate levels may play a role in the risk of breast and colorectal cancers.
- Alcohol may act as an irritant, especially in the mouth and throat. Cells that are damaged may try to repair themselves, which may lead to DNA changes in the cells that can be a step toward cancer.

- In the colon and rectum, bacteria can convert alcohol into large amounts of acetaldehyde, a chemical that has been shown to cause cancer in lab animals.
- Alcohol and its byproducts can also directly damage the liver, leading to inflammation and scaring. As liver cells try to repair the damage, they may acquire mistakes in their DNA.
- Alcohol may act as a solvent, helping other harmful chemicals, such as those found in tobacco smoke, to enter the cells lining the upper digestive tract more easily. This may help explain why the combination of smoking and drinking is much more likely to cause cancers in the mouth or throat than either smoking or drinking alone. In other cases, alcohol may slow the body's ability to break down and get rid of some harmful chemicals.
- Alcohol may raise body levels of estrogen, a hormone important in the growth and development of breast tissue. This may have an effect on a woman's risk of breast cancer.
- Too much alcohol can add extra calories to the diet, which can contribute to weight gain in some people. Being overweight or obese is known to increase the risks of many types of cancer.
- Alcohol may contribute to cancer in other, as of yet unknown ways.

A recent study was published in the American Journal of Public Health. The authors, including Timothy Naimi, a School of Medicine and School of Public Health associate professor, attribute 6,000 American deaths annually to cancer from moderate drinking, which they define as a drink and a half or less per day. Add in alcohol consumption at all levels and the total surges to 20,000 cancer deaths a year, according to the study (For perspective, that 20,000 figure represents 3.5% of all cancer deaths in the country).

For men, lethal alcohol-caused cancer typically affects the mouth, throat, and esophagus, the researchers say. In women, breast cancer is the most common cancer killer linked to alcohol consumption [1].

Whether it is wine, beer or any other alcohol, the evidence is clear, there is no nutritional value that justifies the risk.

Chapter Eighteen: Meat

"When health is absent, wisdom cannot reveal itself; art cannot become manifest; strength cannot be exerted; wealth is useless, and reason is powerless"

—Heterophiles

Ahhh, the smell of the outdoor grill cooking steaks and burgers ... a summertime staple! The way the meat industry portrays it, there is no other way to get protein except through meat. While meat does have the 8 essential amino acids, it also carries a lot of other ingredients. As we are beginning to see, one benefit may not outweigh all of the other detriments. There are other excellent sources of protein that can be consumed without all of the dangerous additions. As challenging as this one may be to read please read it carefully.

The meat that is in the meat departments of our grocery stores has little resemblance to the meat consumed by our grandparents. They ate meat that was fed with grass – not corn; it had been fed no growth hormones, no antibiotics, and no pesticides or herbicides were in its feed. The animals used to roam in the wild grazing on clean grass and drinking pure water. They weren't kept in tight pens or cages. And, they definitely weren't fed the flesh of other animals.

The amount of meat consumed has certainly changed too. There was a time that meat was eaten on special occasions and when it was consumed it was served with lots of fresh vegetables from the gardens. Now meat is the primary food consumed at all meals. Bacon, sausage or maybe something called Spam for breakfast, cold cuts of turkey or ham at lunch (which are all processed by the way) or maybe a burger followed by some kind of steak, pork chop or chicken for dinner. More meat is consumed by an average person in a week than used to be consumed by people in an entire year.

Where has all of this meat consumption gotten us as a nation? Are we healthier today than we were 100 years ago?

The number of studies linking meat consumption to cancer has been increasingly easier to find. There have been more studies performed and the results are unequivocally strong in the assessment that meat consumption has a strong connection to cancer.

T. Colin Campbell Ph.D, research scientist and professor at Cornell University conducted an extensive study on the connection between meat consumption and cancer. The book is called *The China Study*. His findings have dramatically changed the way people have viewed meat consumption. What he found was that a slight increase in animal protein consumption resulted in a significant increase in the incidences of cancer. You will find that more recent studies continue to confirm his findings and strengthen the concern that meat causes cancer. These are just a few of the many studies that are now available to read regarding the connection between meat and cancer.

A study was written that searched through cohort studies on Medline, EMBASE, and the Cochrane Library from their inception through April 2013 evaluating case-control studies, which assessed the association between red and/or processed meat intake and gastric cancer risk. Twelve cohort and thirty case-control studies were included in the meta-analysis. Their findings indicated that consumption of red and/or processed meat contributes to increased gastric cancer risk. They added a caveat that said further investigation is needed especially for red meat [1].

The National Cancer Institute conducted a rather large multi-ethnic cohort study published in 2005. They followed 478,040 men and women from 10 European countries that were free of cancer at enrollment between 1992 and 1998. Information on diet and lifestyle was collected at baseline. After a mean follow-up of 4.8 years, 1329 incident colorectal cancers were documented. They examined the relationship between intakes of red and processed meat, poultry, and fish and colorectal cancer risk using a model adjusted for age, sex, energy (nonfat and fat sources), height, weight, work-related physical activity, smoking status, dietary fiber and folate, and alcohol consumption. The results indicated that red and processed meat intakes were associated with an increased risk of colon and pancreatic cancer. Carcinogenic substances related to meat preparation methods might also be responsible for the positive association [2].

Another study attempted to look at the risk factors of meat and fat as well as cholesterol associated with pancreatic cancer. This was a multi-ethnic cohort study. There were 190,545 cohort members. During the 7 years of follow-up there were 482 incidences of pancreatic cancer that occurred within this group. A dietary questionnaire was submitted determining quantity and type of food ingested. The strongest association was with processed meat. Those who ate pork and red meat were both associated with 50% increases in risk. Those who had great amounts of total fat and saturated fat from meat had a statistically significant increase in pancreatic cancer risk [3].

Fruits and vegetables are high in water content and are fiber-filled allowing them to move quickly throughout the body. It takes as little as 30 to 45 minutes to digest most fruits and vegetables. The water hydrates the cells while the fiber acts like a broom keeping the intestines clean removing waste from the body as it moves through the colon.

Meat on the other hand has little water and no fiber. These factors cause the meat to take as long as 72 and even up to 96 hours to transit through the body's digestive system. In fact, some red meat could "hang" on the internal colon pathway for months! Imagine if you left a steak just sitting on the kitchen counter for 3 days. It would begin to putrefy and rot. The smell alone would be rather repulsive. The same putrefaction process takes place within the body. As this happens, various toxins are released contributing to the toxic load within the body.

Many consider meat to be the most toxic food that we consume. They feel that it is the greatest contributor to cancer of all of the other toxins that we are exposed to on a daily basis. While there are many studies that correlate the connection between meat consumption and cancer, there are no studies that have been performed to try to understand the "why."

Is it because of the lack of fiber? Or, that the meat today is produced in such an unnatural way. While all the answers aren't readily available, the connection between meat and cancer is obvious and action must be taken to reduce the risk.

Some try to say that poultry and fish are better options than red meat or pork. Don't be fooled! If commercially produced it could actually be worse. Poultry are no longer free range unable to eat natural foods such as bugs but are kept in small, tight cages and have been fed unnatural feed. Fish are now raised in man-made ponds "farm raised." In both of these situations, a large amount of antibiotics are administered so a virus doesn't come in and wipe out the entire farm. More antibiotics are given to the animals than is used on humans. We eat these antibiotic laden meats and wonder where these "superbugs" came from that are resistant to antibiotics.

Growth hormones are also given to the poultry and fish to accelerate their growth and shorten the time necessary to get them mature enough to slaughter. It once took 16 weeks for a baby chick to reach maturity. Now it takes only 8. We consume these growth hormones when we eat these foods and then they have an impact on our health. Why are American girls going through puberty at 8, 9, 10 and 11 instead of 14, 15 or 16?

You might think that wild is better – think again. Our rivers, lakes and oceans are loaded with toxins. So many lakes now have signs warning against the consumption of the fish if pregnant. If it isn't good for a little baby then it must not be good for an adult either. Fish caught out of our oceans are full of mercury and other harmful toxins that have accumulated over the years. Wild game such as deer are now battling the equivalent to HIV in their species as they consume GMO crops. There just are no longer meats of any source that can be considered safe to eat.

When the American Cancer Society begins discussing the risks associated with meat and the relationship to certain types of cancer, then it is a certainty that the evidence is irrefutable and there is a connection between meat consumption and cancer. The American Cancer Society has finally succumbed to science and has now been more inclined to view food choices as possible reasons for cancer. This has taken a very long time to happen.

We have made multiple trips to Nigeria over the last couple of years. Nigerians haven't been experiencing cancer for many years but it is now becoming quite common, especially among the people who are rich. Meat has become a status symbol and if meat isn't consumed then you must not have much money. For people of means, meat is served for breakfast, lunch and dinner (sound like America?) The people who are poor don't have the money for meat, are much healthier and don't experience the same incidences of cancer. As we started to teach people that eating like Americans wasn't healthy, they began to realize that their parents and grandparents didn't eat much meat and they didn't have much cancer. Since our visits, we've had many people write to us indicating that by changing their diets, they were able to heal from cancer.

Chapter Nineteen: Dairy

"A man's health can be judged by which he takes two at a time
- pills or stairs."

—Joan Welshl

Growing up I was always told to drink my milk to build strong teeth and bones. On the television I saw commercials featuring attractive movie stars with their white mustaches. Little did I know that those ads were paid for and sponsored by the milk and dairy industry. Of course the farmers want us to drink more milk.

I grew up in Wisconsin, also known as cow country and never stopped to think for a minute "Where do cows get their calcium?" Nature often provides the answers to so many questions in life. The more I began to think about drinking milk, the more I realized that consuming cow's milk was unnatural.

Man is the only animal in nature that once weaned from its mother, begins to drink milk from the cow. The milk from the cow is meant for cows, milk from pigs is meant for pigs and milk from humans is meant for humans. You don't see any other mammal go from their momma to another animal for milk. Man somehow has gotten confused about the purpose and source of milk.

Cow's milk is designed to take a baby calf and grow it into a 2,000 pound full-grown cow. All of the fats, proteins and other nutrients in cow's milk are designed for cows not humans. I don't know about you but I don't want to be a 2,000 pound human.

Add to that, man pasteurizes the milk before it is consumed. This process changes the structure of the milk and alters the nutrients making it virtually a foreign substance within the body. During pasteurization, enzymes like lactase, galactase, and phosphatase are destroyed. Without these enzymes, milk is especially difficult to process in our bodies, especially since the human pancreas cannot always create these enzymes on its own.

Pasteurized milk becomes acid forming requiring calcium from the body to neutralize this acidity. Did you know that the United States with all of its milk consumption has one of the highest rates of osteoporosis in the world? Singapore, Hong Kong, Japan, and certain parts of South Africa (with low milk consumption) have historically had very low rates of osteoporosis.

Cow's milk, and all other dairy sources from any animal other than humans contain increased amounts of fats, calcium and protein that the human body cannot assimilate properly. Continuous consumption of dairy products has been found to increase risks of several forms of cancer in both males and females.

Other factors to consider with dairy consumption are the hormones, the dietary phosphates, IGF-1-an insulin growth factor and lactose. All of these have been studied as possible cancer influences.

The following studies support these concerns:

A study reviewed several epidemiological studies that had indicated an increased risk of prostate cancer with long-term, high intake of dairy products in male U.S. physicians and males in Sweden. This relation has been formerly associated with the higher dietary intake of calcium in dairy products. However, the high dietary phosphate of dairy products affects much larger fluctuation in serum phosphate and may be a more likely source of prostate cancer risk as men consume high amounts of dairy products [1].

Prostate cancer has been linked to dairy products in several other studies. In Harvard's Physicians Health Study, including male physicians, those who consumed more than two dairy servings daily had a 34% higher risk of developing prostate cancer than men who consumed little or no dairy products. Several other studies have had similar findings.

Dairy product consumption increases levels of insulin-like growth factor I (IGF-1) in the bloodstream. IGF-1 is a potent stimulus for cancer cell growth. High IGF-1 levels are linked to increased risk of prostate cancer and breast cancer.

Recent scientific studies have suggested that dairy products may be linked to increased risk for not only prostate cancer, but testicular cancer, and possibly for ovarian and breast cancers. For ovarian cancer, galactose, a component of the milk sugar lactose, has been under study as a possible instigator. A recent analysis of studies examining a relationship between dairy product consumption and ovarian cancer risk found that for every 10 grams of lactose consumed (the amount in one glass of milk), ovarian cancer risk increased by 13% [2][4].

Most cows' milk will contain a significant number of cancer viruses, primarily those responsible for leukemia and lymphoma, two of the most common diseases in cattle. The meat from cows also has numerous carcinogenic viruses. Hence, another reason to avoid meat [3].

Cow's milk is extremely mucus forming within the body and contributes to many issues within the body like allergies and asthma. In actress Alicia Silverstone`s book *The Kind Diet,* Silverstone recalls growing up with bronchitis three or four times a year; she was on regular allergy medication and relied on an inhaler for her asthma. It wasn't until she gave up dairy that her allergies went away. "Very soon after becoming vegan, I stopped experiencing allergies or any asthma-type symptoms," says Silverstone. "They just disappeared."

It's obvious that cows milk was never intended for humans and science has confirmed that there is a connection between its consumption and cancer. Any substance that makes the body work harder, in this case cow's milk, contributes to the toxic load making it more difficult for the body to maintain proper health.

Many alternatives to cow's milk include:
- Almond milk
- Rice milk
- Hemp milk
- Coconut milk
- Avoid soy milk as most soy is GMO

Use these like you would cow's milk in recipes, on cereals or by the glass.

Chapter Twenty: White Sugar

"You are what you eat. What would YOU like to be?"
—Julie Murphy

An average person will eat 170 pounds of sugar in a year. That is about 22 teaspoons of added sugar every day! This is over 11,000 pounds in 70 years. It is a serious problem that needs to be addressed. Between fat, sugar and salt, the food industry has created a situation where people's taste buds have been tarnished and tainted whereby eating a fresh, succulent apple doesn't arouse any taste sensation any longer. And fruit, itself has been shown to have been increased in sugar content at least 30% in the last several years.

Since sugar has become the new, legalized cocaine in terms of addiction and even in terms of life-threatening consequences, we will show studies of how sugar has become carcinogenic and deserves the name "poison."

The case against sugar is so compelling that, in 2009, the American Heart Association (AHA) released guidelines suggesting people limit its intake. According to the AHA women should eat less than 6 teaspoons a day; men are to keep their intake to 9 teaspoons. But if I had cancer, and I knew that sugar would make the cancer stronger, I would do everything I could not to feed the cancer and eliminate as much sugar from all sources from my diet until the cancer has been defeated.

Researchers at Huntsman Cancer Institute in Utah were one of the first to discover that sugar "feeds" tumors. The research published in the journal, Proceedings of the National Academy of Sciences said, "It's been known since 1923 that tumor cells use a lot more glucose than normal cells. Our research helps show how this process takes place, and how it might be stopped to control tumor growth," according to Don Ayer, Ph.D., a professor in the Department of Oncological Sciences at the University of Utah.

Dr. Thomas Graeber, a professor of molecular and medical pharmacology, has investigated how the metabolism of glucose affects the biochemical signals present in cancer cells. In research published on June 26, 2012 in the journal Molecular Systems Biology, Graeber and his colleagues demonstrate that glucose starvation – that is, depriving cancer cells of glucose (sugar) – creates an accumulation of reactive oxygen species (ROS) that results in cancer cell death [1].

Since refined sugars are strongly linked to cancer, not only as a cause of it but also as something that feeds the cancer cells once a person has the disease – nothing could be more important to consider in the attempt to improve the outcome of cancer treatments. The kinds of sugar so prevalent in today's standard American diet lead to cancer directly by causing inflammation throughout the body and in some places more than others depending on the individual and their constitution.

Another study confirming the link with sugar and cancer was conducted by Drs. Rainer Klement and Ulrike Kammerer as a comprehensive review of the literature involving dietary carbohydrates and their direct and indirect effect on cancer cells. It was published in October 2011 in the journal Nutrition and Metabolism, and concluded that cancers are so sensitive to the sugar supply that cutting that supply will suppress cancer [2]. This study went on to declare that as you increase sugar consumption, you will increase the likelihood of the cancer spreading, creating a larger tumor and essentially creating a situation that is harder to overcome.

Also, eating white sugar (or white anything) causes magnesium mineral deficiencies because the magnesium has been removed in the processing, making sugar a ripe target as a major cause of cancer because deficiencies in magnesium are not only pro-inflammatory but also pro-cancer [3].

Heavy refined carbohydrate intake causes more than just magnesium mineral depletion with other minerals depleted as well. It will also lead to dehydration, which after a time can lead to diabetes, heart disease and ultimately cancer. Dehydration creates inflammation and thus sets the stage for cancer [4].

A UCLA study found that tumor cells consume both fructose and glucose and these findings that were published in the journal Cancer Research, linked fructose intake with pancreatic cancer. This study also helped explain other studies that have linked fructose intake with pancreatic cancer. The researchers concluded that anyone wishing to curb their cancer risk should start by reducing the amount of sugar they consume. This is the first time a link has been shown between fructose and cancer proliferation. "In this study we show that cancers can use fructose just as readily as glucose to fuel their growth," said Dr. Anthony Heaney of UCLA's Jonsson Cancer Center, the study's lead author. While this study was done on pancreatic cancer, these findings may not be unique to that cancer type, Heaney said. "These findings show that cancer cells can readily metabolize fructose to increase proliferation" [5].

Foods that cause a sharp rise in blood glucose (i.e. foods with a high-glycemic index ranking) trigger the secretion of insulin and insulin growth factor (IGF-1), two hormones that also promote cancer growth [6].

Dr. Otto Warburg's 1924 paper, on Metabolism of Tumors, stated, "Summarized in a few words, the prime cause of cancer is the replacement of the respiration of oxygen in normal body cells by a fermentation of sugar."

Since Oncologists have not been trained in nutrition therapy for cancer patients, it is not surprising that you will find drawers with sugar-laden foods and drinks in the IV rooms where patients are receiving their chemotherapy treatments. As we watched the IV of chemo go into our son, we also watched him eat a snack bar and wash it down with a soda pop provided free of charge by the hospital. It seems, that if it is available in the doctor's office, it must be okay to consume. Doctors wouldn't feed people food that would hurt them! Oncologists don't appear to know that the food their patients are eating is making their job harder and more complicated. Their patients will need more chemo treatments to try to overcome the stronger cancer cells that are being fed by the sugary foods they are consuming.

Let's take a stand and change the outcomes of many of the four million cancer patients being treated in America today. Let's create a ribbon that looks like a sugar cube or place it in the shape of a piece of candy or a donut and place it everywhere depicting the dangers of sugar and it's relevance to cancer. When people stop eating the foods that the food industry is creating, then the incidences of cancer will reduce significantly as will the cost of health care and maybe even begin the slow transition to teaching Americans that what we place in our mouth has a direct correlation to our recovery.

Chapter Twenty-One: White Flour

"Man is more miserable, more restless and unsatisfied than ever before, simply because half his nature– the spiritual– is starving for true food, and the other half– the material– is fed with bad food."

—Paul Brunton

Everyone loves pies, bagels, cookies, breads, doughnuts and desserts. These are fun comfort foods. Although they tantalize the taste buds, the effect bakery has on our bodies is devastating. Not only do the sugars and the oils contribute but also the flour that is used in these baked goods is especially harmful.

Everyone loves spongy, white bread. Even the Wonder Bread commercials years ago said it was good for growing strong bones. Unfortunately, that is not close to what really is happening.

Grain that comes from the plant must go through many steps to get to the beautiful, smooth, white flour that you can pick up in 5-pound bags in the grocery store.

Take a look at the process to make white flour:
1. Remove the wheat seed's bran – its six outer layers
2. According to the USDA, during the process of removing the bran, you have also removed:
    – 76% of vitamins and minerals
    – 97% of dietary fiber
3. The flour is bleached, preserved and aged with chlorine dioxide

4. It is further whitened by adding chalk
5. Alum and ammonium carbonate improve the look and feel for consumers
6. Emulsifiers are added – these make the bread appear softer and hide the real age of the bread. These emulsifiers don't prevent bread from rotting, they just hide the signs so you do not know whether or not you are in fact eating bread that is still "good."
7. Alloxen is added to make it look clean to the consumer. This additive has been known to destroy beta cells in the pancreas. It has often been given to laboratory rats to induce diabetes.
8. Sorbitan mono-saturate, an anti-salting agent, is added in the final stages.
9. A few synthetic nutrients are added back into the white flour and it is then called "Enriched."

Turning grain into white flour is quite a process. There are numerous chemicals, additives and preservatives required to create that rich, soft, white texture.

White flour when mixed with water becomes sticky. Because the fiber has been removed, baked goods made from white flour move slowly through the colon. When the colon is slowed down it becomes more difficult for the body to rid itself of toxins. Toxic buildup is a contributing cause of cancer.

When you eat a product that was created from white flour you are consuming what is known as a high glycemic index food. The body reacts to this food consumption exactly as it would if it were consuming refined sugar. It will release Insulin-like Growth Factor (IGF) to all the glucose to enter the cells to stimulate growth. Insulin and IGF promote cell growth (cancer cell growth) as well as trigger inflammation in the body. These will all set the stage for tumor growth.

An interesting study was done that showed that after injecting breast cancer cells into mice, the cells were less susceptible to chemotherapy once the mouse's insulin system had been activated by the presence of sugar (or refined flour) [1].

Baking with "whole" wheat flour retains fiber, bran, germ and nutrients. Vitamin E is retained and acts a natural preservative.

Gluten, a naturally occurring protein found in wheat, has gained a lot of attention by health experts over the last several years. Gluten causes inflammation within the body and is responsible for many of the symptoms people realize today from swelling of the midsection to snoring. It will most likely be many years before any research is done to see if there is a connection between gluten and cancer. It stands to reason though that anything that causes inflammation is putting additional strain on the body and should be eliminated while battling cancer. Anyone with a thyroid issue should also avoid all sources of gluten.

As much as our culture loves breads, pastas, bagels, donuts, croutons, cakes, pies, etc, we must remember, that eating white flour causes the same damage to our bodies as if it were sugar.

Chapter Twenty-Two: High Fructose Corn Syrup

"Remember, too, that at a time when people are very concerned with their health and its relationship to what they eat, we have handed over the responsibility for our nourishment to faceless corporations."
—Lynne Rossetto Kasper

High fructose corn syrup was introduced in the late 1950's but didn't become introduced into the consumable food world until the late 1970's and early 1980's. It is an inexpensive flavor enhancer that tastes sweet. Since it has corn in it, one would conclude that it is safe. Before we discuss its safety, it is important to note that since it became so prevalent in sweetened drinks and processed foods like corn and tortilla chips, the amounts consumed by Americans has sharply risen. Earlier, we learned that regular sugar consumption has reached an annual amount of 170 pounds a year. The U.S. Department of Agriculture estimates the average American consumes more than 65.6 pounds of high fructose corn syrup per year. The third National Health and Nutrition Examination Survey reported that more than 10% of America's daily calories come from fructose – of which the largest part comes from sweetened drinks and processed foods [1].

From the time period when high fructose corn syrup was introduced through today, obesity rates have more than tripled and diabetes incidence has increased more than seven fold. There have been other variables introduced as well, but this is a notable possibility for the cause of the increase. These two factors are precursors to pancreatic cancer which epidemiological studies have reported a remarkable increase in the past 20 years [2][3][4].

When one 20 ounce HFCS sweetened soda, sports drink, or tea has 17 teaspoons of sugar (and the average teenager often consumes two drinks a day) as Dr. Mark Hyman says, "We are conducting a largely uncontrolled experiment on the human species. Our hunter gatherer ancestors consumed the equivalent of 20 teaspoons per year, not per day."

So what are the dangers of high fructose corn syrup and how can they be connected to increased cancer growth?

High fructose corn syrup (HFCS) causes cancer in a unique way because much of it is contaminated with mercury due to the complex way it is made. High fructose corn syrup causes selenium deficiencies because the mercury in it binds with selenium, driving selenium levels downward. Selenium is crucial for glutathione production and its deficiency in soils tracks mathematically with cancer rates. Selenium and mercury have a strong affinity to bond with each other.

Fructose can promote cancer growth by a number of mechanisms, including altered cellular division, change in oxygen assimilation, DNA damage, and inflammation [5]. The metabolism of fructose differs from that of other carbohydrates. Fructose is the preferred food choice for cancer cells. It seems that cancer prefers it to glucose. The enhanced protein synthesis caused by fructose appears to promote a more aggressive cancer [6].

Data collected for 14 years from The Singapore Chinese Health Study using a 648,387 person cohort found that individuals who consumed 2 or more soft drinks per week were twice as likely to develop pancreatic cancer [7]. Similarly, a paper published in the American Journal of Clinical Nutrition, using a cohort of 77,797 people followed for 7 years revealed a 93% increase in the occurrence of pancreatic cancer in those who drank 2 or more soft drinks per day [8].

However, data regarding the intake of fruits and vegetables indicates a reduced risk of pancreatic cancer [9]. Despite the fact that naturally occurring fructose (in fruits and vegetables) is chemically identical to high fructose corn syrup and agave (in sweets and soft drinks), there is a marked difference in the delivery systems. Fruits and vegetables contain quantities of fiber and antioxidants that seem to have an inverse effect on pancreatic cancer risk [10].

High fructose corn syrup is an excellent reason to avoid all sweetened beverages and processed food. It is not a food ingredient. It is an industrial ingredient that found its way into the American consumable food supply. The longer it stays in the food supply, the more likely that the health of each generation will slowly deteriorate.

As you fight the cancer, you must not introduce anything into your body that will feed the cancer and inhibit the process of recovery and immune enhancement. High fructose corn syrup should never be introduced into anyone's body. If it is, there will definitely be deadly results.

"Doubt and confusion are the currency of deception, and they sow the seeds of complacency."

Chapter Twenty-Three: Artificial Sweeteners

"About eighty percent of the food on shelves of supermarkets
today didn't exist 100 years ago."
—Larry McCleary

Aspartame

Artificial sweeteners have been in the American food chain for over 30 years. The most common one, aspartame (known as NutraSweet and Equal) which is the most common form of sweetener found in soda, yogurt, flavored water, and many other sugar-free foods has an interesting history. After 16 years of trying to get FDA approval, it was finally given the green light in 1981.

A review of industry backed studies done in 1996 found 100% of industry studies (74 of 74) found aspartame to be safe, while over 90% of independent researchers' studies (84 of 91 studies) found at least one potential health problem related to consumption of aspartame. Even though it was finally approved, an FDA review called out the many irregularities in the industry studies, identified evidence of data manipulating and even some of these studies were called "... sloppy at best." Since its introduction, there were more complaints to the FDA regarding reactions to aspartame than all other food additives combined. What was strange that despite those complaints, the FDA stopped taking any more complaints on aspartame, and determined that it was considered GRAS (generally regarded as safe). Typically to be given this distinction there are a number of studies that have been legitimately performed and executed under strict standards.

One primary concern about aspartame is that it is not heat stable in liquids. When it gets warm or is exposed to heat it will break down into three carcinogenic chemicals including methanol, formaldehyde and diketopiperazine (DkP) the tumor agent! Dr. Russell Blaylock, neurologist, has speculated that a potential cause for the increase in brain tumors in this country could be the warming of aspartame filled beverages that have been heated. You can actually taste the difference because it will not have as sweet a flavor once it is left in the heat.

- A study from Harvard links diet soda and blood cancers (leukemia, non-Hodgkins lymphoma, and multiple myeloma). Just one soda with aspartame per day in men and women gave rise to a significant 40% increased risk of leukemia [1]. This is really the only long-term study that has ever been done on aspartame in people. This included a prospective study from the Nurses' Health Study and Health Professional's Follow-up Study at Harvard.

Splenda

Splenda is a sugar that has been modified with 3 chlorine molecules. Despite the advertisement, there is nothing natural about Splenda. Before it came on the market there were only 6 human trials. Technically there were only two trials before it was approved. In the course of the approval process, only 23 people took Splenda for 4 days. What the researchers were looking for was tooth decay outcomes, not safety or tolerance of the product.

Since Splenda has been on the market, researchers have found that at least 15% of it cannot be excreted out of the body. The number of people who have had severe negative reactions to Splenda has been significant.

It is evident that there have been few studies done on this product. No one knows the true dangers this product can have on the body. The irony is that although it has been touted as beneficial for weight loss issues, in fact the use of artificial sweeteners has not ever been helpful with weight loss and, there are more cases where it has promoted weight gain instead.

Today, even though cancer has increased by leaps and bounds

since the introduction of artificial sweeteners, you will be hard pressed to find strong studies that will objectively evaluate the carcinogenic properties of various artificial sweeteners. It is uncertain as to why the medical and scientific community has not pursued the path of these non-foods as potential causes for cancer. There is evidence that the manufacturers have been able to control or hide the true evidence of the dangers of these products.

However, if we were to wait for science to catch up, then most people would likely find themselves and their health in a dangerous place. Since all of the "artificial" sweeteners are not 'food', then it makes logical sense to avoid them totally not just while fighting cancer but also to avoid cancer. Whether the studies are available or not, it takes common sense to recognize that only whole, unprocessed foods are what the body can use without harm and artificial sweeteners are not considered whole foods.

Chapter Twenty-Four: Salt

"Get Health. No labor, effort nor exercise that can gain it must be grudged."
—Ralph Waldo Emerson

Salt is used extensively in the food industry to make foods taste good so people buy more. It is found in nearly everything processed whether in a can, box or package. Even in the fresh made foods at the deli counter, salt is used abundantly. Go to a restaurant and most food served has had salt added and there are even saltshakers at the tables just in case enough wasn't added in the kitchen. Our taste buds have become so addicted to salt that we consume it at almost every meal. More than 75% of the typical American's daily sodium comes from processed foods, to which salt is added as an inexpensive flavor enhancer and preservative. But, what is all of this salt doing to our health?

Most people know that consuming too much salt in their diet can increase blood pressure and heart disease risk. But salt can also increase risk for cancer, specifically stomach cancer. There have been several studies that have confirmed it. This may be due to stomach lining damage. Another factor to consider is that salt has been correlated with Helicobacter pylori (H pylori) infection, so the two factors may act synergistically to promote the development of stomach cancer.

Salt intake was first reported as a possible risk factor for stomach cancer in 1959. In some early studies, using refrigeration for food storage, thereby potentially reducing the amount of salt required for food preservation, was found to be correlated with a reduction in stomach cancer rates. This led researchers to hypothesize that salt intake must

135

play a role in stomach cancer. Today, the evidence is overwhelming that salt is a major factor. Studies have been performed throughout various regions in the world and have proven unequivocally the direct correlation.

Stomach cancer is the fourth most common cancer and is the third leading cause of cancer death worldwide [1]. Based on the considerable evidence that is available, limiting salt intake is an important strategy for preventing gastric cancer.

Do I need salt?

Sodium is important for proper body functions. It is needed to control blood pressure and blood volume. Sodium is also needed for muscle and nerve function. It will balance the amount of water that exists within and outside of the cells. The body requires about 500 milligrams of sodium a day. That is equivalent to 1/10th of a teaspoon.

The US Department of Agriculture (USDA) recommends that adults consume no more than 2,400 milligrams (mg) of sodium a day, although our body is capable of handling up to 3000 milligrams of sodium per day.

As we get older, especially after we pass 45 years of age, our risk for high blood pressure rises. The USDA recommends that people middle-aged and older consume no more than 1,500 mg of sodium a day. That's the amount of sodium found in approximately one level teaspoon of salt. On average, according to the Center for Science in the Public Interest, Americans consume about 4,000 mg of sodium daily.

Excess salt is generally excreted through the urine. When this happens more calcium than normal is pulled from the bloodstream to assist in neutralizing the excess sodium. While this leads to a weakening of the bones it may also contribute to kidney stones. According to the Linus Pauling Institute, more than one study has concluded that limiting salt intake for someone with a history of kidney stones reduces the likelihood he will develop the problem again.

Natural, unrefined salt contains 84 different minerals. Table salt has had all minerals removed except for two – sodium and chloride. These two minerals when isolated and combined become toxic to the body and should be avoided as much as possible.

To create table salt an extensive refinement process is needed. It is first treated chemically to remove the calcium and magnesium. Then it is processed through a multiple-effect vacuum evaporator, which removes all other minerals leaving nearly pure (99.9) sodium chloride. Then magnesium carbonate, calcium silicate, calcium phosphate, magnesium silicate, or calcium carbonate (all additives) are added to make it free-flowing. This processing removes all of the rest of the beneficial minerals leaving a toxic substance.

Don't be fooled by "Sea Salt." All salt comes from the sea and though it looks like it might be healthier it still has gone through a similar processing as regular table salt. If it is white in color it has been highly processed.

Are there any healthy options?

Celtic sea salt and Himalayan salt are two excellent choices to replace the traditional saltshaker. Each contains a wide variety of minerals making them extremely healthy. Most people find that these salts have a better taste than traditional table salt. They also find that less is required because they are higher quality. Many have seen the benefits listed below from using these types of unrefined salts:

- Controlling the water levels within the body, regulating them for proper functioning
- Promoting stable pH balance in the cells, including the brain
- Encouraging excellent blood sugar health
- Aiding in reducing the common signs of aging
- Promoting cellular hydroelectric energy creation
- Promoting the increased absorption capacities of food elements within the intestinal tract
- Aiding vascular health
- Supporting healthy respiratory function
- Lowering incidence of sinus problems, and promoting over-all sinus health
- Reducing cramps
- Increasing bone strength
- Naturally promoting healthy sleep patterns
- Creating a healthy libido
- Circulation support

• Promotes kidney and gall bladder health when compared to common chemically-treated salt [2]

If you want a good book on the subject, read David Brownstein, MD's, *Salt: Your Way to Health*. In this book, the author relates to salt as a misunderstood nutrient.

Another excellent way to get the health benefits of sodium is to eat more whole foods. Foods like beets, celery as well as many other vegetables have naturally occurring sodium.

Chapter Twenty-Five: Fats and Oils

"Appetite has really become an artificial and abnormal thing, having taken the place of true hunger, which alone is natural. The one is a sign of bondage but the other, of freedom."
—Paul Brunton

There are numerous benefits to having fat in the diet:

Fats provide energy. Fats are the most efficient source of food energy. Each gram of fat provides nine calories of energy for the body, compared with four calories per gram of carbohydrates and proteins.

Fats build healthy cells. Fats are a vital part of the membrane that surrounds each cell of the body. Without a healthy cell membrane, the rest of the cell couldn't function.

Fats help communicate. Fat provides the structural components not only of cell membranes in the brain, but also of myelin, the fatty insulating sheath that surrounds each nerve fiber, enabling it to carry messages faster.

Fats help the body use vitamins. Vitamins A, D, E, and K are fat-soluble vitamins, meaning that the fat in foods helps the intestines absorb these vitamins into the body.

Fats make hormones. Fats are structural components of some of the most important substances in the body, including prostaglandins, hormone-like substances that regulate many of the body's functions. Fats regulate the production of sex hormones.

Fat provides healthier skin. One of the more obvious signs of fatty acid deficiency is dry, flaky skin. In addition to giving skin its rounded appeal, the layer of fat just beneath the skin (called subcutaneous fat) acts as the body's own insulation to help regulate body temperature. Lean people tend to be more sensitive to cold; obese people tend to be more sensitive to warm weather.

Fat forms a protective cushion for your organs. Many of the vital organs, especially the kidneys, heart, and intestines are cushioned by fat that helps protect them from injury and hold them in place. As a tribute to the body's own intelligence, this protective fat is the last to be used up when the body's energy reserves are being tapped into.

Most people understand the differences between the good (unsaturated fat), bad (saturated fat) and dangerous (trans-fat) fats. We know that oils derived from animal fat are not good for our health due to their high levels of saturated fat and cholesterol, and that oils derived from some plants are generally good for our health due to their unsaturated fat content.

However, not all unsaturated fats are healthy. Many plant seed oils such as sunflower, safflower, peanut and corn oil are rich in inflammatory polyunsaturated fatty acids (PUFAs) and devoid of anti-inflammatory PUFAs. On the other hand, some plant seed oils such as olive oil have balanced PUFAs and are considered healthier. Therefore, it is important to distinguish between the types of PUFAs in dietary oils for optimal health.

Omega 3 and omega 6 are two types of polyunsaturated fatty acids. They are both required for the body to function but have opposite effects when it comes to inflammatory response which is a known pre-curser to cancer. Too much omega 6 (which is common on the standard American diet) and too little omega 3 are implicated as a cause for certain cancers.

Animal studies as early as 1959 clearly demonstrated that mice and rats that were fed high fat diets were far more susceptible to skin and breast cancer than animals fed diets low in fat [1]. These studies got very little attention for nearly 20 years until epidemiological data demonstrated the prevalence of various types of cancer was much higher in countries with high fat diets as compared to those with low fat diets [2].

Since that time, abundant experimental data has shown that feeding rats or mice a variety of high-fat diets increases susceptibility to cancer of the breast, skin, colon, pancreas and prostate. Much of the evidence relating dietary fat to cancer has been presented and discussed in more recent reviews [3].

Cancer of the breast and colon account for a large proportion of the total number of cancers in Western populations. Both show a strong positive correlation with fat consumption in multi-country studies.

There is abundant data showing that animals fed high-fat diets develop tumors of the mammary gland, intestine, skin and pancreas more readily than animals fed low-fat diets. This data is consistent with the multi-country correlations linking dietary fat with cancer of the breast, colon, pancreas and prostate [4].

It is evident that although fat is beneficial, the quantity and quality is very important. A panel of nutritionists and scientists at the National Institute of Health recently recommended that the ratio of omega 3 to omega 6 fatty acids consumed should be 1 to 4 or less. The usual ratio in the United States is much higher at 1 to 10-20 [5].

As a person fighting cancer, it is best to avoid nearly all forms of fat until the situation with the cancer has been resolved. Later, you will see how much fat is recommended as well as the types of fat. A person really doesn't need as much fat in their daily diet as they think they do.

Chapter Twenty-Six: Toxin Synergy

"Until man duplicates a blade of grass, nature can laugh at his so-called scientific knowledge. Remedies from chemicals will never stand in favour compared with the products of nature, the living cell of the plant, the final result of the rays of the sun, the mother of all life."

—T.A. Edison

As Dr. Russell Blaylock points out in his book, Natural Strategies for Cancer Patients, there have been no studies done on what happens when two carcinogens are combined.

- What if we eat food that has a combination of additives and pesticides?
- Or food that has food coloring and neurotoxins?
- Or food that has added hormones and is genetically modified?
- What happens to the person who consumes or inhales tobacco and consumes sugar?
- What about the person who uses over the counter drugs and already has heavy metal toxicity in their body?

One carcinogen alone cannot cause cancer but more than one can. How many of us have experienced more than one toxin at a time? Since there are no studies on the toxic synergy of these known carcinogens, it would appear that if we continue down this path we are taking a big gamble with our health.

Here are some interesting facts:

First, toxins can make each other more toxic.

A small dose of mercury that kills 1 in 100 rats and a dose of aluminum that will kill 1 in 100 rats, when combined have a striking effect: All The Rats will Die. In other words, doses of mercury that have a 1 percent mortality rate will have a 100 percent mortality rate if some aluminum is there [1].

- Mercury will kill 1 out of 100 rats.
- Lead will kill 1 out of 1000 rats.
- Combine mercury and lead – 100% of exposed rats will die.

This was such an interesting phenomenon that another study was done on the effects of both female and male hormones on the neuro-toxicity of thimerosal (a form of mercury). The results were stunning!

For example, small amounts of thimerosal causes less than 5% neuron deaths within the first three hours incubation and small amounts of testosterone causes no significant death within this time frame. However, mix these two together and 100% neuron death was observed at the earliest time checked. This represents a severe enhancement of thimerosal toxicity. So, testosterone and mercury are deadly when combined!

To add to that study, at 12 hours the neuron death affected by a small amount of thimerosal alone could be reversed by a small amount of estrogen. Estrogen significantly reduced the testosterone enhanced toxicity of thimerosal [2].

Second, people are continuously exposed to a wide variety of chemical substances, biological agents, physical agents, and other stressors.

Each stressor has the potential to cause a physiological effect. A few examples of stressors are:

• Automotive exhaust
• Cleaning products
• Chemicals in treated water
• Consumption of alcohol or tobacco
• Cosmetics
• Environmental pollution

- Food
- Insect repellents
- Noise
- Prescription drugs
- Psychological stress
- Social stress
- Solvents
- Ultraviolet radiation
- Whole-body vibration

Third, exposures can happen one after the other, or all at once. Combinations can produce:

- Consequences that are significantly different than would be expected from individual exposures.
- A range of combined acute and chronic effects.
- Effects that can appear immediately or sometime later.
- Increased or unexpected harmful effects – including entirely new kinds of effects.

The possible combinations of exposure are huge and knowledge is limited about the effects that mixed exposures will have on the body. Individual susceptibility adds to the complexity of exposure and resulting outcomes [3].

Here are examples to help illustrate synergistic toxicity:
- Exposure to noise and the solvent toluene results in a higher risk of hearing loss than exposure to either stressor alone.
- Common food colors are synergistically neurotoxic with flavor enhancers at levels you can get from a typical snack and drink.
- Exposure to carbon monoxide and methylene chloride produces elevated levels of carboxyhemoglobin that reduce the blood's ability to carry oxygen.
- Aluminum, copper, lead, mercury, and cadmium can be found in mussels at levels that, individually, are considered below the threshold of toxic harm. But these metals act synergistically with low concentrations of the

mussel's own acid to kill cells.
- Viruses can increase susceptibility to heavy metals. And vice versa.
- In one study, viral infection increased the uptake of PBDE.
- PBDEs, PCBs, and methyl mercury are each synergistically toxic with the others. Very low exposures combine to induce greater than expected harm.
- In general, metals have synergistic toxicity – and organic metals have synergistic toxicity with organic compounds. Research indicates that low PCB exposure while in the womb, in combination with low exposure to methyl-mercury and lead, results in cognitive impairment [4].
- Exposure to a combination of 1 PCB, 2 dioxins, and 3 pesticides means a person is 38x more likely to develop type 2 diabetes than someone exposed to just 1 of the chemicals.
- Tungsten and cobalt together can be carcinogenic and together have been found to rapidly accelerate the growth of human leukemia cells.
- Rats who drank milk retained 2x more mercury in their bodies than rats that didn't.
- Microscopic particles in diesel exhaust combine with lipids in cholesterol to activate genes that trigger inflammation of blood vessels, in turn leading to atherosclerosis, heart attacks and strokes.

There is significant potential for unexpected 'synergistic toxicity' effects from vaccines, particularly for a susceptible population that may already have high toxin levels due to a lessened ability to excrete toxins. Yet synergistic toxicity of vaccines has not been studied – studies have focused on only individual toxicity of a single component of the vaccines (e.g. mercury or measles virus). Further, the toxicity of an environmental toxin is generally studied independently of other toxins, although the few studies that do exist on combining toxins typically show a strong synergistic toxicity effect.

Although this is not an exhaustive list, it is an extremely strong indicator of how difficult it is in today's world to not become toxic.

Our bodies process those toxins through organs like the liver and kidneys and eliminate them in the form of sweat, urine, and feces. Unfortunately, however, when we continue to subject our bodies to these toxins without continuing to feed the body with constant nutrients to maintain the laborious task of perpetually detoxifying, the organs may not be able to continue with the process and toxins will build up. The result is what is known as the "knocking and pinging" of our bodies that send a clear signal like the warning light on the dashboard of your automobile. If you continue much further in this direction, there will be a definite consequence that will likely be negative.

Cancer is merely a manifestation of our body's deterioration process. Although there are several schools of thought as to exactly what is deteriorating, all can agree that by the time cancer has developed into a diagnosis, the body has definitely experienced enough of a deterioration that the liver, colon, lymphatic system, digestive system, and immune system have become compromised and the cancer is the final indicator that things have been going downhill in the body for several years.

Section Two

❦

Nutritional Deficiency

Today's average restaurant meal is more than four times larger than in the 1950's, and according to the Centers for Disease Control and Prevention (CDC), adults are, on average, 26 pounds heavier. Despite the embarrassing abundance of food and the addition of many so called "healthy" food choices to our diets, many Americans still unknowingly suffer from nutrient deficiencies. Whether from vapid calories (junk food), chemical-induced deficiencies, a lack of variety, or any number of other factors, many of us just aren't getting what we need. We may be heavier as a nation, but as the following report indicates, we are not healthier.

The CDC's Second Nutrition Report, an assessment of diet and nutrition in the U.S. population, concludes that there are a number of specific nutrients lacking in the American diet. Nutrient deficiencies have long-lasting health effects.

The top nutrient deficiencies experienced by many Americans are:

- Vitamin B12
- Vitamin C
- Vitamin D
- Iodine
- Iron
- Magnesium
- Zinc

Up until now this book has covered a large number of toxins that we are exposed to on a daily basis. We began the book suggesting that cancer comes from toxicity and nutritional deficiency. This chapter will discuss what that means, why we are deficient and what the consequences are when we don't have the right materials to build healthy cells.

Our bodies are made up of 100 trillion cells. Everyday, over 300 billion of them die and are replaced with new ones. Over the course of one year every cell in your body will be replaced. A year from now you will have a completely new body. The question is will the new cells be stronger or weaker than the ones they are replacing? Will the body be healthier or sicker?

According to the Oxford Dictionary "nutrition" is "the process of providing or obtaining the food necessary for health and growth."

When we look at this definition we realize that especially in fighting cancer, it isn't just putting the right foods into the body but is a process of the cells "obtaining" the nutrients that are contained in the foods.

To start laying the foundation for this discussion we need to say that we believe in Creation and that our bodies were created by God. In Genesis we see that God made man from the dust of the earth, breathed into him the breath of life and man became a living soul. Then He placed him in the Garden of Eden and told him in Genesis 1:29 what he should eat. Then God said, "I give you every seed-bearing plant on the face of the whole earth and every tree that has the fruit with seed in it. They will be yours for food." New International Version (NIV).

It appears that God's original intention for the nourishment of people was raw fruits, vegetables, seeds and nuts. While there are certainly scriptures later in the Bible that allow for the consumption of certain meats and other animal products, we see in Genesis 1:29 what His original plan was. As you think back to the Garden, you envision that the plants were grown in nutrient-rich soil and their fruits were consumed in their natural state (raw) since fire hadn't been discovered. There was no sickness and people lived exceedingly long lives. God never makes mistakes and His original plan for nourishing the body is what many have found has brought them great success with overcoming their physical ailments including cancer.

Did you know?

Fruits are the greatest source of vitamins and the second greatest source of minerals. Vegetables are the greatest source of minerals and the second greatest source of vitamins. Enzymes are the "life-force" within the food.

Enzymes

Most people understand that vitamins and minerals are important for the body's health but few understand the importance of enzymes. Enzymes are naturally occurring elements that are found in all fruits and vegetables.

Enzymes are the power of life. They are living forces that conduct and direct every activity in your body. Enzymes "digest" or break down raw foods. More and more research suggests eating enzyme-rich food helps digestion. According to Dr. Gabriel Cousens, M.D., "Enzymes can even help repair our DNA and RNA."

Enzymes are heat sensitive and destroyed at temperatures above 108 degrees. When we eat cooked foods, we need to use enzymes from within the body to compensate for the enzymes that were killed through the cooking process.

Our bodies have only a limited number of enzymes through which we digest and assimilate nutrients. When the supply has been depleted, which can go quickly depending on how many enzymes are required for each meal, our bodies can no longer break down food efficiently which leads to several areas of concern.

Other reasons for nutritional deficiency?

Those that have chosen to eat more foods at home and may even incorporate more raw vegetables and fruits still have potential for nutritional deficiencies because the produce they purchase today has been grown in soil that is already deficient in many nutrients. The produce may have travelled quite a distance before it was purchased. The growers may have used pesticides, fertilizers, and other chemicals to prevent bugs, inhibit mold or increase growth size. All of these factors can influence the end result where most people have deficiencies in their diets. After several years, the weakened immune system can no longer provide the support to fight back and the weakened cells begin to lose the battle.

Does nutrition really make a difference in the fight against cancer?

Dr. Russell Blaylock has an exceptional book called *Natural Strategies for Cancer Patients* that details the various types of minerals and nutrients that affect health if they are deficient in the diet. His excellent and easy descriptions clearly provide scientific basis for the importance of consuming a pure vegetable, fruit and seed based diet.

Other experts weighing in on this topic include:

Dr. Francisco Contreras states in his book, *Beating Cancer*, that, "Diet and nutritional factors represent 60% and 40% of all cancers in women and men, respectively".

The Children's Hospital Oakland Research Institute estimates "Diet contributes to about one-third of preventable cancers – about the same amount as smoking. Inadequate intake of essential vitamins and minerals might explain the epidemiological findings that people who eat only small amounts of fruits and vegetables have an increased risk of developing cancer. Recent experimental evidence indicates that vitamin and mineral deficiencies can lead to DNA damage. Optimizing vitamin and mineral intake by encouraging dietary change, multivitamin and mineral supplements, and fortifying foods might therefore prevent cancer and other chronic diseases" [1].

While the last chapter focused on the many toxins that we are exposed to through our environment and in the foods we consume, we want to turn our attention now to how the foods we consume help to offset the deficiency of nutrients our bodies have experienced for many years. The recommended changes are not difficult to make. A companion recipe book called *Unravel the Mystery: Simple, Effective, Nutritious Recipes to Fight Cancer* has been created to assist in you in applying the principles of eating outlined throughout this next section of the book.

As you continue on through this book, you will see how easy the changes will be and with the right information and support, you can change your outlook, your future and your health.

Section Three

❧

The Recovery Program

The body is truly miraculous and it was given the inherent ability to heal. Each and every one of us has seen this self-healing ability at one time or another in our own lives. So how do we activate this self-healing when dealing with a disease as aggressive as cancer?

Since most disease is caused by toxicity and/or nutritional deficiency it seems logical that both of these issues must be addressed simultaneously to give the body the best chance of recovering.

In the first section of this book we outlined the many toxins that interfere with normal bodily functions. Although it is unrealistic for anyone to completely remove every toxin from his or her environment great effort must be given to reducing our exposure to as many of these toxins as possible. While it might not be feasible to relocate your house because it is near power lines or in the middle of the city where smog is prevalent you need to focus on the ones that you can change, like what you put in your mouth and on your body.

Because most bodies have been devoid of sufficient nutrition for many years, which is why the cancer was able to take hold, we need to focus our attention on getting maximum nutrition to our cells (not just in our bodies) in the shortest time possible. This chapter will focus on providing the information and instruction on how to supercharge our bodies with nutrients. It will also introduce you to the concept of how to balance your life, the importance of juicing, the best foods to consume, and the benefits of BarleyMax®. You will learn the value of living food and why dead food is addictive. You will identify the areas in your life that need more balance such as rest, stress, hydration, diet, fresh air, exercise and emotional/spiritual health.

Nutrition is a major player when it comes to fighting cancer and winning the battle. Science, testimonies, even the Bible all point to the value of consuming foods that will support and revitalize the immune system which holds the supreme army that will win the war. Even as far back as the 1800's and 1900's medical doctors such as Hippocrates used food as a form of medicine recognizing the value and benefits of it. There are many ways to kill cancer cells so they don't develop and in their various stages of development. Antioxidants from vegetables are one powerful way.

Stop Feeding the cancer cells!

Cancer cells feed on two substances: Sugar and Fat

Sugar increases the growth and rapid reproduction of cancer cells. Alternative treatments now include giving a person fighting cancer, sugar followed by low doses of chemo. As the cancer cells open up to consume the sugar they also take in the chemo more directly. This technique is explained further in a later chapter.

Cancer cells are non-discriminating when it comes to sugar. In other words, even though fruit is good for a healthy person to consume, most fruit contains high concentrations of sugars and should be avoided to a large extent when fighting cancer. Obviously, all other kinds of sugars, refined carbohydrates and foods that break down into sugar (such as white flour products, white rice, white potatoes, white pastas, etc.) must be absolutely avoided.

The goal is to starve the cancer cells so they become weakened. This allows the immune system with its NK (natural killer) cells to work on killing them off entirely. There are a few fruits that are low in sugar and high in antioxidant capacity that will be discussed later.

Fats, even healthy ones can also fuel cancer cells. This includes healthy nuts, nut butters, avocados and almost all oils. While fats have the tendency to feed cancer cells, the body still needs some fat for proper body and brain function. With this in mind, a small amount of "healthy" fat should be consumed on a daily basis.

Daily Fat intake while fighting cancer:
– 1/4 avocado daily in a salad dressing or just cut it up on the salad.
Other essential fats include:
– 1 teaspoon of Pharmax Fish Oil (necessary for the Omega 3 and DHA)
– 2 teaspoons of Flax Oil (Omega 3). However, ground flax seeds should be used instead of flax oil if dealing with prostate cancer.

Remember, consume some fat, but keep the amounts to a minimum.

Since this is the diet most people consume daily, you will find a complete recovery diet laid out in this chapter to assist you in eating only the most highly nutritious foods.

Do Not Eat:

We must stop consuming those foods that are contributing causes to the problem, especially, when someone is dealing with cancer. The following foods should be totally removed from the diet:

- All forms of meat (pork, chicken, fish, beef — includes all wild game)
- Animal by-products — eggs, broth, gelatin, etc.
- Refined table salt
- All forms of sugar — including most fruits, corn syrup
- Artificial sweeteners
- White flour, white rice, white pasta, etc.
- All dairy products including milk, cheese, cottage cheese, butter, sour cream, yogurt, etc.
- All nuts, nut butters, some seeds, any food that is fat to the body (may have a few walnuts)
- All fats and oils with exception of small amounts of flax oil (except if fighting prostate cancer), small amounts of fish oil and small amount of avocado.

Section One, Toxicity, provided extensive research and an in-depth explanation as to why most of these foods are harmful and should never be consumed whether you have a disease or are trying to stay healthy.

While removing all of these foods may look daunting and unrealistic, it is easier to come to terms with this when we realize that the above items are partially responsible for our current sickened state.

What SHOULD Be Eaten?

Lots, and lots, and lots of raw vegetables — these are the super foods that will provide the body with the vitamins, minerals, trace minerals, antioxidants, phyto-chemicals, carotenoids, and enzymes that are vital to health and healing. You will want the largest variety of vegetables possible to ensure an array of all of these elements.

Dr. Russell Blaylock M.D. recommends a healthy person consume at least 10 servings of vegetables each day. If 10 servings is what a healthy person should consume then how much should someone trying to rebuild the body need? The simple answer is "the more the better" — 15 or 20 servings!

We will discuss in detail how to consume the large amounts of raw vegetables. The dark green leafy vegetables are of utmost importance as they are nutrient dense and have the added benefit of large amounts of chlorophyll.

The goal of the recovery program is to create an environment within the body that encourages and facilitates healing. To do this optimally, the body should be given nutrition, in the form of juice, throughout the day, every hour, every day.

Again, this may seem like a daunting task, but when compared to the side effects of chemotherapy, radiation and surgery, one would find this task to be easy and manageable with the only side effects being a bit of detoxification and improved health.

The Recovery Diet is a plant-based diet in which you consume 85% of your food in a whole, unprocessed, uncooked way. They are consumed mostly in juices, smoothies and salads that may be blended for greater nutritional absorption. It's not enough to get the nutrients into the body. What is vital is getting most of the vitamins and minerals to the cellular level so it can rebuild stronger cells. Remember, you have 100 trillion cells in your body. Every day, over 300 billion of them are dying off and new ones will be created. Each cell has the potential of being stronger or weaker than the one it is replacing. The strength of each cell is dependent on the nutrition it receives.

15% of the food consumed is cooked which can be in the form of cooked beans, steamed greens/vegetables, stir-frys, soups, and stews among others.

The most food you will be consuming every day will be in the form of freshly extracted vegetable juice.

The primary foods you will consume each day are leafy greens and vegetables, with small amounts of fruit and oil.

As we move through this chapter and the remainder of the book we'll share more of what can be eaten. There is a great variety of food options and although you may miss your former foods, you will find that when you become nutritionally "full" you will not crave those former foods. Additionally, we have developed a companion recipe book, *Unravel the Mystery, Simple, Effective, Nutritious Foods to Fight Cancer,* where you will find a large variety of recipes that were specially created with high levels of nutrients, low sugar and low fat in mind to enhance the immune system and assist the body in the healing process.

As important as diet is, we will show you how you must regain control over your life. This includes stress, rest, emotions, exercise and much more. To restore your health, you will need to look within.

> *"The best six doctors anywhere*
> *And no one can deny it*
> *Are sunshine, water, rest, and air*
> *Exercise and diet.*
> *These six will gladly you attend*
> *If only you are willing*
> *Your mind they'll ease*
> *Your will they'll mend*
> *And charge you not a shilling."*
>
> — Nursery rhyme quoted by Wayne Fields,
> What the River Knows, 1990

Chapter Twenty-Seven: Introduce Life Balance Concept

Our bodies are complex. Our mind, body and spirit work synergistically to make a complete being. Our goal is to create an environment for healing, so we must look at the situation holistically. Cancer and other diseases occur because the body becomes unbalanced. Perhaps the stress in our life has outweighed our ability to manage it; maybe workload requires less opportunity to eat well and rest; perhaps living from paycheck to paycheck is taking its toll; or the marriage is undergoing severe testing. Once these areas have been identified, they must be reversed to bring the body back into harmony. As incredible as the body is, the continuous assault will lead to impaired function setting the body up to develop disease.

Let's identify all of the areas of health and use a wagon wheel as an analogy. If any one or more of the spokes on the wheel is short or missing then it impacts the way the wagon of health will move.

When one area of the body is impaired, then the other areas try to compensate for it, but they will fail. Each organ is designed to accomplish one task and despite of all of its efforts, it cannot effectively do what another organ can do. If our physical body is strong, but we are mentally unstable, it will not be long until the body will weaken.

Below you will find ten areas of health that must stay in balance for the body to remain in vibrant health. Many of these areas will be discussed in more detail in other parts of this section but this gives an overview of them. As you review this list, evaluate your areas of health to see if you are out of balance in any of them.

1. Living Foods – Raw foods are the foods that God originally intended us to feed our bodies. We find

this in the book of Genesis. We call "raw foods" "living" because they still have their life force (enzymes) intact. These enzymes are required in the digestive process to ensure the nutrients are completely assimilated into the cells of the body. Cooking destroys

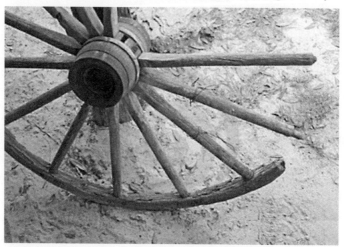

these heat sensitive compounds requiring the body to exert more energy through the digestive process. We believe that living bodies require living foods – ones that are still enzymatically alive. The goal should be to maintain a daily diet where 85% of the food you consume is raw, fresh, and whole in an uncooked state.

2. Dead Foods – If living foods are foods that contain enzymes then it is logical that foods without enzymes are "dead." But the real definition of "dead" food is if the food has been packaged or processed in any way. There are few exceptions, but nearly all food in a jar, can, box or package is "dead." If the ingredient list has more than one ingredient (the actual food!) then it would be considered "dead" food. Packaged and processed foods not only have no living enzymes, but worse, they include added sugars, fats and chemicals that require the body to work harder to not only digest the so called "food" but now it has to store or remove the additional toxic burden and begin repair

in all of the areas that this "food" damaged.

3. Cooked Foods – While cooking diminishes or destroys a percentage of vitamins and enzymes, it can also activate certain phytochemicals such as lycopene, lutein and carotenoids. Some proteins and starches are more readily available in cooked foods. It is best to consume digestive enzymes whenever we consume cooked foods to assist in the digestion of the food. Cooked food will comprise 15% of our daily food intake. Adding a cooked meal each day will prevent rapid weight loss and will help avoid headaches and fatigue, two of the side effects associated with detoxing too quickly. While cooked foods have many benefits consuming a predominately raw fruit and vegetable diet will provide the body with incredible healing abilities.

4. Stress – Stress increases the body's consumption of B vitamins as well as other important minerals. This level of depletion will set the stage for new cell growth that is not as healthy. Do you know how to manage your stress? Are there measures you can take to reduce any of the daily stress that is impacting your health? No one can live in a stress-free environment, but to recover fully, you must take steps to either learn to manage it or find ways to reduce it.

5. Rest – Never underestimate the power of sleep. The old saying, "I'll sleep when I'm dead," doesn't take into account that death could be sooner than intended if sleep isn't respected. As part of your evaluation, determine how many hours of uninterrupted sleep you get each night, how many of those hours are before midnight, and do you maintain your typical sleep routine even during the weekends? Try to sleep at least two or three hours before midnight so you can benefit from those hours. Every hour of sleep before midnight equates to two hours of sleep after 12:00 am. The hours between 1 and 3 am are important, as this is when the body does its deep cleansing of the

liver and kidneys. It is during sleep when the body cleanses, rebuilds and re-sets itself. If sleep is elusive, there is a separate section in this book with suggestions for improving sleep performance. Improved diet, daily exercise, and fresh air will likely improve sleep performance.

6. Sunlight – Vitamin D3, which is really a hormone, is created in the body when it has been exposed to adequate sunlight. Many people have been conditioned by the media and health care practitioners to avoid the sun. Unfortunately, by doing that, they have the potential for developing a vitamin D3 deficiency. Enriched food products do not provide the raw material the body needs to create the true vitamin D3. The research that links vitamin D3 to cancer has become quite prolific. In regions where you can get as much skin exposure to the sun as possible daily, for at least 30 minutes, the benefits will be evident. People tend to develop skin cancer due to dietary deficiencies and over exposure to the sun. The brief time we recommend in the sun along with the extensive nutrient rich diet that you will be on is a winning combination. Health experts agree that vitamin D3 supplementation is required for everyone who has cancer.

7. Emotional/Mental Health – People must take control over what they think. Especially those with a cancer diagnosis. First, they cannot let fear overcome their thought process. Second, if there are relationships that result in negative thinking, it is best to confront those immediately and repair them, not for the sake of the other person, but for your own sake. It is difficult for the body to heal when fear, anger, resentment, rage, self-pity and feelings of inadequacy are present.

8. Cleansing – The toxins that have accumulated over the years must be removed from the body for the body to heal. The elements of the recovery program will help facilitate the cleansing process. The juices, living foods and supplements are powerful cleansers

inside your body. Another way to describe cleansing is detoxification and sometimes there can be a little discomfort associated with this process. A separate section entitled Healing Reactions will prepare you for any potential discomfort you may experience while your body is purging the toxins and the waste. It will also give tips on how to accelerate the detoxification experience. Emotional and spiritual cleansing is vitally important in this process as well.

9. Pure air – Take a moment and watch how you breathe. Do you take quick, short breaths or is your diaphragm moving up and down quite regularly? How often are you taking deep breaths? Oxygen is vital to the person fighting cancer. Cancer doesn't like oxygen. So, learn how to breathe to get oxygen deep into the cells of your body as often as possible. If stress and fear are causing you to breathe shallow, then find ways to reduce or eliminate these factors. Make a concerted effort to breathe deeply throughout the day. Also, ensure that you are breathing in pure, quality air that is not stale, contaminated by exhaust, smoke or other elements that your body will have to expend energy to defuse.

10. Pure water – Cell dehydration causes great damage to the body and its cell formation. Many people who develop cancer are dehydrated. Most of the substances that people drink throughout the day are dehydrating instead of hydrating. These include sodas, coffees and teas. Drinking plenty of fresh, pure water will not only hydrate your cells but aide in the detoxification process that your body needs to go through as it rebuilds. Tap water is detrimental to your recovery. So is any bottled water that is in a flimsy, BPA lined plastic bottle. The best water you can drink is either steam-distilled water that is not in a gallon plastic jug or alkalized, ionized water. Additional information on these types of water is available in a separate chapter.

11. Spiritual – For complete balance, you must begin the process of examining your life in the spiritual component. This book is based on the biblical belief that God has created life and in abundance. To rely on oneself during this time (or any other time) is a great mistake. To recognize that you are weak and He is strong is a major step in creating that much needed balance in your life. Going to Him with your fears, concerns and needs will guide you into a relationship with the One who created you. This will result in a greater sense of peace, awareness and likely increased health.

The wagon wheel is comprised of each of these components. If one of them is lacking or there is an overage of another, there is no way the wagon can move smoothly. The wheel relies on each spoke so it can move the wagon.

Take a look at your life; use this guide to help balance your priorities, which right now the first one is your health.

"Sorry, there's no magic bullet. You gotta eat healthy and live healthy to be healthy and look healthy. End of story."
—Morgan Spurlock

Chapter Twenty-Eight: Juicing

"Health is the natural condition. When sickness occurs, it is a sign that Nature has gone off course because of a physical or mental imbalance. The road to health for everyone is through moderation, harmony, and a 'sound mind in a sound body'."
—Jostein Gaarder

Juicing is the most efficient way to get large amounts of nutrients to the cells of the body. If we consume a whole, raw carrot and our digestive system is working optimally, we will assimilate at the most, only about 30% of the nutrients. Most people who are sick are suffering from a weakened digestive system and are not receiving much nutrition from the foods they eat. But, if we take that same carrot and run it through a juicer and then consume the juice from that carrot over 90% of the nutrients will reach our cells. We call juicing the "secret sauce" that helps the body recover. The importance of juicing cannot be over stressed. When trying to create an environment for healing within the body, vegetable juice is vital.

There are many reasons consuming fresh vegetable juice assists in creating an environment for healing within the body:

1. More nutrients reach the cells – Fresh vegetable juice is nutrient dense!

Digestion normally starts in the mouth where we are "supposed to chew" foods 30 to 50 times (not many people do) to start breaking down the food into small particles. Chewing starts the process of releasing the nutrients (juice) that are locked in the fiber of the food.

167

The process of digestion involves the separation of the juice (nutrition) from the fiber (carrier of the nutrients). All of the nutrients contained in the plant are in the juice; the fiber is only the carrier for the nutrients. When we look at maximizing nutrition we utilize juicing to separate the juice (nutrition) from the fiber (carrier) so the body is able to more efficiently absorb the vitamins and minerals at the cellular level.

When consuming juice the body doesn't have to work so hard on digesting the food which conserves energy allowing more of the nutrition to reach the cells rather than being burned up through the digestive process. Think about how you feel after eating a large meal. Most people feel tired and want to take a nap. This is because the body has to divert blood and energy to assist in the digestion of the foods. With juicing, the digestion is virtually done by the juice extractor allowing the body to use its energy to heal rather than digest.

2. Consume more vegetables!

Imagine eating 2 pounds of carrots each day, chewing each bite 30 to 50 times. Two 8-ounce glasses of juice equal 2 pounds of carrots and can be easily consumed. In fact, many people who are battling cancer drink 6 to 8 glasses of carrot juice per day. That is equivalent to 6 to 8 pounds of whole carrots. Talk about a daunting task to undertake each day. This is one of the keys to the amazing results that many people have experienced on the Hallelujah Recovery Diet. Many people have consumed as much as 1/2 gallon or more of fresh juice a day to help them regain their health. An abundance of fresh vegetable juice is often the key to rebuilding health and maintaining a high level of energy while the body is rebuilding and under stressful conditions.

Important Note: Avoid drinking fruit juices as they are high in concentrated sugars. We discussed in an earlier section that cancer feeds on sugar but even if someone is healthy and doesn't have cancer they shouldn't consume much fruit juice because of the sugar content. Even when someone is healthy we say to "Eat your fruits and juice your vegetables."

3. Nutrition gets to the cells faster – in just minutes!

Digestion of foods can take hours as the body doesn't really start absorbing the nutrients until the food has been digested and enters the small intestine. When juice is consumed the nutrients start to reach the cells within minutes as the juice is in a sense pre-digested through the juicing process. The body's digestive system is bypassed.

4. Juicing is great for detoxification!

Juicing is filled with living enzymes that help the body build healthy new cells and push the old, diseased ones out. This is a continuous process that needs time; therefore consistent, daily juicing is important.

What Makes a Great Juicer?

All juicers are not created equally. As discussed previously, enzymes are the life force essential to fully utilizing the nutrition in the vegetables. Enzymes are sensitive and can easily be damaged by exposure to oxygen or heat. While the process of juicing involves separating the juice (nutrients) from the pulp (carrier) it must be done with care to preserve as much of the enzymes and nutrients as possible. There are three primary types of juicers on the market today:

Centrifugal Force Juicer – This type of juicer is common and relatively inexpensive as compared to all the juicers on the market. They have a spinning basket that rotates at speeds up to 4000 revolutions per minute (RPM). Because of the way this type of juicer extracts the juice, the enzymes are significantly damaged because the juice is exposed to a lot of oxygen while spinning in the fast moving basket. Because of the reduced enzyme activity found in the juice after using this type of juicer, it is not recommended that these types of juicers be used for people trying to rebuild their bodies while fighting cancer. As price is always a consideration and these juicers are the least costly, if this is the only option, then one should ensure they consume the juice as soon after juicing as possible (within 10 to 15 minutes) since the enzymes continue to break down rapidly. It is not recommended that juice from a centrifugal force juicer be stored for any period of time after being prepared. Typical prices range from under $100 to $200. The one that seems to maintain the enzymes the best in this category is the Juice Man Jr. These types of juicers work well in juicing carrots, beets, celery and other hard vegetables. They don't work well with greens like collard, Swiss chard or kale.

Pros:
– Easy to use
– Few parts to clean
– Low cost
Cons:
– Doesn't retain the enzymes effectively
– Doesn't juice greens like collard greens, swiss chard or kale well
– Juice can't be stored and must be consumed immediately

Masticating – This type of juicer has a spinning knife blade that rotates at approximately 1700 RPM's. The Champion juicer is the one that is most common in this category. Significantly more enzymes are preserved through the juicing process since the juice isn't pressed through a spinning basket but rather a stationary strainer. The juice from the Champion can be stored for up to three days though it typically tastes the best when it is consumed within 48 hours. The Champion juicer produces excellent carrot and beet juice. It doesn't do as well with greens like collard greens, Swiss chard or kale. There is a greens attachment that can be purchased separately to facilitate the juicing of greens. When juicing celery it is best to cut the stalks into one-inch strips so the celery strands don't become wrapped around the blade creating heat from the motor of the juicer. The heat generated from this friction will cause the juicer to heat up resulting in lost enzymes in the juice. The Gerson Clinic uses the Champion juicer in its cancer clinic in Mexico. You can expect to pay about $300 for the juicer and about another $90 for the greens juicing attachment. The Champion juicer is easy to use producing good quality juice.

For a little extra cost, the commercial version of the Champion juicer may be a better option if you know the juicer will be running daily and making large amounts of juice. The commercial version has a larger motor and a stainless steel shaft.

Pros:
– Easy to use
– Easy to clean

– Increased enzymes are retained
– Works well with most vegetables like carrots, beets, celery, etc.
– Proven to be effective when rebuilding the body
– Juice can be stored for 48 hours
Cons:
– Celery must be cut into short lengths
– Doesn't juice greens like kale, collard greens or kale well
– Greens attachment is an additional cost
– Gets warm with use

Slow Single Auger – As a single auger moving at a slow speed between 47 and 85 RPM this juicer makes great quality juice. The enzyme activity is very good as the juice is pressed out of the vegetables. There are two primary models the Hurom and the Tribest SlowStar. Both are nearly identical in how they function. They do equally well on both hard and soft vegetables. The big advantage to these juicers is that pushing the produce through the feeding shoot is virtually effortless. The down side to these juicers is they are not as efficient (pulp stays moist) and more fiber gets into the juice. The price for these units is around $400.

Pros:
– Easy to use
– Juices greens and carrots well
Cons:
– Less juice from produce
– More fiber gets through to the juice

Twin Gear Juicers – These types of juicers have slow turning gears that press the juice out of the vegetables. The gears/augers rotate between 85 and 110 RPM's depending on the specific one being used. The enzyme activity found in the juice is exceptional because the produce goes through a pressing process where the juice is actually squeezed out of the vegetables. Our model of choice is the Green Star Elite. Though there are other brands and models available on the market, we have found the Green Star to be dependable, producing consistent results. When stored properly, the juice from the Green

Star can be stored for three full days while maintaining good enzyme activity. The Green Star not only does well juicing hard vegetables like carrots, beets and celery but is excellent for greens too. Typically, a Green Star Elite sells for a little over $500. With this type of juicer, more effort is required to push the carrots into the unit. If the person using the juicer is frail, then it would be best to select the Champion juicer. Cleaning can take longer as there are more pieces that need to be cleaned. Many consider the Green Star Elite to be the Cadillac of juicers.

Pros:
– Pulls the greens through easily
– Outstanding juice quality
– Juice can be stored for 72 hours
Cons:
– Requires more effort to juice carrots
– Harder to clean

Juice, Juice, Juice – Juicing takes a concerted effort and it's not always easy. Here are some tips that you might find helpful with whatever juicer you choose to use:

1. Get into a juicing routine. The more consistent you can be with juicing, the easier it will be to fit it into your busy life. Plan to spend a couple of hours making enough juice to last three days.
2. Use the freshest produce possible. This produces better quality juice that retains its freshness longer.
3. Keep the vegetables cold before juicing.
4. Keep the juice cool throughout the juicing process. Consider putting a bag of ice in the juice to keep the juice chilled.
5. Consider purchasing a box of 8 oz. Mason jars to store the juice. It's best to drink 8 oz at a time and not to store the juice in containers that are larger than the amount that will be consumed at one time.
6. Immediately place the juice into the refrigerator.
7. Don't store the juice in the refrigerator for more than 3 days. Bacteria begins to develop after the 3 days.

8. Juice can be frozen to extend the shelf life. Understand that about 15% of the enzymes are lost through the freezing process. Consume all frozen juice within 2 weeks.
9. Wash the produce in cool or cold water before juicing.
10. Clean the juicer as soon as possible after juicing. This makes it easier to clean, especially the screen.
11. Don't be too concerned with only using organic produce. 85% of the pesticide residue stays with the pulp leaving only 15% in the juice. Of course, if organic is available and practical this would be the absolute best.
12. Peeling carrots is purely a personal decision. Unlike other produce like apples or grapes, there aren't more nutrients in the carrot peel. People usually note that juice made from peeled carrots tastes sweeter than if the carrots are just washed.
13. Ensure that splits are cut out of the carrots as bacteria usually hides in these crevices.
14. It's ideal to have a combination of carrot and greens in the juice. About 70% carrots and 30% other vegetables.
15. Remember "Food Synergy." This will be discussed in a later section of this book.

How many variations of greens and veggies do I juice each day?

At least 2 different leafy greens
At least 3 different vegetables (one will always be carrot)
1 fruit

Our companion book *Unravel the Mystery: Simple, Effective, Nutritious Recipes to Fight Cancer* has 29 different juice recipes that were specially created for people who are fighting cancer.

You may want to choose different leafy greens and vegetables each week or twice a week. The flavor will change for variety, but more importantly, the nutrition will change so your body will get different minerals, vitamins and other important nutrients.

Have fun making different combinations of juice. Remember, using a variety of vegetables helps to provide variety of flavor and nutrients.

- Kale
- Collard
- Swiss Chard
- Dandelion
- Spinach
- Bok Choy
- Watercress
- Beet Greens
- Cabbage
- Broccoli stems
- Zucchini
- Jicama
- Parsley
- Cilantro
- Bitter or hot greens such as turnip greens, arugula, mustard greens, daikon greens (Use sparingly as they make the juice a little bitter)
- Carrots
- Cucumber
- Celery
- Beet (Start with small amounts then increase. Beets are a great liver detoxifier but can cause headaches if too much is used too quickly)
- Ginger
- Garlic
- Brussels sprouts

The only fruits we recommend a cancer patient add to their vegetable juices are below. If the juice is too bitter there is a great possibility that it won't be consumed.

- Granny Smith apple – in small amounts to help make the juice palatable.
- Lemons

- Limes
- Cucumbers
- Tomato (use sparingly as it is a fruit with a high amount of sugar)

Adding a small amount of jalapeño pepper, onion, garlic, red pepper, lemon, lime or ginger works well to enhance the flavor.

Some people only juice carrots, while others exclusively juice all green vegetables. You decide what you prefer.

The most important factor in selecting a juicer is picking one that will actually be used. Many people buy a juicer, use it a few times then put it away and don't use it much. Having freshly extracted juice is paramount to supporting the body's healing and every effort should be made to use whatever juicer is selected. Great value is received when consuming juice from even the cheapest and least effective juicer. Don't use the fact that the better juicers are too expensive to keep you from consuming any juice. Every bit of juice makes a difference.

What about blood sugar issues?

Many people who fight cancer have severe blood sugar issues. Those who do, will need to monitor their blood sugar and begin to drink the carrot/green juice blend slowly, perhaps introducing less carrot and more greens. This gradual approach has assisted many people in their recovery and soon they find that their blood sugar has begun to normalize and they can increase their carrot juice intake without compromising their blood sugar levels.

Carrot juice has an excellent source of beta-carotene that turns into the powerful vitamin A when ingested that has been validated as an excellent antioxidant to fight cancer. It is a tremendous tool in the battle.

Storing the Juice

After the juice is prepared it should be strained an additional time with a hand strainer to ensure that as much of the fiber as possible is removed. If storing the juice, it should be put into containers the same size as you would normally drink at one time – 8 oz. These containers should be filled as full as possible so there is no air remaining. If the juice is put in a larger container, like 16 oz. and only 8 oz. is consumed then there will be a lot of air or oxygen in the bottle with the juice. This will start to break down the enzymes in the remaining juice.

If storing juice in freezer, use the same size jars but only fill them to about a half inch from the top to allow for expansion. Freeze juice for two weeks.

Many health experts recommend that a "healthy" person consumes 10 servings of raw vegetables every day. Imagine how much is needed for a person who is dealing with something like cancer. 15 to 20 servings wouldn't be excessive. The only way to consume this much produce is through juicing and blended salads.

Note: There are no juices on the shelves of the grocery stores that will provide the living enzymes, vitamins, minerals or other nutrients that freshly extracted juices will. That is because those juices on the shelves have been pasteurized. Though they may look inviting and much easier, they will never provide your body with the building blocks it needs to fight the cancer.

Blending vs. Juicing

Both blended smoothies and freshly extracted vegetable juices offer an abundance of nutrients and enzymes. Although some people refer to high-powered blenders as "juicers", blenders retain the fiber, whereas juicers are specially designed to separate the fiber, leaving only the liquid, bypassing the digestion process. Blended ingredients still need to go through the human digestion process because of the fiber content.

When the juice is separated from the pulp, you can easily consume a much larger volume of vegetables than you could by drinking a smoothie containing pulp.

Juicing does not replace salads and smoothies. A diet solidly grounded in whole foods filled with fiber is foundational to a healthy diet. Smoothies, blended soups and blended salads are excellent meal replacements. Because they are filling and substantial due to their fiber content, they keep us from desiring so much cooked food. They are encouraged on the Hallelujah Recovery Diet, but they cannot replace juicing. If we consume both smoothies and juices, we are receiving the best of both worlds. The best vitamin and mineral complement to a whole food diet is plenty of freshly extracted vegetable juice especially when attempting to combat a serious illness.

Chapter Twenty-Nine: BarleyMax®

"Life is a tragedy of nutrition"
—Arnold Ehret

The cereal grasses (barley, alfalfa, wheat, oat, rye) are an amazing part of a healthy diet. They provide an amazing array of nutrients that nourish and promote health and healing within the body. For years they have been studied as scientists tried to fully understand the mechanism within the plants that provide such wonderful benefits. Why are they so powerful in maintaining and restoring health? The term Grass Juice Factor has been established to represent the unique characteristic these cereal grasses provide.

Here is a timeline of studies performed using cereal grasses:

1930 – Summer milk vs. winter milk – rats and guinea pigs thrived on summer milk but became sick and died on winter milk.

1931 – Research on chickens found that by adding 10% cereal grasses to the hen's standard feed realized the following results:
– Winter egg production increased from 38% to 94%
– Stronger shells
– Hatched healthier chicks
– Hens were free of degenerative diseases common to poultry production

1940 – Enhanced fertility of laying hens, supports growth of beneficial bacteria, blocked the development of scur-

vy
1950 – Promotes healing of peptic ulcers
1960 – Improves utilization of vitamin A
Source – *Cereal Grasses: Natures Greatest Health Gift* by Ronald L. Seimold.

The grains must be consumed in their young, grassy state. This valuable nutrition is only in their grass, not in their berries. Typically grain causes an acid residue when introduced to the body. But, if harvested at a young, tender age when the leaves are small and tasteful, the benefits are astounding.

Dark green leafy vegetables are "blood-building" foods as they provide essential vitamins and minerals for the synthesis of healthy blood. They help improve the immune system as they are rich in folate, vitamin C, potassium and magnesium, as well as containing a host of phytochemicals, such as lutein, beta-cryptoxanthin, zeaxanthin, and beta-carotene.

Dr Yoshihide Hagiwara, a Japanese researcher with extensive research into barley grass corroborated early research on the Grass Juice Factor. Dr. Hagiwara tested over 150 green leaved plants and concluded – "Of all the plants I tested, the young leaves of barley and certain other cereal grasses proved throughout my testing to have the most remarkable quantities of active ingredients."

Chlorophyll is another powerful element found within barley and alfalfa. H.E. Kirschner, M.D. said, "Chlorophyll, the healer, is at once powerful and bland – devastating to germs, yet gentle to wounded body tissues. Exactly how it works is still Nature's secret; [but] to the layman, at least, the phenomenon seems like green magic."

Rev. Malkmus, founder of Hallelujah Acres grew his own wheat grass in trays on the window sills of his home for years. He would harvest the grass and run it through a juice extractor. He never thought that barley grass that had been harvested in the field, then juiced and dehydrated into a powder could ever be as good as the fresh wheat grass juice he was consuming.

Then one day someone sent him a bottle of dehydrated barley juice powder. At first he didn't even want to try it. Eventually, he became curious and decided to give it a try. What he discovered was that the dehydrated powder gave him more energy and clearer thinking than what he had experienced through the juice grass he had been growing himself. This is what prompted Hallelujah Acres to start making BarleyMax®.

Many people have experienced its remarkable benefits, but making a barley grass juice product like BarleyMax® that preserves the delicate whole food synergy found in the cereal grasses is truly rare. It is a powerhouse of nutrition and vitality! We believe that it must be a part of the Hallelujah Recovery Diet.

Superior Drying Method

To appreciate the superior, proprietary drying method used to create BarleyMax®, it is important to understand the other three main juice-drying methods in the nutritional juice powder industry:

Standard Spray Drying - Juices are dried to powder quickly, however there is heat involved that reaches over 150 degrees F, which kills the living enzymes and heat sensitive nutrients. As the juice dries and the heat is turned up, the nutrition of the juice is compromised.

Freeze Drying - Typically touted as a higher quality drying process, freeze-drying still involves heat that kills live enzymes (130 degrees F). Depending on how much infrared heat is used; it can take from 12 to 72 hours to dry a batch of juice, which causes additional nutritional degradation. If dried too quickly (requiring high heat), freeze dried products can actually taste burned. Not to mention, freeze-drying requires that the liquid be concentrated before drying, which again involves heat and/or pasteurization.

Refractive Window Drying - This is a relatively new process in the industry, but it still involves enzyme-killing heat. Hot water in excess of 160 degrees F is used to quickly warm the liquid juice to dry it. Unfortunately, juice in its liquid form is most susceptible to nutritional degradation. Even though this is a quick process, it still subjects the juice to conditions that destroy its enzymatic, nutritive components.

The BarleyMax® Process – By contrast, the barley used for BarleyMax® is harvested, juiced, and dried all within a few hours (the fastest, freshest method in the industry) all without significant heat. BarleyMax® is not subjected to harsh sanitization processes that damage the beneficial bacteria and vital nutrients, as is the case with other processes.

When the young, highly nutritious leaves of barley are near the first jointing stage, they are cut without the grass ever touching the ground. The grass is then washed, ground, juiced, and chilled to stabilize the nutrients. Using a temperature of only 104-105 degrees F, the juice is then dried within two minutes into a stable powder with typical moisture of less than 7%.

Care is also taken to protect the fragile juice nutrients from oxidation. Carbon dioxide (CO_2) is injected into the juice prior to drying; this becomes CO_2 gas that surrounds the juice particles at the top of the dryer. The CO_2 dissipates as the drying particles fall to the bottom of the drier, but not until they have protected the juice during its wettest, most vulnerable state. So, the vitamins, minerals, and other nutrients are not oxidized when they reach the consumer.

Because the enzymes are so important for absorption of the nutrients and they are extremely fragile, testing enzyme levels in juice powders helps to understand the quality of the product and assures us heat sensitive nutrients have not been affected.

In June 2013, Dr. Michael Donaldson, PhD and director of research for Hallelujah Acres performed a test on BarleyMax® and other juice powders. He purchased 5 different green superfood powders from America's largest organic grocery chain. Some of these superfoods claim to be "raw," so he tested them for live enzyme activity to see if they really contained live enzymes.

Acid phosphatase was chosen as a marker enzyme because it is always found in abundance in raw foods (fruits, vegetables, nuts, and seeds) and its activity is representative of other enzymes as well.

When there is plenty of acid phosphatase detected, you can be certain that the other enzymes are present as well. But if the acid phosphatase is gone, or greatly diminished, then the rest of the enzymes have likewise been deactivated.

For comparison Dr. Donaldson also used an expired container of BarleyMax®. In fact, it had been expired since December 2012 (this test was performed in June 2013). An expired container was selected to reflect the worse case scenario for BarleyMax®.

In Figure 1 below, you can see the results. The closest competitor, who claims to be a raw food product, has only about 28% of the enzyme activity that you find in BarleyMax®. A few of the products had less than 2% of the activity found in BarleyMax®.

Figure 1.

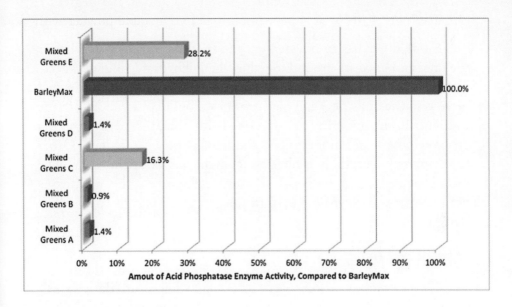

Amout of Acid Phosphatase Enzyme Activity, Compared to BarleyMax

Attention to Detail

Another key difference with the BarleyMax® process is timing. Exactly when the heat is applied makes a significant difference in the quality of the juice and resulting juice powder. If fresh barley juice was poured on to a warm stove top, the heat would significantly degrade enzymatic activity, chlorophyll content and other delicate nutrients. If the same thing were done with powder, the nutritional degradation would be substantially less. This example illustrates how the chemistry of juice is much more active and susceptible to degradation than a stabilized powder. Under the same principle, any unrefrigerated (unstabilized) fresh juice will begin to rot and grow mold. A powdered juice with low moisture (stable) will keep for years as long as it's kept cool and dry. When water is added, the moisture reactivates the chemistry of the liquid juice.

The science behind this example is the reason why the BarleyMax® process was designed to ensure that the majority of the drying process occurs when the temperature is relatively low (65F). Keeping the temperature low while the juice is still in liquid form locks in the nutritional integrity of the original, fresh juice before the heat peaks at

104-105 degrees F when the juice is closer to its powder form.

No Pulp, No Fillers

Some other barley powders on the market contain pulp; that is, the fiber and juice are ground together, then dehydrated and packaged. This is obviously not ideal. The reason pulp is removed in the first place is so the body does not have to digest fiber in order to absorb the nutrients in the juice. Juice that is free from fiber, then dehydrated, is far more potent and more easily assimilated at the cellular level. Other barley grass juices, though fiberless, contain maltodextrin to stabilize the nutrients. Again, with the BarleyMax® process this additive is not necessary. BarleyMax® is 100% juice carefully dried to a powder... that's it!

Whole Food Benefits

The proprietary process used to dry barley juice into BarleyMax® is unmatched. By taking extra care to preserve the vitamins, minerals and enzymes in barley, these synergistic co-factors operate in harmony as a stabilized whole food -- a true superfood -- which benefits the body more than any one nutrient could by itself.

Other Significant Factors

Specially selected barley grass seeds are grown in a mineral-rich, volcanic lakebed at an elevation of 5,000 feet. Slower growth at this elevation allows the plant to absorb maximum nutrition from the incredibly nutrient-rich soil. Harvested at just the right moment for peak nutrition, the barley grass is cut, washed, juiced, and dried with a patented drying process that retains the living nutrients -- all in just a few hours.

In the end, each 8.5 oz container of BarleyMax® contains the gluten-free, dehydrated juice of 15 pounds of freshly harvested barley grass, a much more nutrient-dense and better tasting alternative than freeze dried products or even freshly harvested "indoor" wheat grass.

A Complete Food

The rich scent, vibrant color, and delicious, fresh taste of Bar-

leyMax® are living proof of its pure nutrition and health promoting power — there's nothing else like it.
- Vitamins
- Minerals
- Essential amino acids
- Chlorophyll
- Flavonoids
- Trace elements
- Antioxidants
- Live enzymes

Plus, with its living enzymes and countless micronutrients, BarleyMax® offers one of the widest spectrums of naturally occurring nutrients in a single source.

BarleyMax® has been shown to protect human cells from DNA damage, the "biological rust" that plays a large role in aging and disease. As an added bonus, a study involving extract of barley leaf has shown to decrease LDL (bad) cholesterol!

Why Alfalfa?

An added ingredient in BarleyMax® is alfalfa. The Chinese have used alfalfa since the sixth century as treatment for many health conditions. It is considered the richest source of land source trace minerals because of its extensive root system. It has been noted that the benefits include supporting kidney problems, assisting with auto-immune disorders, supporting arthritis, nourishing the digestive, skeletal, glandular and urinary systems, cleansing the blood, liver and bowels, assisting with cholesterol, strokes, whooping cough as well as assisting to help maintain an overall sense of well being. BarleyMax® combines the juice of the young plants of alfalfa and barley in a way to maximize the benefits of both variety of cereal grasses.

People who regularly consume the Standard American Diet may find the flavor of BarleyMax® (original flavor) a little strong. Berry and Mint flavors are also available but there is about 15% less of the barley and alfalfa juices in these varieties to make room for the organic flavorings.

Because the juice from young barley and alfalfa plants are so nutrient dense and include the amazing "Grass Juice Factor," BarleyMax® should be a regular part of anybody's daily routine whether dealing with a serious physical problem or just trying to maintain vibrant health.

Study Reveals that BarleyMax® Protects DNA from Oxidative Damage

A recent test revealed that BarleyMax® prevents DNA damage. A Comet assay of colon cancer cells found that a diluted solution of BarleyMax® was able to protect the cells from DNA damage induced by hydrogen peroxide [1].

Throughout this book we have discussed that DNA damage is one of the initiating steps of many disease processes, including cancer. Our bodies have a three-fold defense against DNA damage – enzymes that disarm free radicals, small molecules that absorb free radicals (like uric acid), and dietary antioxidants to boost protection of DNA, lipids, and proteins.

The cells of our bodies are constantly bombarded with free radicals produced from the "fire" of oxygen-based metabolism. These free radicals cause biological "rust," making the systems of the body seize up and grind to a halt. Free radical damage plays a major role in disease and untimely deaths.

In this study, the HT29 cell line, a human colorectal adenocarcinoma cell line widely used as a colon cancer model, was selected. HT29 cells were incubated with BarleyMax® at various concentrations along with hydrogen peroxide for 1 hour. After thorough rinsing the cells were mixed with agarose gel and laid onto a microscope slide. Cells were then lysed, electrophoresed, the DNA was stained, and then individual cells were scored. Damaged DNA is shorter than intact DNA and moves quicker under the electrophoresis field, forming a tail that appears like a comet when visualized with fluorescent dye. The amount of DNA in the tail is quantified compared to the amount remaining within the cell nucleus. A bigger tail indicates greater DNA damage.

As shown in Figure 2, BarleyMax® at 0.03% significantly reduces DNA damage. At 0.25% BarleyMax® or higher the cells were almost completely protected; damage was reduced to about 10% of the negative control value.

This was an in vitro experiment, so the data cannot be directly

Figure 2, Effect of BarleyMax on H₂O₂-induced DNA damage in HT29 cells in Comet assays#

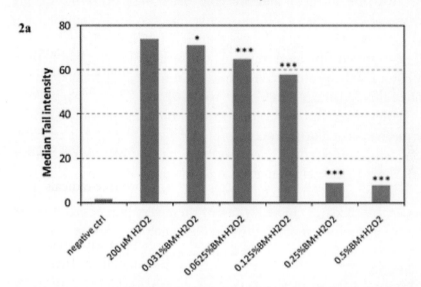

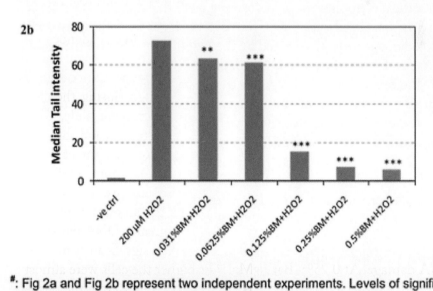

#: Fig 2a and Fig 2b represent two independent experiments. Levels of significant difference between H_2O_2 treated controls and asterisk sign indicated BarleyMax/H_2O_2 treatments: * = $p < 0.05$, ** = $p < 0.01$, *** = $p < 0.001$, in Mann-Whitney test.

applied to DNA protection in people. The Comet assay is widely used and accepted as a very sensitive method to detect DNA damage in single cells. In vitro results like these with BarleyMax® do correlate well with DNA protection of white blood cells in volunteers who consume kiwifruit juice [2], and broccoli sprouts [3]. Also, the Comet assay was able to detect DNA protective effects of eating spinach and tomato puree [4], and blood orange juice [5]. Whole diet effects can even be captured. The fecal water of volunteers who ate a diet high in fat and meat, when compared to a low-fat, low-meat diet, caused twice as much DNA damage in a Comet assay [6].

BarleyMax® has DNA-protective properties, possibly by multiple mechanisms. For maximum protection an optimal diet and lifestyle must be followed. BarleyMax® can be part of that protection. BarleyMax® is the dehydrated juice from young barley grass and alfalfa. It is the juice from a whole food, replete with all of the vitamins, minerals, antioxidants, and enzymes of these very potent green foods. It has been carefully processed so that as much as possible of the vibrancy, taste, and life of the fresh juice is preserved for convenient consumption.

Damaged DNA is shorter than intact DNA and moves quicker under the electrophoresis field, forming a tail that appears like a "comet" when visualized with fluorescent dye. A bigger tail indicates greater DNA damage; this is indicated by the height of the bar on the graph; the taller the bar, the more DNA damage.

The first column is a negative control, a "vehicle" control; the experiment procedure itself does not induce noticeable DNA damage.

The second column is a positive control, where the cells are incubated with hydrogen peroxide. Concentration of the hydrogen peroxide is 200 micromolar. Clearly there is a lot of DNA damage.

The next columns are cells incubated with the same amount of hydrogen peroxide and increasing amounts of BarleyMax®.

As the amount of BarleyMax® was increased the cells were protected more and more until there was almost no damage of the DNA, compared to the "vehicle" control.

Each treatment with BarleyMax® is twice as much as the next column on the left.

Chapter Thirty: Living Food

"The doctor of the future will be oneself."
—Albert Schweitzer

The term live food refers to raw, uncooked, and sprouted vegetables, fruits, seeds and nuts, not heated above approximately 108 degrees Fahrenheit, consumed for optimizing health, reversing disease, as well as delicious taste. The terms "live" or "living" food are used to differentiate the inclusion of sprouted and growing plants from simply raw harvested plants such as leaves, fruits, and vegetables. Kristine Nolfi, MD is credited with creating the term "living food" in the 1940's to describe the diet when writing about healing herself of breast cancer with raw vegan foods. Live, raw, living foods are not cooked, microwaved, or irradiated, and ideally are organic, that is, grown without the use of chemical pesticides, herbicides, fertilizers, or genetic modification. Heating above 108 degrees destroys the beneficial enzymes, micronutrients, chemistry, and life force of plants crucial to human health.

Why Live Food?

Living plant material is the ultimate nutrient delivery system for the body because it contains much more than just vitamins and minerals; it contains complex living energies that plants absorb from nature. While there is much talk about why raw plant material is restorative to the body and mind, science is showing that uncooked plants contain enzymes, phytonutrients, structured water, micro-clustered elements and minerals, and other nutrients that are perfectly designed to operate within our human physiology and optimize its functions.

187

Plants take water, air, and nutrients from the soil, and convert sunlight into their physical matter. Living food plant material contains exactly what our bodies need, and when we eat it we are consuming solidified solar energy. A live vegan diet and balanced lifestyle work to regain and maintain health where other approaches fail.

A Short History of Live Food

Although often presented in the media as a new fad diet, the concept of eating uncooked food is not new, predating the discovery of cooking by fire. Humans are the only creatures on this planet that cook their food, and consequently, we have far more disease than wild animals.

We believe the living food diet and lifestyle started in the Garden of Eden as stated in Genesis 1:29. God gave Adam and Eve a garden and told them the fruit of the trees was their food. It has also been found with the Essenes over 2000 years ago, with detailed descriptions in the Dead Sea Scrolls for healing and optimizing health. The ancient Greek biographer Diogenes Laertius noted that 500 BC, philosopher and mathematician Pythagoras forbade his followers to eat meat, and espoused a raw vegetarian diet to "derive health of body and acuteness of intellect." Ancient Greek physician Hippocrates, father of medicine whose name and principles are the foundation for modern medicine's Hippocratic Oath, used a live vegan diet for healing. Socrates, Plato, and Aristotle also promoted vegan diets.

As evidenced historically, many people have found living foods to be instrumental in the process of restoring their health.

Not All Produce is Created Equal

When we go the grocery store and look at the produce we have to ask ourselves a few questions:

1. What type of soil were the vegetables grown? Soil that has been depleted of nutrients will have limited vitamins and minerals because they weren't available to the plant's root system. Commercially grown produce is commonly lacking in many nutrients, especially, trace minerals.
2. How long has it been since the produce was picked?

As produce begins to age the enzymes that are naturally present begin to break down the plant resulting in less nutrition.

3. Was the product ripe when it was harvested? Many fruits and vegetables are picked unripe so they last longer in the supermarket before going bad. Some vegetables and fruits like tomatoes are harvested green then artificially ripened when they get close to their destination.

4. Were pesticides, fertilizers, and other chemicals designed to prevent bugs, inhibit mold or increase growth used?

When we realize that the foods we consume is used by the body as medicine we start looking at the quality of the produce to ensure that we are getting maximum nutrition (value) for our dollars and efforts.

Here Are Some Tips for Purchasing Produce:

1. Shop locally as much as possible. Use the farmers markets or local produce stands throughout the year. Ask the local growers how the plants were grown. Did they use pesticides? You can usually tell if the vegetables are grown naturally as they will have more blemishes, little worms and be less perfect. Lettuce leaves might have little holes. Squash and tomatoes might have bug marks. These are naturally occurring.

2. Focus on foods that are in season. They will most likely be fresher as they didn't have to travel across the country to get to the market.

3. Consume a variety of produce. Include many different colors of vegetables into your diets.

4. Dark leafy greens are the feeders – lots of Swiss chard, collard greens, kale and spinach.

While it isn't necessary to only use organically grown produce the nutritional level will be greater and the chemical residue will be less. We would typically say that the health benefits of consuming fruits and vegetables far outweighs the risks from pesticide exposure however, when the body is working so hard to heal, even small amounts of pesticide residue will cause it to work harder.

Organic foods are typically more expensive than conventionally grown produce. Below you will find a list of the fruits and vegetables with the most amounts of pesticides. If available, these items should be purchased organically. The smaller the number in this list the greater the pesticide residue.

1. Apples
2. Strawberries
3. Grapes
4. Celery
5. Peaches
6. Spinach
7. Sweet Bell Peppers
8. Nectarines - Imported
9. Cucumbers
10. Potatoes
11. Cherry Tomatoes
12. Hot Peppers
13. Blueberries
14. Lettuce
15. Snap Peas

Below are the fruits and vegetables with the least amount of pesticides residue. The lower the number indicates the least amount of pesticides.

1. Sweet Corn
2. Onions
3. Pineapples
4. Avocados
5. Cabbage
6. Sweet Peas
7. Papayas
8. Mangos
9. Asparagus
10. Kiwi

11. Grapefruit
12. Cantaloupe
13. Sweet Potatoes
14. Mushrooms
15. Watermelons

The Environmental Working Group generated the above lists after analyzing pesticide residue testing data from the U.S. Department of Agriculture and Food and Drug Administration [1].

Genetically modified plants, or GMOs, were discussed in the toxicity section but it is important to consider GMO when purchasing produce. GMO isn't often found in the produce section of grocery stores. Field corn, nearly all of which is produced with genetically modified seeds, is used to make processed foods like tortillas, chips and corn syrup. It is also used heavily in animal feed and biofuels. Soy is another heavily GMO crop that makes its way into processed food.

The genetically modified crops likely to be found in produce aisles of American supermarkets are yellow crooked neck squash, zucchini, Hawaiian papaya and some varieties of sweet corn. Most Hawaiian papaya is a GMO. Only a small fraction of zucchini and sweet corn are GMO. Since U.S. law does not require labeling of GMO produce, it is advised that people who want to avoid it to purchase the organically grown versions of these items [1].

Chapter Thirty-One: Cooked Food

"Healthy citizens are the greatest asset any country can have."
—Winston Churchhill

Eating raw food is absolutely necessary when battling cancer and for regaining health. Raw foods are the foundation for an optimal diet and are necessary for effective digestion and proper bowel movements. They must be the foundation of any healthy diet. But should one's entire diet consist of only raw food? Eating an entirely raw food diet has many drawbacks and is not the healthiest way to live.

Eating many cooked foods will have negative impacts on our health but there are some foods that when steamed or made into soups will add significant value and enhance one's overall level of health. The inclusion of cooked foods, that are prepared properly, is necessary to regain and maintain health.

When food is baked at high temperatures and especially when it is fried or barbecued toxic compounds called acrylamides are formed. Another result of high heat is that most of the vital nutrients are lost. Many vitamins are water-soluble, and a significant percentage can be lost with cooking, especially when overcooked. Also, most of the plant enzymes that function as phytonutrients in our body are destroyed by overcooking.

Exposing foods to high temperatures through baking, browning, barbecuing and other methods should be avoided.

When cooked for shorter periods of time and in small amounts of liquid, only small amounts of nutrients will be lost and many nutrients will actually have increased absorbability.

Making soups and steaming vegetables are the healthiest forms of cooking. Don't overcook. Remove from the heat when the vegetables become soft but when they still have some crunch. Boiling vegetables is less desirable because many of the nutrients will be discarded with the water after the vegetables are removed.

Sometimes, cooking can actually destroy some of the harmful anti-nutrients that bind minerals in the gut and interfere with the utilization of nutrients. Destruction of these anti-nutrients increases absorption. Steaming vegetables and making vegetable soups breaks down cellulose and alters the plants' cell structures making digestion easier.

Roasted nuts and baked cereals reduces the availability and absorbability of protein and should be avoided. Certain foods, especially fruit, avocado and nuts undergo significant change with cooking and are best eaten raw.

Studies verify that significantly more of the beneficial anti-cancer nutrients (carotenoids and phytonutrients – especially lutein and lycopene) are absorbed when consuming cooked vegetables as compared with raw. There may not have been as much absorption if they had been consumed raw.

Digestibility and absorption of many beneficial nutrients are significantly increased when we cook beans. Eating beans in soups increases the plant protein in the diet, this is especially important. Even most essential nutrients in vegetables are made more absorbable after being cooked in a soup. And water-soluble nutrients are not lost because the liquid portion of the soup is consumed too. A benefit of eating steamed vegetables and soups is that it expands nutrient diversity.

Beyond the many health benefits of cooked food there are also psychological benefits too. It is difficult being all-raw, especially in cold winter months. Having a bowl of hot soup can calm the nerves and emotions.

So, keep the salad as your main dish and then enjoy the benefits of healthy, cooked foods prepared the healthiest way.

Chapter Thirty-Two: Cleansing

"Poor health is not caused by something you don't have; it's caused by disturbing something that you already have. Healthy is not something that you need to get, it's something you have already if you don't disturb it."

—Dean Ornish

Cleansing is the process of removing waste, toxins, sludge, hormones, and so on that have taken up residence in the body but with healthy eating the body has finally mustered up enough energy to do some major housecleaning. There are several routes that the toxins can be removed, but all of the pathways must be open and ready for the removal. There are the primary routes and the secondary routes.

Primary Routes

The primary routes of elimination all have direct access to the outside of the body. They are a transition point between normal bodily processing and excretion. Ensuring optimal function of all six primary routes is essential to regaining health.

1. Bowels – This is a major route of elimination of toxins from the body. As food is ingested, it passes through the digestive tract and is continually broken down. Nutrients are absorbed along the way. What the body cannot utilize is then eliminated in the stool. Toxins and waste are eliminated in the stool, thus protecting the body from toxic accumulation. You should empty

your bowels not once but two or three times every day – there should be an urge after every meal. A healthy stool should break up easily and not be a strain to pass. It should resemble a long broomstick that can easily break into shorter pieces. Don't be surprised if the color resembles the color of your food.

Here are some of the negative impacts and possible indicators of colon dysfunction due to clogging:

- Obesity
- Body odor
- Fatigue and lethargy
- Constipation
- Chronic halitosis (bad breath)
- Unclear thinking
- Diarrhea
- Fibromyalgia
- Digestive pain
- Depression
- Grinding teeth
- Nervousness
- Drooling while sleeping

2. Bladder – The main function of the bladder is to store and release urine. The complex urinary system filters blood through the kidneys as a means of maintaining health and proper pH within the body. The urinary system is the primary system responsible for excretion of metabolic waste. Uric acid and nitrogen, from protein breakdown, are the major metabolic bi-products excreted in the urine. Consume adequate amounts of liquids so the urine is a pale yellow to nearly clear color. This will help to keep the toxins moving through the urinary system.

3. Skin – Elimination of toxins and carbon dioxide from the skin is achieved through sweating. Sweat stimulated by exercise, fever, environment (i.e. summer weather, saunas, steam room etc.) is a way for the body to rid itself of toxins that are stored in fat

tissues.

– This is our largest single organ.

– Eliminates over twice as much by weight as the bowels - each day.

– Bathing washes away residues (use only natural moisturizer such as cold-pressed organic olive oil, coconut butter or avocado oil)

4. Breathing – The lungs are responsible for the elimination of carbon dioxide with every breath. Carbon dioxide in a naturally occurring toxin in the body. The lungs are the largest and most important internal elimination organs. They exchange over 12,000 quarts of air every day. Breathing is a major way for the body to maintain homeostasis. The pH balance in the body is achieved through breathing and optimal kidney function.

5. Voice – The voice is an important way for the body to eliminate emotional toxins. The expression of true emotions and organic feelings through voice allows the body the opportunity to express and release emotions. The proper release of emotions whether positive or negative is an important part of detoxification and elimination for the body.

6. Menstruation – Menses is a primary route of elimination for women. Monthly, women are awarded an additional opportunity to detoxify and eliminate toxins from the body. As blood and uterine lining are shed the body can eliminate unwanted waste. Dark, heavy painful menstruation is a sign of excess toxins in the system. Menstruation should be a natural, pain-free process that the body cycles through every 28 days.

For the first 90 days on the Recovery Program, FiberCleanse is used to facilitate the removal of toxins from within the body. With its 28 herbs, psyllium based FiberCleanse works synergistically within the body to perform a complete, full body detox. It helps to mobilize toxins from within and between the cells. As these toxins make their way to the colon, FiberCleanse acts like a broom sweeping the colon walls encouraging the removal of toxins that may have built up in the colon over the previous years.

One tablespoon taken in the morning followed with 2 to 3 large glasses of pure water will begin the process. If two to three healthy bowel movements aren't realized within the first several days consider taking twice daily. It will elicit a gentle, reaction that will not propel you to spend most of your day in the bathroom. FiberCleanse is not recommended for pregnant or lactating women. Always consult a physician or pharmacists if taking medications to ensure there are no contraindications.

Secondary Routes

Secondary routes of elimination are utilized when the primary routes are overburdened with toxins. The body attempts to shed unwanted toxins from the system by utilizing the secondary routes. Optimal functioning of all primary routes and minimal toxic exposure will prevent the body from utilizing the secondary routes of elimination. Secondary routes of elimination include nasal discharge, earwax, tears, hair, excess vaginal secretions, phlegm, mucus or blood in stool, mucus in the eyes in the morning and throughout the day, mucus and draining in the nose or sinuses, and sneezing.

Cleansing is an on-going situation. Even after you have eliminated the sickness and restored your body, you will continue to take measures to keep it cleansed. The daily impact from unhealthy air and environmental toxins will always need to be addressed. Healthy foods, daily exercise, selective supplementation and stress management are all beneficial ways to keep the toxins at a reasonable level.

Chapter Thirty-Three: Stress

"You may tend to get cancer from the thing that makes you want to smoke so much, not from the smoking itself."
—Williams Saroyan

According to Webster's New Collegiate Dictionary, the definition of stress is "a physical, chemical, or emotional factor that causes bodily or mental tension and may be a factor in disease causation." There is, however, a difference between negative and positive stress.

Positive stress would involve a healthy internal response to the pressures and tensions of life. When one has a settled sense of purpose in life, the pressures associated with change are more likely to be viewed as opportunities for growth.

In contrast, negative stress that seems to appear daily, will wear the body out through negative internal responses. Anger, for example, will trigger the body's stress response. When we become aware and realize the adverse consequences to our health that anger can produce, that knowledge could help us respond a little differently.

Another example of negative stress is when individuals see themselves as powerless victims and fear they could be easily replaced in their jobs. Negative internal responses are primarily the ones that are upsetting the delicate checks and balances in our bodies and are costing so many of us the health we need and want.

Many physicians today treat more and more illnesses that are stress related. What is contributing to this increase?

How many on this list of situations and events apply to your life now or have within the past twelve months?

- Death in the family
- Job loss
- Financial burdens
- Severe illness or health challenge
- Going back to school
- Problems with children
- Deadlines at work
- Increased responsibilities at work
- Moving yourself and/or your family to a new location

It is believed that the top three stress producing situations are: the death of a spouse, divorce, and a death in the family (other than a spouse).

Many cancers surface within one year from one of these major life events. They become the trigger for the cancer. As the body reacts to the uncontrolled stress it becomes completely out of balance because the messaging system is so overloaded from the stressor.

The more of these situations you are currently facing, or have experienced recently, the greater chance there is that you might not have been able to handle them constructively or in a healthy way, thus setting your body up for some damaging responses.

The body's response to bad stress:
1. The whole body becomes strained.
2. Energy is depleted.
3. Your hormones (the chemical messengers in your body) become out of balance.

When our hormonal balance (the messenger system) becomes upset it affects the:

- Emotions
- Brain
- Body temperature
- Muscles
- Energy level

Stress comes not only from what we do but how we react to the external world. Our body often responds to stress with a fight or flight (run) response.

1. Muscles contract to provide you with a "hard coat" of protection.
2. Metabolism speeds up to give you more energy to react.
3. Breathing increases to give you more oxygen to function.
4. Digestive system begins to shut down to divert more blood and energy to the large muscles needed to operate.

When improper response to stress occurs it can cause elimination organs to hold on to toxicity and metabolic waste. This leads to the acceleration of illness and disease. For the chemical messengers in our bodies to function optimally requires management of our responses to the stresses in our lives.

There are many foods that help to either alleviate stress or help to rebuild after being exposed to major stressors:

1. Fresh living food and juices:
   a. Our body is a living organism made of living cells that require living food (raw food) to function properly.
   b. The most abundant source of nutrients that can be used by our bodies is from raw vegetables.
   c. Drinking the freshly extracted juices of vegetables is the fastest way to obtain the nutrients necessary to restore the human body to health
   d. Living food raises the alkalinity of the body.
   e. Living food helps soothe nerves and calms the body as it loosens the constriction of body tissues.
2. Dark green vegetables like kale and broccoli are packed with vitamins and minerals that help replenish the body when it has been stressed out.
3. Oranges, along with Brussels sprouts, broccoli, red and green peppers and strawberries contain lots of vitamin C, which boost your immune system and fights

brain-cell damage resulting from constant exposure to cortisol.

4. Spinach, Swiss chard and kale are loaded with magnesium, which has been credited as a major stress fighter, helping to relax muscle fibers and put you at ease.

5. Omega-3 – A 2011 study from Ohio State showed a 20% reduction in anxiety among medical school students who took omega-3 supplements.

6. Oatmeal, though not a raw, living food contains complex carbohydrates that help to increase serotonin production. The oats have calming magnesium and potassium. Don't add additional sugar and purchase only steel cut oats.

7. Cooked foods – While void of living enzymes, cooked foods can have a greater calming effect on the body than raw food can. Understand the consumption of the cooked food in this case is for comfort rather than nourishment.

8. Supplements
    a. Vitamin B6 – Vitamin B6 helps produce serotonin in your body, which is a calming neurotransmitter.
    b. Vitamin B12 also helps relax the body. It helps form GABA, a type of calming neurotransmitter.
    c. Folic acid helps create dopamine in the body, which is a neurotransmitter associated with pleasure.
    d. Magnesium stimulates the production of GABA and dopamine in the body, both of which help you to feel calm and happy.
    e. Melatonin is a great supplement to help you sleep better. Stress can become worse when you are unable to sleep well.
    f. Kava is a plant known to Pacific islanders for centuries and has long been used as a mood elevator. Studies show that Kava has demon-

strated effectiveness in helping people who are suffering from panic attacks and other psychological disorders including obsessive – compulsive disorder. Kava has shown to be an effective means of anxiety relief. However, this supplement should be used with the supervision of a doctor due to its effects on the liver.

g. Celery Seed – This supplement is known to be very helpful for many health problems. Celery seed also proves to be beneficial for treating anxiety and stress symptoms. Its active compound known as phthalides provides sedative effects making it helpful for people with anxiety and stress.

h. Niacin/Niacinamide – This supplement provides effects similar to benzodiazepine drugs that are often prescribed to people with anxiety, depression and stress. This supplement has to be taken with food.

i. Valerian is another common supplement being used for people who are afflicted with insomnia and other symptoms brought about by anxiety. Valerian slows down the central nervous system to provide relief from anxiety. However, if you have plans of undergoing any surgery you should stop taking Valerian at least two weeks before. Avoid taking valerian along with any other sedatives.

9. Herbal Supplements – There are many herbal supplements that claim to fight stress.

a. St. John's Wort is one of the best studied. It has shown benefits for people with mild-to-moderate depression. The herb also appears to reduce symptoms of anxiety.

b. Maca root in its unprocessed form contains a phyto nutrient that helps ward off anxiety and depression. Some studies have found that maca root is just as useful at fighting depression as prescription antidepressants.

Various methods of managing stress:

1. Deep breathing:
   a. The brain uses 1/3 of oxygen we breathe. The air we breathe coordinates with all our movements and mental actions to help us work, play, and think more efficiently.
   b. Short, shallow breathing keeps body and mind rigid and uptight.
   c. To calm yourself, take a few slow, deep breaths to relax. As you do, think happy thoughts and your mind will relax. Your body will begin to relax in response to this and the tension and stress will fade.
2. Laughter:
   Humor is an excellent way to reduce tension. Some health care practitioners recommend their patients turn to humor as a source of relief from various conditions.
3. Stretching:
   a. Strengthens muscles
   b. Tones muscles
   c. Increases flexibility
   d. Relaxes large muscle groups in legs and back
   e. Relieves mental stress
   f. Makes joints loose and supple
   g. Slow, gentle stretching relieves stress in the body and in the mind
   h. Improves your mental focus and clarity
      i. Reducing worry and anxiety
      ii. Strengthening your overall well-being
      iii. Creating a sense of inner peace
4. Exercise – one of the best stress-busting strategies is to start exercising
   a. Aerobic exercise boosts oxygen circulation and spurs your body to make feel-good chemicals called endorphins. Aim for 30 minutes of aer-

obic exercise three to four times a week.
   b. Walking is beneficial in many ways to relieve
      stress especially if walking with a companion
      in a beautiful park or other natural setting.
5. Crunchy raw vegetables can help ease stress in a purely
   mechanical way. Munching celery or carrot sticks helps
   release a clenched jaw, and that can ward off tension.
6. Eat small meals throughout the day, which will keep
   your blood sugar stable (when blood sugar is low, mental, physical, and emotional energy decreases, and stress
   increases).

Having stress in our lives is inevitable and it seems with the faster paced lives we live today and the pressures that come from everywhere there is more of it now than there ever was. By recognizing the negative impact stress can have on our lives and taking steps to alleviate as much as we can while incorporating methods to manage the stress we aren't able to avoid we will be able to support our bodies in its journey toward improved health.

Over the years there have been many stories of people with terminal cancer who decided to leave their homes to go enjoy their last days on the beach or hiking in the mountains only to have their cancer go away. Could it be that they left behind the stress that was causing the problem in the first place?

Chapter Thirty-Four: Rest

"There is no illness that is not exacerbated by stress."
—Allan Lokos

Why do we sleep? Is sleep important to healing and the health of the body? In our hectic lives, sleep seems to be one of those things that we figure we'll get to one day. We treat it like it is a luxury. But, if sleep isn't important, then why is it that all animals in nature ... sleep?

The purpose of sleep remains one of the most perplexing biological riddles. Aristotle thought that we sleep because of cooling of the vapors of the head. Freud thought sleep was a symbolic journey back to the security of the womb. Pavlov thought of it as a conditioned response. Others have argued that we sleep to repair the ravages of the day, or to purge our brains of extraneous information, or to conserve our energy. Sleep has also been called maintenance time for our bodies.

Perhaps none of these explanations is correct. Perhaps they all are, for it may well be that sleep, like waking, has many functions. We may be making an enormous and costly mistake by assuming that our nights are any less significant or complex than our days.

Our bodies are constantly repairing the wear and tear of living, but when we sleep, those energy hungry machines like muscles and digestive system, even lungs and heart, take a break and free up blood flow and energy (nutrients) for other things like – recovery and repair.

The key to understanding this is to realize that the body has limited resources. There's only so much blood, so many white blood cells, so much flow through the liver and kidneys, so much energy for use in cellular functions. If you're moving around, eating, and generally being active, more resources go to those activities, so less are available for repair. When you rest, or sleep, your body redistributes the resources to repair functions.

It could be said that the primary purpose of sleep is for generating nerve energy or low-level electricity. But, many other beneficial activities are also accomplished during sleep. The physiological rest obtained during sleep is extraordinarily valuable. During the prolonged rest of sleep, the body replenishes its cells and organs with fuel, replaces cells that have lost their vitality and rids itself of extra toxins that may not have been eliminated the previous day.

This is also when the body's immune system is rebuilt to continue the fight against infection and to maintain health.

The benefits of sleep may be chronicled as follows:
1. The regeneration of nerve energy
2. Refueling the liver and cells with glycogen
3. Destruction of old cells and replacement with new cells (multiplication of cells occurs during sleep at a rate of more than twice that during waking hours).
4. The body expels more debris and waste during sleep and rest than when active

Here are some things that happen to the human body while sleeping:
- Brain – The activity in the cortex drops by about 40% while in the first phase of sleep. This reduces the blood flow required for brain activity and the blood is redirected to the muscle to restore energy. The brain does become more active through later phases as it does interesting activities like reevaluate memories, shift short term to long term storage, link thoughts to one another, and more.
- Digestive System – During sleep the digestive system slows down. For this reason, eating late at night is not recommended because the enzymes and stomach acid which is used to convert food into energy is not running at normal levels, thus resulting in poorer digestion and reduced nutrient uptake.

- Hormones – During our waking hours, the body burns oxygen and food to provide energy. This is called catabolic rate and is dominated by stimulation of adrenal hormones and corticosteroid. But during sleep, the hormone system will switch on anabolic phase, energy conversion for improvement and growth. At this stage, the adrenalin hormone level and corticosteroids drop and the body begins producing human growth hormone (HGH), melatonin, as well as sex hormone testosterone, fertility hormones, FSH (follicle-stimulating hormone) and LH (luteinizing hormone). HGH encourages growth, maintenance and muscle repair.
- Immune System – While you sleep, your body produces hormones called cytokines. Cytokines are made to help the immune system fight against certain diseases and infections. That is why getting enough sleep can help fight infections. A cancer killer called Tumor necrosis Factor (TNF) is also pumped through the blood vessels during sleep.
- Blood – Heart rate is decreased between 10 and 30 beats per minute during sleep. This results in a decrease in blood pressure, which occurs in deep sleep. During rest, blood flows from the brain, relaxes the arteries and enlarges the limbs. The cells and tissues that break down to produce toxins also become less active during sleep. This gives an opportunity for damaged tissue to be rebuilt.
- Body temperature – At night, the body temperature along with the adrenalin begin to fall.
- Muscle – Even when people change sleep positions 35 times a night, the muscles remain relaxed. This gives an opportunity for body networks to be repaired and restored.
- Skin – During deep sleep, metabolism rates accelerate and many body cells show increase in production and reduced damage to proteins. This is why sleep can beautify the skin.

Chronic sleep deprivation leads to numerous health problems like depression, high blood pressure, obesity, irritability, irregular hormone production, decreased concentration and memory, and weakened immune system.

Scientists are realizing more and more the physical implications of not getting enough sleep. In a study done at the University of Chicago, Dr. Eve Van Cauter found that, after four hours of sleep for six consecutive nights, healthy young men had blood test results that nearly matched those of diabetics. Their ability to process blood sugar was reduced by 30%, they had a huge drop in their insulin response, and they had elevated levels of a stress hormone called cortisol, which can lead to hypertension and memory impairment [1]. Such physical effects were unheard of before this study, and as a result, scientists are now looking into connections with lack of sleep and obesity.

How much sleep do we need?

The amount of sleep that a person needs varies according to the individual's body and his or her sleeping conditions. Some people fare nicely on five or six hours of sleep daily, while others require eight or nine hours daily. Why the difference? Sleep needs vary with every individual and every circumstance.

- People sleep more in winter than in summer.
- Mental workers sleep more than physical workers.
- People who work outdoors get by with one to two hours less sleep than those who work equally arduously indoors.
- To answer the above questions, one must understand the intricacies of nerve energy expenditure and the conditions that enable the body to most efficiently regenerate it.

The most efficient sleep can be termed sound sleep, slow-wave sleep, delta sleep, stage four sleep and deep sleep. It produces about twice the amount of recuperation as does lighter stages of sleep.

Since most Americans are toxic, it is doubtful that sleep researchers have examined the sleep of very many truly healthy people. The data the researchers have charted as normal really reflects the average of unhealthy people.

Truly healthy people sleeping under ideal conditions require less sleep than less healthy individuals. This is due to several factors. First, a healthy person needs less recuperation due to less energy expenditure. Second, a healthy person is capable of a greater proportion of very sound sleep because of less internal body disturbance. Third, a healthy individual can regenerate nerve energy faster due to the increased efficiency.

The ideal conditions of sleep are determined by both internal and external circumstances. The more comfortable the sleeper, the sounder their sleep will be. Pure air affords less sleep and quiet surroundings promote deeper sleep. Also, the less light in the sleeping area, the less disturbed will be the sleep.

Certain internal conditions determine quality of sleep. A person with a toxin-free body sleeps more readily and more soundly than a toxin-laden individual.

For example, insomnia will often result from drinking coffee. The distress and stimulation from the caffeine may inhibit sleep; especially sound sleep. The body must expend energy in expelling the caffeine. At the same time, it generates less nerve energy because of lack of sound sleep.

Another condition that interferes with sleep is eating at bedtime. The primary reason for sleep is to regenerate nerve energy. However, if a person eats before sleeping, his/her body will direct much of its energies towards the digestion of the food. Since the brain is involved in digestion, less sound sleep will result.

Additionally, the body will suffer a deficit of nerve energy because less was regenerated during the digestive process than would have been if the food had not been eaten.

Anything that is in the sleeper's environment or body that disturbs the senses or uses more nerve energy than normal interferes with sleep, thus making it less efficient and effective.

The book *Better Sleep for a Better Life* details specific conditions that interfere with sleep.

Those who sleep in fresh air invariably report better sleep and a lesser need for sleep than those who sleep inside their homes. Why should this be so? Stated very simply, any improvement in sleeping conditions improves sleep. When a person sleeps in fresh air, the body receives its oxygen needs in a relatively pure state. Air inside homes is likely to have less oxygen and more pollution than fresh air. Impure air provides less of our needs and gives the body more problems than does fresh air.

It is beneficial to sleep by open windows in a quiet environment so that fresh air flows freely during sleep. If the environment is noisy, it is wise to have the house ventilated so that fresh air is continuously funneled to and through the bedroom. Even polluted air from the outside is better than stale air trapped indoors. Sleeping is also improved by working in a fresh air environment during the day.

Exercise is a blessing that we should indulge in regularly. Optimally, we should exercise daily, but certainly not less than four times weekly. Performed as much as possible within our limitations, exercise creates only benefits and no liabilities.

Exercise in the form of jogging, calisthenics, gardening, bicycling, swimming, brisk walking, etc., up to about half an hour daily, takes no time from our waking moments! Sleep needs are reduced by about that amount!

Exercise "fine-tunes" the body. Elimination is so accelerated by exercise that extraordinary body cleansing occurs. The body not only eliminates extra carbon dioxide generated during vigorous exercise, but it also assists with the removal of accumulated toxins ingested from nonfoods and drugs and toxins created as a result of overeating, eating wrong combinations, eating under stress, etc.

Foods that require less digestion and assimilation use less nerve energy. Foods that are associated with toxic materials, such as most cooked foods, meats, animal products, condiments, additives, etc., give the body eliminative problems.

Eliminative problems require a great deal of nerve energy to be properly dealt with. For example, a single drink of alcohol can exhaust the body for a day or two. The need for sleep is greatly increased so that the body may recuperate its energy.

Here are some principles you should keep in mind relative to diet and sleep requirements:

1. The healthier the food, the less nerve energy is required to digest and use it. Healthy food lessens sleep needs and increases sleep efficiency.

2. The more unfit the foods eaten, the more nerve energy is expended and the more sleep is required. Moreover, sleep will be less efficient when unhealthy foods are consumed.

3. Fasting individuals require only three to five hours of sleep daily after fasting for a short time. People who eat meat, condiments and cooked foods and who overeat require inordinate amounts of sleep. Despite the extra sleep, they are usually not well rested because they have a perpetual deficit of nerve energy due to their unhealthy practices.

4. You should not eat for at least two hours prior to bedtime. Though meals do sometimes cause drowsiness and sluggishness, due to the redirection of blood supply to the digestive organs, we should not expect to sleep well while the body is at working digesting and assimilating.

5. Eating beyond the body's need imposes an extra task upon the body. Processing and disposing of food requires a great deal of energy. Unhealthy foods usually end up in a pathogenic state that drains the body's resources in eliminative efforts. This drain of energy results in poor sleep and in a correspondingly greater need for sleep. A person who over tasks his digestive system and sleeps 12 hours a day may be less rested than a healthy person who gets only six hours!

Sleeping Conditions

In America, bedding usually consists of an innerspring mattress over box springs, sheets, a pillow with pillowcase and blankets and/or quilts.

For body comfort, the softer the mattress, the better the quality of sleep. Of equal benefit is airiness. A soft innerspring mattress meets these conditions ideally. A thin cotton mattress on top of a foam, air or waterbed mattress works well too. Pressure points, hot spots, cold spots, and areas where air is deprived disturb the body. The body, like the lungs, will suffocate without fresh air. Although the skin requires only a fraction of the air required by the lungs, it requires it nevertheless. Plastic materials deny the body air.

Fabrics that breathe, such as cotton, are ideal (organic if possible). Sleep should be conducted on cotton surfaces with lots of circulation underneath. Cotton sheets, blankets or materials should be used for cover.

Sleep is more efficiently experienced when the body is comfortable in temperature and when it is physically at ease.

Sleeping on concrete or a hard surface would provide very few contact points between the body and the concrete (or hard surface). The body's weight would rest on these points, thus creating pressure points that interfere with blood circulation and skin respiration. Distress of the areas in contact would soon occur and thus rouse the brain into a lighter stage of sleep in order to perform a body movement.

On the other hand, a very soft bed permits the underside of the body to make more even contact with the sleeping surface.

Some Sleep Conditions

Insomnia is an inability to sleep. Obviously, this interferes with the body's ability to recover the nerve energy it needs for the following day's activities. Taking sleeping pills or tranquilizers will ultimately make the problem worse by adding to the body's toxic load.

Rather than immediately searching for methods to induce sleep, you should first look for the causes of the problem. Insomnia results when an individual is assaulted by too much stimuli. Stimuli can result from improper sleeping conditions or stress, but are usually due to body toxicity. This toxicity results from both external sources and from ingested materials. Drugs and drug-like substances are major offenders. These include caffeine, condiments, chocolate, soft drinks, cooked foods, wrong foods, dead foods, allergenic foods, over-the-counter and prescription drugs, etc. The solution to insomnia is simple: Discontinue causes! Remove the conditions that interfere with sleep, and implement the conditions that promote it.

Insomnia is usually overcome in a few days during a fast and will not recur if a regimen of healthful practices is adopted. A good night's sleep can be had by almost anyone who discontinues body-disturbing practices and institutes healthful practices.

Snoring is not normal! A multitude of conditions can be responsible for snoring. Enlarged tonsils or adenoids may block the air passage sufficiently to cause the loud "flutter" of snoring. Most snoring occurs because the soft palate, when relaxed, flutters in the diverted current of air. Diverted air may be due to growths, fatty tissue in the throat, nasal deformities or other swelling. My husband found that when he avoids gluten he no longer snores. Food allergies and sensitivities may likely be a problem people never would have considered.

Most fasting people who have previously snored are surprised when the condition disappears. The condition does, however, speedily return if the person returns to its causes – an unhealthy diet. But many have overcome it permanently.

Healthy Sleep Tips

1. Eat Healthy Foods – no caffeine, meat, dairy, condiments, and soft drinks.
2. Eat at least two hours before going to bed
3. Get to sleep between 9 and 10 PM
4. A warm shower just before retiring, followed with a good back rub, especially in the middle of your back, will likely generate positive effects after relaxing the nerves and muscles.
5. A hot soaking for your feet will draw any blood from your brain and is effective in helping you relax
6. Make sure the bed is comfortable
7. Include fresh air in the room
8. Ensure there are no lights on in the room – and keep it dark all night long. Exposure to light will reset the sleep process significantly impacting the quality of sleep
9. Keep the mind free of the worries of the day. Should they impose on your thoughts, block them out by saying soothing sentences or recite a short poem. One particular good strategy should be to close the left nostril by pressing it with a finger, then to take four deep breaths through the right nostril. After that, close the right nostril and take 4 deep breaths through the left. Do this repetition four times. Breathe slowly on both nostrils, yet count your breaths. You'll rarely

have to count a lot before drifting off to sleep.

10. Slowly count backwards from 100 when trying to fall asleep.

11. Before falling asleep, tell yourself repeatedly that you will sleep through the night waking up feeling rested and refreshed.

"Sleep deprivation has effects on the body much like stress, including weight gain, increased cortisol levels, distorted thyroid hormone levels, and elevations in glucose and insulin that increase the risk for insulin resistance and diabetes,"
—Robert Sack, Ph.D.

Chapter Thirty-Five: Sunshine

"Healing is a biological process, not an art. It is as much a function of the living organism as respiration, digestion, circulation, excretion, cell proliferation, or nerve activity. It is a ceaseless process, as constant as the turning of the earth on its axis. Man can neither duplicate nor imitate nor provide a substitute for the process. All schools of healing are frauds."
—Herbert M. Shelton

Most health messages of the past century have focused on the hazards of too much sun exposure. UVA radiation (95–97% of the UVR that reaches Earth's surface) penetrates deeply into the skin, where it can contribute to skin cancer indirectly via generation of DNA-damaging molecule. Sunburn is caused by too much UVB radiation; this form also leads to direct DNA damage and promotes various skin cancers. Both forms can damage collagen fibers, destroy vitamin A in skin, accelerate aging of the skin, and increase the risk of skin cancers. Excessive sun exposure can also cause cataracts and diseases aggravated by UVR-induced immunosuppression such as reactivation of some latent viruses.

However, excessive UVR exposure accounts for only 0.1% of the total global burden of disease, according to the 2006 World Health Organization (WHO) report, The Global Burden of Disease Due to Ultraviolet Radiation. They measure how much a person's expectancy of healthy life is reduced by premature death or disability caused by disease. Coauthor Robyn Lucas, an epidemiologist at the National Centre for Epidemiology and Population Health in Canberra, Australia, explains that many diseases linked to excessive UVR exposure tend to be relatively benign – apart from malignant melanoma – and occur in older age groups, due mainly to the long lag between exposure and manifestation, cumulative exposures, or both. Therefore, sun-induced exposures don't appear to be extremely globally burdensome.

In contrast, the same WHO report noted that a markedly larger annual disease burden of 3.3 billion worldwide might result from very low levels of UVR exposure. This burden includes major disorders of the musculoskeletal system and possibly an increased risk of various autoimmune diseases and life-threatening cancers.

The best-known benefit of sunlight is its ability to boost the body's vitamin D supply; most cases of vitamin D deficiency are due to lack of outdoor sun exposure. At least 1,000 different genes located in virtually every tissue in the body are now thought to be regulated by vitamin D3, the active form of the vitamin, including several involved in calcium metabolism and neuromuscular and immune system functioning.

Although most of the health-promoting benefits of sun exposure are thought to occur through vitamin D photosynthesis, there may be other health benefits that have gone largely overlooked in the debate over how much sun is needed for good health. As for what constitutes "excessive" UVR exposure, there is no one-size-fits-all answer. Lucas suggests, "'Excessive' really means inappropriately high for your skin type under a particular level of ambient UVR."

Other Health Links Associated with Low Vitamin D3

- Various studies have linked low vitamin D3 levels to diseases other than cancer, raising the possibility that vitamin D3 insufficiency is contributing to many major illnesses
- Poor bone-mineral density in older people
- Multiple Sclerosis
- Type 1 Diabetes in children
- Metabolic Syndrome – a cluster of conditions that increases one's risk for type 2 diabetes and cardiovascular disease
- Hypertension
- Atherosclerosis

- Rheumatoid arthritis (RA)
- Asthma
- Infectious diseases
- Influenza
- Bronchitis
- Gastroenteritis
- Bacterial infections such as tuberculosis and septicemia
- Collagen-induced arthritis
- Lyme arthritis
- Autoimmune encephalomyelitis
- Thyroiditis
- Inflammatory bowel disease
- Systemic lupus

The first reports of an association between sun exposure and skin cancer began to appear in dermatology publications in the late nineteenth century. It was not until the 1930's that the U.S. Public Health Service began issuing warnings about sun-related health risks. People were cautioned to avoid the midday summer sun, cover their heads in direct sunlight, and gradually increase the time of sun exposure from an initial 5–10 minutes per day to minimize the risk of sunburn.

In the decades that followed, the skin cancer hazards of excessive sun exposure would be extensively studied and mapped. Today, the three main forms of skin cancer – melanoma, basal cell carcinoma, and squamous cell carcinoma – are largely attributed to excessive UVR exposure. Skin cancers became the most common form of cancer worldwide, especially among groups such as white residents of Australia and New Zealand.

Australia was among the first countries to spearhead large-scale sun protection programs, with the Slip-Slop-Slap initiative (short for "slip on a shirt, slop on some sun-screen, and slap on a hat") introduced in the early 1980's. As a result of increased use of hats, sunscreen, and shade, the incidence of malignant melanoma has begun to plateau in Australia, New Zealand, Canada, and Northern Europe among some age groups.

Whereas skin cancer is associated with too much UVR exposure, other cancers could result from too little. Living at higher latitudes increases the risk of dying from Hodgkins lymphoma, as well as breast, ovarian, colon, pancreatic, prostate, and other cancers, as compared with living at lower latitudes. A randomized clinical trial by Joan Lappe, a medical professor at Creighton University, and colleagues, published in the June 2007 issue of the American Journal of Clinical Nutrition, confirmed that taking a daily dietary intake of 200–600 IU vitamin D3 and calcium resulted in a 50–77% reduction in expected incidence rates of all cancers combined over a four-year period in post-menopausal women living in Nebraska.

This study is suggesting an older amount of recommended daily diet intake. Today recommended daily diet intake of vitamin D3 for someone with cancer has increased to 10,000 IU. There are health care practitioners that believe this is still too low.

Although excessive sun exposure is an established risk factor for malignant melanoma, continued high sun exposure was linked with increased survival rates in patients with early-stage melanoma in a study reported by Marianne Berwick, an epidemiology professor at the University of New Mexico, in the February 2005 Journal of the National Cancer Institute. Most melanomas occur on the least sun-exposed areas of the body, and in fact, occupational exposure to sunlight actually reduced melanoma risk in a study reported in the June 2003 Journal of Investigative Dermatology.

According to Krause, who was head of the Heliotherapy Research Group at the Medical University of Berlin, a serum vitamin D3 level of at least 40 ng/mL should be adequate to protect against hypertension and other forms of cardiovascular disease (as well as cancers of the prostate and colon).

How Much Is Enough?

One problem with the literature is that everyone recommends something different, depending on the studies with which they are most aligned.

These days, most experts define vitamin D3 deficiency as a serum blood level of less than 20 ng/mL. Holick and others assert that levels of 29 ng/mL or lower can be considered to indicate a relative insufficiency of vitamin D3. Using this scale and considering various epidemiologic studies, an estimated 1 billion people worldwide have vitamin D3 deficiency or insufficiency, says Holick, who adds, "According to several studies, some forty to one hundred percent of the U.S. and

European elderly men and women still living in the community [that is, not in nursing homes] are vitamin D3 deficient." Holick asserts that a large number of infants, children, adolescents, and postmenopausal women also are vitamin D3 insufficient. "These individuals have no apparent skeletal or calcium metabolism abnormalities but may be at much higher risk of developing various diseases," Holick says.

In the context of inadequate sunlight or vitamin D3 insufficiency, some scientists worry that the emphasis on preventing skin cancers tends to obscure the much larger mortality burden posed by more life-threatening cancers such as lung, colon, and breast cancers. Many studies have shown that cancer-related death rates decline as one moves toward the lower latitudes (between 37°N and 37°S), and that the levels of ambient UVR in different municipalities correlate inversely with cancer death rates there. "As you head from north to south, you may find perhaps two or three extra deaths [per hundred thousand people] from skin cancer," says Vieth. "At the same time, though, you'll find thirty or forty fewer deaths for the other major cancers. So when you estimate the number of deaths likely to be attributable to UV light or vitamin D3, it does is not appear to be the best policy to advise people to simply keep out of the sun just to prevent skin cancer."

To maximize protection against cancer, Grant recommends raising vitamin D3 levels to between 40 and 60 ng/mL. Research such as that described in Holick's August 2006 Journal of Clinical Investigation article indicates that simply keeping the serum level above 20 ng/mL could reduce the risk of cancer by as much as 30–50%.

Cedric F. Garland, a medical professor at the University of California, San Diego, says that maintaining a serum level of 55–60 ng/mL may reduce the breast cancer rate in temperate regions by half, and that incidence of many other cancers would be similarly reduced as well. He calls this "the single most important action that could be taken by society to reduce the incidence of cancer in North America and Europe, beyond not smoking." Moreover, these levels could be readily achieved by consuming no more than 2,000 IU/day of vitamin D3 at a cost of less than $20 per year and, unless there are contraindications to sunlight exposure, spending a few minutes outdoors (3–15 minutes for whites and 15–30 minutes for blacks) when the sun is highest in the sky, with 40% of the skin area exposed.

Holick, Vieth, and many other experts now make a similar daily recommendation: 4,000 IU vitamin D3 without sun exposure or 2,000 IU plus 12–15 minutes of midday sun. They say this level is quite safe except for sun-sensitive individuals or those taking medications that increase photosensitivity.

Gilchrest says some sunlight enters the skin even through a high-SPF sunscreen, so people can maximize their dermal vitamin D3 production by spending additional time outdoors while wearing protection. "Without the sunscreen, this same individual would be incurring substantially more damage to her skin but not further increasing her vitamin D3 level," she says.

Creating a Balanced Message

A growing number of scientists are concerned that efforts to protect the public from excessive UVR exposure may be eclipsing recent research demonstrating the diverse health-promoting benefits of UVR exposure. Some argue that the health benefits of UVB radiation seem to outweigh the adverse effects, and that the risks can be minimized by carefully managing UVR exposure (e.g., by avoiding sunburn), as well as by increasing one's intake of dietary antioxidants and limiting dietary fat and caloric intake.

Antioxidants including polyphenols, apigenin, curcumin, proanthocyanidins, resveratrol, and silymarin have shown promise in laboratory studies in protecting against UVR-induced skin cancer, perhaps through antimutagenic or immune-modulating mechanisms.

Many experts are now recommending a middle-ground approach that focuses on modest sun exposures. Gilchrest says the American Academy of Dermatology and most dermatologists currently suggest sun protection in combination with vitamin D3 supplementation as a means of minimizing the risk of both skin cancer and internal cancers. Furthermore, brief, repeated exposures are more efficient at producing vitamin D3. "Longer sun exposures cause further sun damage to skin and increase the risk of photo-aging and skin cancer, but do not increase vitamin D3 production," she explains.

Lucas adds that people should use sun protection when the UV Index is more than 3. As part of Australia's SunSmart program, "UV Alerts" are announced in newspapers throughout the country whenever the index is forecast to be 3 or higher. U.S. residents can obtain UV Index forecasts through the EPA's SunWise website (http://epa.

gov/sunwise/uvindex.html).

In the near future, vitamin D3 and health guidelines regarding sun exposure may need to be revised. But many factors not directly linked to sun protection will also need to be taken into account. "Current observations of widespread vitamin D3 insufficiency should not be attributed only to sun protection strategies," says Lucas. "Over the same period there is a trend to an increasingly indoor lifestyle, associated with technological advances such as television, computers, and video games." She says sun-safe messages remain important – possibly more so than ever before – to protect against the potentially risky high-dose intermittent sun exposure that people who stay indoors may be most likely to incur.

Serotonin, Melatonin, and Daylight

We humans are programmed to be outdoors while the sun is shining and home in bed at night. This is why melatonin is produced during the dark hours and stops upon exposure to daylight. This pineal hormone is a key pacesetter for many of the body's circadian rhythms. It also plays an important role in countering infection, inflammation, cancer, and auto-immunity, according to a review in the May 2006 issue of Current Opinion in Investigational Drugs. Melatonin also suppresses UVR-induced skin damage, according to research in the July 2005 issue of Endocrine.

When people are exposed to sunlight or very bright artificial light in the morning, their nocturnal melatonin production occurs sooner, and they enter into sleep more easily at night. Melatonin production also shows a seasonal variation relative to the availability of light, with the hormone produced for a longer period in the winter than in the summer. The melatonin production caused by exposure to bright morning light has been effective against insomnia, premenstrual syndrome, and seasonal affective disorder (SAD).

The melatonin precursor, serotonin, is also affected by exposure to daylight. Normally produced during the day, serotonin is only converted to melatonin in darkness. Whereas high melatonin levels correspond to long nights and short days, high serotonin levels in the presence of melatonin reflect short nights and long days (i.e., longer UVR exposure). Moderately high serotonin levels result in more positive moods and a calm yet focused mental outlook. Indeed, SAD has been linked with low serotonin levels during the day as well as with a delay in nighttime melatonin production. It was recently found that mammalian skin can produce serotonin and transform it into melatonin, and that many types of skin cells express receptors for both serotonin and melatonin.

With our modern-day penchant for indoor activity and staying up well past dusk, nocturnal melatonin production is typically far from robust. "The light we get from being outside on a summer day can be a thousand times brighter than we're ever likely to experience indoors," says melatonin researcher Russel J. Reiter of the University of Texas Health Science Center. "For this reason, it's important that people who work indoors get outside periodically, and moreover that we all try to sleep in total darkness. This can have a major impact on melatonin rhythms and can result in improvements in mood, energy, and sleep quality."

For people in jobs in which sunlight exposure is limited, full-spectrum lighting may be helpful. Sunglasses may further limit the eyes' access to full sunlight, thereby altering melatonin rhythms. Going shades-free in the daylight, even for just 10–15 minutes, could confer significant health benefits.

Other Ways the Sun Can Benefit Us:

The sun may be best known for boosting production of vitamin D, but there are many other UVR-mediated effects independent of this pathway.

- It may help prevent autoimmune diseases.
- It will help in limiting DNA damage and increase gene repair, thus reducing melanoma risk, as reported 15 May 2005 in Cancer Research.
- It may help treat skin disorders such as psoriasis
- It will increase blood levels of natural opiates called endorphins according to the June 2003 Journal of Investigative Dermatology, and a study published 24 November 2005 in Molecular and Cellular Endocrinology

Research Challenges

Growing evidence of the beneficial effects of UVR exposure has challenged the sun-protection paradigm that has prevailed for decades. Before a sun-exposure policy change occurs, however, we need to know if there is enough evidence to infer a protective effect of sun exposure against various diseases.

Only through well-designed randomized clinical trials can cause-and-effect relationships be established. However, most sunlight-related epidemiologic research to date has relied on observational data that are subject to considerable bias and confounding. Findings from observational studies are far less rigorous and reliable than those of interventional studies. But interventional studies would need to be very large and carried out over several decades (since most UVR-mediated diseases occur later in life). Moreover, it is not at all clear when, over a lifetime, sun exposure/vitamin D is most important. So for now scientists must rely on the results of well-conducted observational analytic studies.

This research clearly implicates that the sun should be a vital part of your recovery process. The synergistic effects from combining sunlight with the other antioxidants and phytochemicals in the Hallelujah Recovery Diet although not studied, will likely produce significant results in the body as it continues to fight the battle against cancer [1].

Chapter Thirty-Six: Water

"The First wealth is health."
— Ralph Waldo Emerson

Second to oxygen, clean water is our most important nutrient. The beauty of clean water is the many benefits it provides us. It helps stabilize (and cool) our body; it transports nutrients; it dilutes and carries away wastes; it bathes every cell and hydrates our skin; it works intimately with air and sunshine to promote life and growth. Just as it cleans and refreshes our outsides, so it freshens us throughout.

And the perfect water for us is the biologically active water found in the cell structure of raw plant foods. In general, fruits contain the highest amount of this structured water, approximately 88%, and vegetables contain slightly less, although some, like cucumbers, contain up to 96% water. Obviously, as we begin to enjoy more and more of these foods, our need for additional outside water is reduced.

Conversely, the more we cook our vegetables, the more we will thirst for additional water, since cooking removes or de-structures this valuable, biologically active source.

The real beauty of clean water is in the many benefits it provides us:

- It helps stabilize (and cools) our body by providing the-cooling medium for our sophisticated respiration/persp ration/evaporation processes
- It transports nutrients. No nutrients are available to our bodies unless they are in a liquid state, ready to then be transported with the aid of water
- It dilutes toxins and carries away metabolic waste

The water we have available to us now has little resemblance to the water they drank in The Garden or even as recently as a hundred years ago. Contamination and pollutants get to water supplies from every direction and have been found in municipal water systems in every part of our own nation. It is only prudent to take special care about the water we supply to our cells. Many types of ground water are available from wells, springs, lakes, and rivers but even these are either polluted or the body has a difficult time assimilating the minerals. Rainwater is no longer a good option due to environmental toxins picked up in the atmosphere.

Of the types of water available, "pure" distilled water is a preferred choice, although most filtered waters help guard against the toxins and pollutants that unfortunately continue to run through our water systems. Steam distilled water not only cleans the water but has a molecular structure that assists the body in the removal of toxic buildup – detoxification. The cost for a good distiller is around $300.

Another excellent option is alkaline/ionized water. Using a special machine that filters out most impurities creates this water. While the water is not quite as pure as distilled, it has other benefits that may prove beneficial in the fight against disease. The machine that make the alkaline/ionized water breaks water molecules into smaller parts (called micro-clustering) so that they are more absorbable through the membrane in your body's cells; this makes the water more hydrating and helps to escort nutrients into the cells and toxins out. Hydrogen is pumped into the water that then adds oxygen into the cells (Cancer doesn't like an oxygenated environment).

Additionally, the minerals are ionized allowing them to be more easily utilized within the body. As the name implies, the water is alkaline. Disease has a difficult time thriving in an alkaline body. The resulting, oxygenated, hydrogen rich, alkaline water assists the body in maintaining a healthy, alkaline state. After extensive research on the top alkaline producing water machines, we have found that the Enagic Company with the Kangen water machine has the greatest capacity for producing quality water consistently. While there are other manufacturers with similar products on the market, we have tested their units against the Kangen and have found them to be inferior.

It is unknown the long-term impact of the use of water that is alkaline. There are some who say that a person could become too alkaline. Others say that we are exposed to too many toxins (internal and external) and becoming too alkaline would be nearly impossible. We may never know the truth but for someone with a chronic disease, the body would greatly benefit from this type of water. If becoming too alkaline becomes a concern in the future then there are options on the machines to reduce alkalinity, so the other benefits of the water (hydrogen, ionized minerals and water structure) can be enjoyed. None of these are inexpensive units so don't waste your money on one that is inferior. One of the best countertop units will cost around $4,000.

Reverse osmosis, activated carbon, and ceramic drip systems are an example of the other filtering systems available. While these units will do a decent job of removing most of the impurities (depending on manufacturer and model) they won't provide the benefits of either distilled or Kangen for removing toxins and rehydrating the cells.

Bottled water is an option but buyers beware. Unless you know the source and processing method used in the purification system it is better to find a way to purify your own water at home. Remember, glass containers are generally better than any of the plastic jugs, although the harder plastics are less likely to leach into the water than the softer plastic bottles. Look for BPA free on the plastic jug.

Consider a whole-house water filtration system to remove chlorine, fluoride, pesticides, prescription drugs and other toxins from the water when it initially enters the house. While distilled water and reverse osmosis do an outstanding job of removing these chemicals, there is a slight residue that could remain from an alkaline unit. Additionally, using a whole-house system ensures that the water used to bathe, shower, brush teeth and wash vegetables are free of chlorine and other toxins.

Chapter Thirty-Seven: A Typical Day

"No disease that can be treated by diet should be treated with any other means."

—Maimonides

So what will a normal day on the Hallelujah Recovery Diet look like? You will find below, in clear, easy terms what you will eat, how many juices to drink and where to find the list of supplements.

A Typical Day on the Recovery Diet includes:

1. Many Juices
   • Consume six 4 ounce glasses of BarlyMax® every other hour throughout the day.
   • Consume six 8 ounces glasses of freshly extracted vegetable juice every other hour throughout the day.

These 12 hourly juices will flood the body with a broad spectrum of naturally occurring vitamins, minerals, and trace elements consistently throughout the day which the body uses to rebuild its immune system to fight the cancer.

A schedule of juices that need to be taken daily is in Appendix A. You can find it for download on the website *www.UnravelTheMystery. com/downloads.* Print off a copy and tack it to your refrigerator and check off each juice you have consumed. At the end of the day count the number of juices you consumed that day. Try to get to the 12 juices per day as often as possible.

2. Two large salads that are consumed at lunch and at dinner. They can be eaten in a salad form or they may be blended in a high powered

blender so they can be partially digested which allows the body to work less in digesting the salad. People who eat a blended salad have a greater likelihood of absorbing more nutrients since they don't need to totally rely on their own digestive systems. Most digestive systems of people with cancer are weakened which doesn't allow for optimal nutrient processing of foods.

If weakness or reduced appetite creates an inability to eat a dinner plate filled with various colors of vegetables and greens then blend the contents and serve in a soup bowl.

If the large soup bowl becomes too difficult to consume at one time, the next best thing is to create a smaller amount of blended salads and incorporate them into every other hour after the juices and supplements have been consumed and have had time to digest. Even if the large salad is broken down into 4 smaller meals, the nutrition will be consumed.

You may choose to have a cooked meal after either of the salads has been eaten.

3. A list of recommended supplements while on the Recovery Diet complete with optimal methods to assimilate is available on *www.UnravelTheMystery.com*. A list is in Appendix B and can be downloaded at *www.UnravelTheMystery.com/downloads*.

4. Drink Kangen or distilled water as needed.

Sometimes people have a hard time visualizing each of those spokes on the wagon wheel. What is important is that you spend a little time every day giving attention to each one of those spokes. As you can see from the breakdown below, if you want to spend the first part of your day in prayer, then you will need to make that a ritual. Rituals are not easy to break. You don't often forget to brush your teeth or take a shower, do you? If you turn each of these spokes into specific rituals, including when is the best time of the day to perform them, then it is much more difficult to get out of balance and let the other spokes take over. Use this as a guide, but create your own schedule so you can begin the ritual of staying in balance!

A Typical Day on the Recovery Program includes:

Early Morning
- Meditate or pray. Get your mind in a place of gratitude and peace.
- Forgive those who need to be forgiven (including your-self) and move on knowing that this is a special day. Listen to calming music.
- Stay away from TV shows and any media that portrays sadness, provokes anger or agitation and hopelessness.
- This is good advice for the entire day! Vegetable Juice and BarleyMax® is consumed every hour throughout the day.

Supplements as scheduled.

Mid-day
- Sunshine
- Gentle exercise
- Include several deep breathing exercises to get oxygen to cells
- Rest as needed

Lunch
- Prayer
- BarleyMax®/Salad
- Rest

Resume juices after meal

Mid-day
- Prayer
- Sunshine
- Gentle exercise
- Deep breathing
- Rest as needed

Dinner
- Prayer
- BarleyMax®/Salad
- Cooked Food

Resume juices after meal until 2 hours before bedtime.

Evening
- Experience humor-studies indicate humor and laughter will release a hormone that can help in the battle with

cancer. Watch a funny movie. Read a funny book. Talk
to funny people.
- Complete the juices for the day
- Complete the supplements for the day
- Go to sleep before 10:00 pm

Chapter Thirty-Eight: SuperFoods

"Being healthy is a way of life. It's not just about what you feed your body; it's about what you feed your mind and the social environment you keep. Make healthy food choices, exercise your body and brain, and choose your friends wisely."
—Steve Maraboli

We've all heard of super foods and we see a lot of marketing hype around some of these foods but what makes foods super? In the fight against cancer we need to consider the role that nutrition plays in the healing process. Every mouthful we consume we should consider as medicine. An even better way to see it is that every mouthful is giving the body an opportunity to grow strong healthy cells that once increased in numbers can use their shear number and power to kill off the cancer cells.

This means that with every bite and with every drink, the nutrient and enzyme content must be high and the variety of nutrients as well.

The list we have accumulated is not exhaustive. There are numerous other vegetables and beans that have incredible nutrients that can assist the body in creating healthy cell formation. The following are merely some examples of every day foods that aren't in a fancy bottle with an inflated price that are hard to get. The majority of these superfoods are easily grown or obtainable, not expensive and should be used as frequently as possible in the daily Recovery Diet. Use with other high nutrient vegetables to create a powerful army of new cells!

Super Foods to Eat while on the Recovery Diet:

Broccoli Sprouts

They contain a very high concentration of sulforaphane. This compound originates in the seed and is not created in the plant. One sprout contains all of the sulforaphane that is present in a full-grown broccoli plant. Sulforaphane is especially cancer protective.

Small quantities of fresh broccoli sprouts contain as much cancer protection as larger amounts of the mature vegetable sold in grocery stores, according to researchers at Johns Hopkins University. Just 5 grams (0.17 ounces) of sprouts contain concentrations of the compound glucoraphanin equal to that found in 150 grams (5.2 ounces) of mature broccoli. The compound is a precursor to sulforaphane, proven in animal studies to boost cell enzymes that protect against molecular damage from cancer-causing chemicals.

Sulforaphane has been shown to mobilize, or induce, the body's natural cancer protection resources and help reduce the risk of malignancy. Broccoli is the best source of the chemical precursor to sulforaphane – glucoraphanin. Now, broccoli sprouts are an "exceptionally rich source" of inducers of cellular enzymes for "detoxifying" chemical carcinogens – cancer causing compounds. Some of these compounds are potent enhancers of phase 2 enzymes, which speed the detoxication of electrophiles and reactive oxygen metabolites. Therefore, they say, induction of phase 2 enzymes by these compounds can "... protect cells against mutagenesis and neoplasia."

The researchers calculated how much broccoli one would have to eat in order to produce a significant degree of protection against cancer, based on epidemiologic evidence. They found that one would have to eat about two pounds of broccoli a week in order to reduce, say, one's risk of colon cancer by about 50%.

Three-day-old sprouts have the additional advantage that they're far more uniform in their potency. Broccoli sprouts look and taste something like alfalfa sprouts, according to the researchers. The report also notes that small quantities of broccoli sprout extracts markedly reduced the size of rat mammary tumors that were induced by chemical carcinogens.

The researchers refer to the concept of "chemoprotection" – "deliberate efforts to increase the body's own defense mechanisms to reduce susceptibility to carcinogens by administration of substances that can be precisely identified, and ideally, delivered in the diet. The interesting aspect of chemoprotection strategies is that they're almost never organ-specific. Chemoprotection produces a general cancer protective effect, which blocks multiple steps – a cascade of steps – that are common to cancer formation.

A small amount of sprouts go a long way. A pound of seeds will probably make over ten pounds of sprouts which from the researchers calculations translates to as much cancer protecting phytochemicals as 1000 pounds (half a ton) of broccoli! The other major benefit is that the sprouts don't smell as you don't have to cook them. They are eaten raw, usually as an addition to salad. (Proceedings of the National Academy of Sciences, 1997;94:10367-10372)

Other sprouts (except alfalfa sprouts) would be beneficial to add to the diet as well.

Garlic

Phytochemicals in garlic have been found to halt the formation of nitrosamines, carcinogens formed in the stomach (and in the intestines, in certain conditions) when you consume nitrates, a common food preservative. In fact, the Iowa Women's Health Study found that women with the highest amounts of garlic in their diets had a 50% lower risk of certain colon cancers than women who ate the least. It has also been known to help fight breast, esophageal, and stomach cancers.

Garlic also contains the amino acid L-cysteine, which directly increases the level of glutathione in cells. People with low levels of glutathione have a greater cancer risk.

Onion

Has quercetin, a flavonoid that demonstrates a special ability to protect DNA in cells. A powerful cancer inhibitor.

Leafy Greens

Rich in chlorophyll, they are very effective in binding carcinogens that may come from grilling foods, molds in foods, and other areas. The carcinogen/chlorophyll combination is difficult for the body to absorb so it is essentially removed through the bowels. Chlorophyll also has a chemo-protective effect and the numerous studies have shown significant positive results.

Spinach, kale, romaine lettuce, dandelion greens, beet greens, mustard greens, collard greens, chicory and Swiss chard are excellent sources of fiber, folate and a wide range of carotenoids such as lutein and zeaxanthin, along with saponins and flavonoids.

According to American Institute for Cancer Research's (AICR) Second Expert Report: Food, Nutrition, Physical Activity, and the Prevention of Cancer: A Global Perspective, foods containing carotenoids probably protect against cancers of the mouth, pharynx and larynx. Researchers also believe that carotenoids seem to prevent cancer by acting as antioxidants – that is, scouring potentially dangerous "free radicals" from the body before they can do harm. Some laboratory research has found that the carotenoids in dark green leafy vegetables can inhibit the growth of certain types of breast cancer cells, skin cancer cells, lung cancer and stomach cancer. The Second Expert Report also noted probable evidence that foods containing folate decrease risk of pancreatic cancer and that foods containing dietary fiber probably reduce one's chances of developing colorectal cancer. Green leafy vegetables are rich in all of these and daily intake of them is invaluable when fighting or preventing cancer.

Cruciferous Vegetables (Broccoli, cauliflower, cabbage, bok choy, brussels sprouts)

Have very high concentrations of sulforophane which we discussed above in broccoli sprouts. High intake is required to reach optimal protection. They also contain brassinin; a powerful cancer-fighter. Daily intake of these cancer-fighting vegetables is optimal.

BarleyMax®

BarleyMax® is the dehydrated juice from young barley grass and alfalfa. It is the juice from a whole food, replete with all of the vitamins, minerals, antioxidants, and enzymes of these very potent green foods. See chapter 29 for more information on the superior quality of BarleyMax®.

Vegetable Juices

There are three main reasons why juicing is considered a superfood:

1. Juicing helps you absorb nearly all the nutrients from

the vegetables. This is important because most cancer patients have impaired digestion. This limits your body's ability to absorb all the nutrients from the vegetables. Juicing will help to "pre-digest" them for you, so you will receive most of the nutrition, without your digestive system working so hard. The energy saved in digestion can be directed to fighting the cancer.

2. Juicing allows you to consume an optimal amount of vegetables in an efficient manner. The optimal number of servings of vegetables per day is at least 10 servings. 15-20 is a better goal for someone fighting cancer. A serving size for raw vegetables is 1 cup. Some people may find eating that quantity of vegetables difficult, but it can be easily accomplished with a quick glass of vegetable juice.

3. You can add a wider variety of vegetables in your diet. Many people eat the same vegetable salads every day. This violates the principle of regular food rotation and increases your chance of developing an allergy to a certain food. But with juicing, you can juice a wide variety of vegetables that you may not normally enjoy eating whole.

Flax seed

A more potent source of phytoestrogens than soy. Several studies performed by various researchers have determined that the lignan in the flax seed had significantly positive effect on reducing cancer tumor growth [6].

According the Michael Donaldson, PhD, other studies have found that flax oil, primarily in the case of prostate cancer has not performed as well as ground flaxseeds which contain the most lignans. Some flax oils contain lignan but we still recommend that in cases of prostate cancer, freshly ground flaxseed are the optimal choice [7][8].

Fermented Vegetables

Because there's no heat involved in the fermentation/culturing process, all of the enzymes stay in tact, just like raw foods – but with many added benefits!

1. Cultured foods provide probiotics and more bioavailable vitamins and minerals, B vitamins and omega-3 fatty acids in particular. A good balance of gut bacteria can even influence the expression of genes that determine vitamin absorption and metabolism which can have a profound effect on your ability to stay healthy and trim.
2. Cultured foods can assist in detoxifying, fighting infections, reducing high cholesterol levels, and supporting digestive and immune systems.
3. They're a solid source of amino acids.
4. Cultured foods also increase lactase and lactic acid, and other chemicals that battle harmful bacteria. They even act as antioxidants that may prevent and fight cancer.

Just about any vegetable can be cultured. Some of the most popular cultured veggies are beets, cabbage, carrots, cauliflower, celery, garlic, cucumber, kale, leeks, onions, parsnips, radishes, rutabaga, shallots, turnips, kelp, and various herbs. Consume 1/2 cup daily.

Asparagus

According to the National Cancer Institute, asparagus is the highest tested food containing glutathione, one of the body's most potent cancer fighters. Additionally, asparagus is high in rutin, which is valuable in strengthening the blood vessels. It should be cooked and pureed. Take 4 heaping tablespoons in the morning with breakfast and in the evening with your meal [9].

Watercress

This clover-like veggie looks a bit like tiny spinach leaves. These little greens have been found to reduce DNA damage to the cells, which is what often leads to cancer. They are also known to increase antioxidant levels in the body, which is another great way to fight off cancer and other illnesses. A study done by Norwich Research Centre found that smokers who were given 170 milligrams per day eliminated higher than average amounts of carcinogens in their urine. Smoker or not, it may be worth it to add this to your diet [10].

Additional Great Food choices:

Black and Navy Beans

A study out of Michigan State University found that black and navy beans significantly reduced colon cancer incidence in rats, in part because a diet rich in legumes increased levels of the fatty acid butyrate, which in high concentrations has protective effects against cancer growth. Another study, in the journal Crop Science, found dried beans particularly effective in preventing breast cancer in rats.

Walnuts

Their phytosterols (cholesterol-like molecules found in plants) have been shown to block estrogen receptors in breast cancer cells, possibly slowing the cells' growth, says Elaine Hardman, PhD, associate professor at Marshall University School of Medicine in Huntington, West Virginia.

CAUTION: 3-6 nuts a day is enough due to their high fat content while fighting cancer.

Tomatoes

This juicy fruit is the best dietary source of lycopene, a carotenoid that gives tomatoes their red color. Lycopene was found to stop endometrial cancer cell growth in a study in Nutrition and Cancer. Cooked Tomatoes have more cancer-fighting properties than raw tomatoes. Both contain the molecule lycopene, but heating the tomato changes its chemical structure and makes the benefits more readily available to your body.

Berries

All berries are packed with cancer-fighting phytonutrients. But black raspberries, in particular, contain very high concentrations of phytochemicals called anthocyanins, which slow down the growth of premalignant cells and keep new blood vessels from forming (and potentially feeding a cancerous tumor), according to Gary D. Stoner, PhD, a professor of internal medicine at The Ohio State University College of Medicine.

CAUTION: Due to their sugar content, berries must not be consumed in great quantities while fighting cancer.

Medicinal Mushrooms

Mushrooms have long been used in medicine; the earliest records go back over 4,000 years in China. Medicinal mushrooms come in all shapes and sizes – Maitake mushrooms, Cordyceps, Shiitake, Reishi, Coriolus, Versicolor, etc.

Medicinal Mushrooms contain high levels of glycoproteins and polysaccharides (Beta Glucan Polysaccharide being a particularly active health contributor). Research, including 4 Nobel Prizes, shows that glycoproteins can help cellular communications. So they help your hormones do their job better, they help receptor sites receive the messages they are supposed to receive, and they help your immune system see the rogue cells and differentiate them from the healthy cells. They also help increase levels of the different white cells in your immune system.

Variety is the spice of life! Continue adding these powerful foods to your daily routine while rounding them out with other colorful, health promoting vegetables and the combination will be amazing!

Chapter Thirty-Nine: Food Synergy

"Stretching oneself too thin is the disease of modern life —
letting oneself get too thick, the other."
— Terri Guillemets

Earlier we discussed how two toxins can create more damage than each one individually. By contrast, two foods when eaten together can create a sum of nutritional benefits larger than one eaten alone. For example, when you eat a tomato alone, it will give certain nutritional benefit. When you eat broccoli alone, it will provide other nutritional benefits. But, if eaten together, these two create such a nutritional powerhouse that even prostate cancer tumors have been known to be reduced.

Elaine Magee, author of *Food Synergy* found that like whole food supplements, individual nutrients, whether they are in food or in supplements work better when combined with two or three other nutrients.

Examples of of Food Synergy include:
- Spinach & Vitamin C — Dark green, leafy vegetables like spinach and kale are best eaten in combination with another veggie high in vitamin C like beets, or a portion of an orange because vitamin C helps to improve iron absorption in your intestines.
- Tomatoes & Avocados — Tomatoes are rich in an antioxidant called lycopene, which has been proven to reduce the risk of cardiovascular disease and certain cancers. But lycopene is also fat-soluble, which means

combining it with a healthy, fat like avocodos helps boost absorption even more. Ninety-eight percent of the flavonols (powerful phytochemicals) in tomatoes is found in the tomato skin, along with great amounts of two carotenoids. If you cook the tomatoes and eat them with a little fat or oil, you have increased the absorption of the key nutrients.

- Oatmeal & Orange Juice — The combination of these morning basics has actually been shown to prevent heart attacks and clean arteries twice as effectively as eating either one on its own. The organic compounds known as phenols (found in both) stabilize cholesterol levels when consumed together.
- Broccoli & Tomatoes — Both contain cancer-fighting properties, but a study at the University of Illinois indicates that the tumor-inhibiting effects are greatly enhanced when broccoli and tomatoes are consumed together. This can be found in the Journal of Nutrition.
- Blueberries(Wild) & Grapes — Its been proven, these fruits mixed together actually have a greater antioxidant response than one fruit eaten on its own.
- Superfood expert Dr. Steven Pratt has touted the immense synergy between blueberries and walnuts for brain health. He believes that blueberries combined with almost every other food will produce synergy.
- Good fats and Veggies — Eating a little "good fat" along with your vegetables helps your body absorb their protective phytochemicals, like lycopene from tomatoes and lutein from dark-green vegetables. Recognizing that cancer will feed on fat, the 1/4 avocado or the 1 tsp of flaxseed oil daily should be used in the most optimal way to achieve the greatest amount of nutritional value. This would likely be with the daily salads. A recent study measured how well phytochemicals were absorbed after people ate a lettuce, carrot, and spinach salad with or without 2 1/2 tablespoons of avocado. The avocado-eating group absorbed 8.3 times more alpha-carotene and 13.6 times more beta-carotene (both of which help

protect against cancer and heart disease), and 4.3 times more lutein (which helps with eye health) than those who did not eat avocados. Again, with cancer, the optimal amount of avocados to eat in one day is 1/4 of an avocado. An Iowa State University study that was reported in the American Journal of Clinical Nutrition found that people who ate salads with full- or low-fat dressings were better able to absorb lutein, a carotenoid (pigment-based plant compound) important in vision health. "With fat-free dressing, they essentially saw no evidence of the carotenoid showing up in the blood.

- Grapes and Omega 3 — The polyphenols found in grapes make it easier for your body to absorb omega-3 fatty acids.
- Cruciferous Vegetables (kale, cabbage, Brussels sprouts, cauliflower, broccoli, etc.) — Two phytochemicals naturally found in cruciferous vegetables (cambene and indole 3-carbinol) were more active when combined, according to research that tested the compounds individually and together in rats. The researchers found that the two compounds were able to protect the rats against liver cancer much better together activating enzymes that help the body eliminate carcinogens before they harm the genes. Foods rich in cambene include Brussels sprouts and certain varieties of broccoli. And all cruciferous veggies are rich in indole 3-carbinol.
- Apples consumed with the peel on can kill more free radicals than apple flesh without the skin. It turns out that the bulk of an apple's anticancer properties are hidden in the peel. The phytochemicals in the apple flesh seem to work best with the phytochemicals in the peel to reduce the risk of cancer.
- Apples, Onions, and Berries + Green Tea, Purple Grapes and Grape Juice — Or any combination of the first group of foods with the second, although onions seem to throw a bit of bitter water on this collection, from a taste-perspective anyway (Grape/Onion Juice, anyone?). A recent study found that the phytochemicals

quercetin (found mainly in apples, onions and berries) and catechin (found mainly in apples, green tea, purple grapes, and grape juice) worked together to help stop platelet clumping. Platelets are a component in blood that play an important role in forming clots. Platelets' clumping together is one of several steps in blood clotting that can lead to a heart attack.

- Nutmeg and Mushrooms — These make an unusual combination but since nutmeg is a natural antibacterial it can effectively counter the effects of the bacteria-prone fungus.

These are just a few examples of why combining certain high-density nutritious foods can be of greater benefit. One example above may not be useful to cancer patients since grape juice and even grapes have high sugar content. Please do not consider using this combination until well after your cancer has been eliminated.

Synergy is real. Some of its effects are measurable and quantifiable.

An example of nutritional synergy is:

One-half cup of beans provides the nutritional equivalent (in terms of usable protein) of two ounces of steak, while three cups of whole-wheat flour provide the equivalent of five ounces of steak. Eaten at separate times, the two food items contribute the equivalent of seven ounces of steak. But because they each have different amino acids, if the two substances are consumed together they provide the equivalent of nine ounces of steak, or 33% more useable protein. Here is a case where, literally, the whole is greater than the sum of its parts (Peter A. Corning, Ph.D. Institute for the Study of Complex Systems).

There is still much we don't know about how the components in food work together. Case in point: In the past 10 years, scientists have identified hundreds of biologically active plant-food components called phytochemicals (also called phytonutrients). A decade ago, we didn't even know about phytochemicals like lycopene (the one that has made tomatoes famous) or anthocyanins and pterostilbene (which have propelled blueberries into the news).

The easiest way to take advantage of food synergies is to eat a wide variety of colorful foods with as many meals as possible. Enjoy the endless possibilities!

Section Four

❦

Important Considerations

Important Considerations

Fighting cancer requires additional measures that aren't needed in other illnesses or diseases. However, some of the suggestions here will be beneficial in overall improved health and should be considered a healthy habit to begin.

Digestion

Are you one of those people who can consume a whole meal in less than 10 minutes? When asked how you did that, do you just shrug and say you must have been hungry. The body has to expend considerable extra energy to digest the food that has not been properly chewed and swallowed which ultimately means that less energy is directed toward recovery.

People assume that all of the digestion work is done in the stomach but in fact, the salivary glands, teeth and gums are all important in the digestion process. Digestion begins in the mouth with the salivary glands. Consider approaching the act of chewing in a new way. Every time you put a mouth full of food in your mouth, remember to chew it from 30-50 times until it is a liquid-pulp before you swallow. You produce up to 32 ounces of saliva every day. Chewing your food will help your body absorb vital nutrients more thoroughly and rapidly due to the enzymes secreted in your saliva. After food is liquefied in the mouth, the tongue will recognize the various flavors of each food and then send messages to the brain, which in turn, orders production of the corresponding digestive juices needed to break down that food. Chewing your food well ultimately leads to more effective digestion.

Don't drink any beverage with your meal

Another healthy habit to begin is to refrain from drinking beverages including water while eating a meal. Drink BarleyMax® before the meal and wait at least 30 minutes after the meal before drinking your next juice.

Friends and Family

When your friends and family find out your diagnosis, the first things you will receive are casserole dishes. Although these are well-meaning gestures, you will want to establish boundaries.

Create a list of fresh produce items and create another list of activities. Distribute these lists to them. Ask them if they would be willing to purchase a 5 pound bag of organic carrots for you each week and clean and peel them for you. Perhaps they would be willing to purchase a few other juicing ingredients (vegetables) each week, cleaned and ready for juicing.

If possible, ask them to come to your home and juice fresh vegetables and make fresh salads as often as possible. We are aware of those who have a schedule with friends and family coming in every hour juicing for the sick person.

An example of a produce list to give to them might look like:

Produce List:
- Leafy greens – collards, kale, chard, dandelion, spinach, turnip, mustard, beet, romaine etc.
(This list is according to the most nutrient dense so please try to consume as many of the top four each day in juice and in salad as possible.)
- Organic carrots – we peel them only because they taste sweeter. If they are not organic then we highly recommend they be peeled every time.
- Cucumbers – without wax
- Celery
- Beet
- Ginger
- Parsley
- Cilantro
- Romaine lettuce
- Tomatoes
- Onions
- Garlic
- Root vegetables
- Cabbage

Activities List:
- Juice vegetables
- Create fresh salads (clean, cut, store produce)
- Create fermented vegetables
- Create broccoli sprouts
- Clean house
- Go grocery shopping

Although your friends and family may think this is an unusual way to assist you, you can simply assure them that their efforts in this manner will be of great benefit to you.

Chapter Forty: Sugar and Fat Feed Cancer

For optimal benefit on the Recovery Diet, two particular food types must be significantly reduced or virtually eliminated. They both feed the cancer cells strengthening them making the fight more difficult. These two food items are fat and sugar.

A number of health care specialists in cancer were asked how much sugar and fat a person fighting cancer should consume in a typical day. Their responses are below:

Sugar:

There is ample evidence to support the fact that sugar from any source whether it is processed or from fruit, will enhance the growth of cancer.

A perfect example is when you go in for a PET scan. The IV solution that they are sending through your veins to see the glow of cancer contains sugar. When the cancer tastes the sugar, it will light up and the evidence comes to light.

Since sugar is a cancer feeder, it is best to avoid all sugars and sugar substitutes. Remember, simple carbohydrates break down into sugar so although it may not look as if it has sugar in it, the body will receive it as sugar. Example: bread, even wheat bread breaks down into the body and it uses it as if it was sugar.

Stevia may be used as a sweetener if desired, however, there has not been any significant evidence even to support the use of stevia so it may be best to use it sparingly.

If any sweetener is required, then blue, black or raspberries may be sparingly used since they have the least amount of sugar in all fruit and have a high amount of antioxidants. Berries should be used in very low amounts. Berries may be consumed at a rate of 10-15% of the daily diet. This would look like a small handful on a salad or in a smoothie, but not both.

Fats/Oils:

Cancer tends to become stronger when you consume fats and oils. This is not the result that you are looking for so it is best to avoid them almost entirely.

The best oil to use if you have any kind of cancer EXCEPT prostate cancer is Flax oil. If you DO have prostate cancer, it is best to grind the flax seeds fresh before you consume them and refrain from consuming any other oil. The flax seeds provide the important Omega 3 essential fatty acids.

On a typical day on the Recovery Diet the amount of fats/oils you should consume look like this:

- A few walnuts to get the essential fatty acid of Omega 3
- 2 Tablespoons of flax oil
- 1 teaspoon of fish oil
- ¼ of an avocado a day

The best way to utilize these oils is to create salad dressings for all of the large vegetable salads that you will need to consume daily while on this program.

The 1/4 avocado can be eaten in its entirety, sliced over a salad or used in a blended salad or as an ingredient in a smoothie.

The fish oil can be poured over a salad since it is only a teaspoon or it can be placed in a smoothie or blended salad.

Remember, nuts have fat. Stay away from them.

"Modern drug based medicine is as incomplete as a novel written with three vowels. As discordant as a symphony constructed using only some of the notes. Nutritional therapy is the much needed missing part of our vocabulary of healthcare. The fight against disease needs all the help it can get."

—Andrew W. Saul

Chapter Forty-One: Other Foods to Avoid

"It is easier to change a man's religion than to change his diet."

—Margaret Mead

Alfalfa Sprouts

Dangers of L-Cavanine

Alfalfa sprouts contain a protein called L-Cavanine. This is a toxic, non-protein amino acid and is naturally occurring in the seeds of alfalfa. Its purpose is to defend the seed against herbivores and is a vital source of nitrogen for the growing plant. When consumed by humans, the body mistakenly incorporates it into its own proteins in place of L-arginine, a beneficial amino acid. This produces proteins that may not function properly. Consuming foods with L-Cavanine might trigger a flare-up of lupus in patients experiencing a remission of symptoms, lower blood cell counts and spleen enlargement, according to the Beth Israel Deaconess Medical Center.

Bacterial Contamination

Alfalfa sprouts might contain several forms of deadly bacteria, including E. coli. The Food and Drug Administration, or FDA, recommends that children, the elderly and people with reduced immune function refrain from consuming alfalfa sprouts due to their increased susceptibility to infection. Sloan-Kettering notes case reports of people suffering infections with listeria and salmonella after consuming alfalfa in food and supplement form.

Other Safety Concerns
- • Avoid alfalfa sprouts if you are pregnant or nursing.
- • Alfalfa sprouts also have a high purine content, which might aggravate gout.

Note: The above is referring to alfalfa sprouts only. As the plant matures, the amount of the protein L-Cavanine drops dramatically. It is not a concern when consuming mature plants like what is used in BarleyMax®.

Coconut Oil

Although it may have some benefit for other illnesses, it still is too much fat for a cancer patient and therefore the weakness of the product far outweigh any benefits.

Chapter Forty-Two: Weight Loss and the Recovery Diet

"Be not sick too late, nor well too soon"

—Benjamin Franklin

It is not uncommon for people on the Recovery Diet to lose weight. Most people can afford to lose some weight. At first it will seem like a good thing but after a while friends may start to become concerned because they aren't used to seeing someone so thin.

Let's explore some reassuring facts:

First, most toxins are retained in our body fat. Therefore, when we lose the fat, we can more easily rid ourselves of the toxins. Second, our country doesn't understand the meaning of what "looking healthy" really is. We are so accustomed to seeing people with full faces, full stomachs and bulkier bodies that when we see someone who has visible shoulder blades, collarbones and cheekbones, we tend to think they look "unhealthy." It is better to judge your health through your energy rather than how much you weigh or even how you look.

We must be mindful that when people go through conventional methods to fight cancer, that is, chemotherapy and radiation, they not only lose weight, but they lose their hair, they develop diarrhea, numerous canker sores in their mouth among many other serious side effects. Those people truly do appear unhealthy.

For most people, after they have eliminated the cancer from their body and have been on the Recovery Diet long enough to ensure their organs and digestive system have fully recovered, their body will bring its weight back naturally (without the added toxins!).

If the weight loss is significant and becomes a serious concern for you or for your family there is a way that you can work on re-gaining some of it:

Introduce a little more cooked food. The calories will help to re-gain the weight. We don't recommend too much additional cooked, if possible, because it can interrupt the detoxification process. Ensure that the guidelines found in the "Cooked Food" section of this book are followed. When we say cooked food we're talking about steaming vegetables and eating healthy vegetable/bean soups. Eating traditional types of cooked food add strain on the digestive system which requires your body to expend more energy when the goal is to use that energy to continue to fight the cancer and detoxify the body.

Section Five

❧

Nutritional Supplementation

"Surgeons can cut out everything except cause."
—Herbert M. Shelton

In a survey discussed in the Prescription for Nutritional Healing Book, vitamin and mineral supplementation was found to be higher among people with cancer and with those who had recovered from it than the general population. About 64-81% of cancer patients and cancer survivors take nutritional supplements.

In his book, Natural Strategies for Cancer Patients, Dr. Russell Blaylock emphasizes the importance of nutrition with cancer patients. He also discusses the viability of significantly changing the diet while using conventional methods of cancer treatment like chemotherapy and radiation. This is one of the most well written and comprehensive books on the science behind nutrition and cancer that has been written. It would be a book that can be given to an oncologist if they are against the use of antioxidants with chemotherapy or radiation. I wish we had known about this book when we were trying to convince the oncologist that Joshua should have strong antioxidants while on his chemotherapy treatments. We were not as well prepared to make the case and now, we want anyone reading this book to know how to reach and teach your oncologist the value of taking supplements while using conventional methods to treat cancer.

If you prefer not to give your oncologist an entire book, this chapter will assist you in that effort.

Let's begin by asking the question, with all of the vegetables and juices that a person with cancer must consume on the Recovery Diet, why take supplements too?

The vegetables are only as good as the soil they grow in. The nutrient content of soil has changed exponentially in the last 20 years. With different variations of crop planting, excessive use of numerous types of pesticides, herbicides and fertilizers, and of course, the genetically modified seeds comes a significant decrease in nutrients left in the soil. If fewer are in the soil, then less will be in our vegetables.

There is a school of thought that even though we try as hard as we can to eat more vegetables and fruits, the produce itself can no longer keep our immune systems in peak performance. Even almonds have to be irradiated today, which eliminates their living enzyme capacity. The longer we continue to consume produce that lacks certain nutrients, the more likely our bodies will succumb to disease.

The Recovery Diet ascribes to the theory that selective supplementation each day in addition to juices and raw vegetables can provide the spectrum of vitamins, minerals, nutrients, enzymes, etc. that are needed during this critical time.

It will take a lot of energy to re-build the immune system so it has the capacity to go after the cancer cells and annihilate them. This energy must come from freshly extracted vegetable juices, raw vegetables and supplements.

The Supplements that are extremely important to the Hallelujah Recovery Diet Program are:

BarleyMax®: Young barley and alfalfa leaves that have been grown in the pristine, nutrient rich soil are harvested at their nutritional peak. They are then processed in a way that protects the delicate, fragile enzymes or heat sensitive nutrients. This ensures that Barley-Max® provides the cells of the body with maximum nutrition to keep them strong and vibrant. Using BarleyMax® each day is essential to strengthen the immune system and boost energy. It may well be the most nutritionally dense food you consume on any given day. BarleyMax® is available in three delicious flavors and capsules. For more in-depth information on BarleyMax® read the section under The Recovery Program chapter in this book.

FiberCleanse: For toxin removal. As the body begins cleansing, it is important that the toxins are eliminated timely and efficiently through proper bowel function. FiberCleanse provides a complete, full-body detoxification with a balanced blend of 28 herbs in a psyllium base to help not only cleanse the colon but the other cells throughout the body. It assists in restoring optimal bowel function ensuring the timely elimination of toxins from the body. Removing toxins from cells and achieving good bowel function is imperative to ensure timely and efficient elimination of toxins. Two to three good bowel movements per day are optimal. FiberCleanse is available in three flavors or capsules. Note: Consult your doctor or pharmacists before using FiberCleanse if on prescription drugs. Should not be used by pregnant or lactating women. It is not designed for using more than two or three consecutive months.

Nascent Iodine: Iodine supplementation is essential for thyroid function but is also critical for the proper function of every other gland in the body, from the tear glands, saliva glands, sweat glands, lymph glands, the pancreas, breasts and ovaries in women, and the prostate gland in men. It also enhances the immune system and assists with cell detoxification. Most people are extremely deficient in iodine and with the uncertainty of the impacts of the Fukushima fallout it is wise for everyone to consider iodine supplementation. When iodine combines with amino acids it supports apoptosis, which is essential when battling cancer. Nascent iodine is the best iodine for maximum utilization and uptake into the thyroid gland. This form also has strong anti-viral, anti-bacterial, and anti-germ properties. The optimal way to take nascent iodine is to put one or two drops into a small glass of water and then drink it about 15 minutes before consuming any food. This can be done 2 or 3 times a day when larger amounts are desired. Nascent iodine is active for 2 to 3 hours.

Vitamin D3: The health benefits of vitamin D3 vary depending on research. However, some studies show that vitamin D3, (cholecalciferol), is necessary for retaining bone density and for maintaining the body's immunity against cancers, heart disease, diabetes, weakness, muscle wasting and osteoporosis, among other disorders. Some lab and population studies have shown that vitamin D3 may help reduce the risk of certain cancers. Vitamin D3 may help with reducing the likelihood of skin, breast and colon cancers, among several others. Some studies suggest that vitamin D3 supplements may help treat the symptoms of seasonal affective disorder. Vitamin D3 is actually a hormone, produced naturally in the body. Recent research indicates that servings up to 5,000 - 10,000 IU per day may be needed to achieve optimal blood levels. Optimal blood levels of vitamin D3 are 50 to 80 ng/ml. Other studies have found that even higher doses have been used successfully in the battle with cancer but always under the care of a qualified health care professional. An inexpensive blood test will help determine your vitamin D3 blood level.

Professional Strength Probiotics: Probiotics play a critical role in the development, support and function of the immune system (about 80 to 85% of the immune system resides in the colon). A healthy intestinal tract is host to about 3 pounds of bacteria. About 85% of those should be 'friendly' flora. Most labels on probiotic brands boast a high amount of bacteria (CFU), but very few make it past your stomach acids to your colon, where probiotics are needed most. Hallelujah Diet Professional Strength Probiotic delivers up to 60% of its bacteria all the way to your colon – giving you far more effective results. Suggested serving is 2 probiotics daily for the first 2 to 4 weeks and then 1 daily thereafter.

Bio-Curcumin: Studies suggest that curcumin may be used to support the immune system. As inflammation is an underlying factor associated with cancer, curcumin is a powerful anti-inflammatory agent. Traditional health benefits of curcumin include: antioxidant, natural anti-inflammatory, anti-bacterial, anti-rheumatic, anti-carcinogenic and hepato protective. Based upon the research of Dr. Bharat Aggarwal, who headed the 12-member team of researchers at University of Texas (U.T.) M.D. Anderson Cancer Center, the use of curcumin, the biologically active extract of the turmeric spice can help supply the body with an abundance of free radical fighting nutrients that may help protect the body from various types of cancer. Bio-Curcumin provides the active components of turmeric in the most bioavailable form, delivering up to seven times higher concentrations in the blood than typical curcumin supplements. Take one capsule twice per day.

Digestive Enzymes: When battling cancer Digestive Enzymes are taken to assist in maximizing nutrient absorption from the foods we eat. For the first three weeks of the Recovery Program, take Digestive Enzymes with each juice and meal whether raw or cooked. This is to ensure maximum absorption of nutrients from the foods consumed during the initial adoption of the diet while the body is at its weakest state. After the first three weeks, when you eat cooked foods it is especially important to take 2 Digestive Enzymes to support digestive health in these situations as most of the naturally occurring enzymes are essentially destroyed.

Betaine Hydrochloric Acid (HCL) Pepsin & Gentian Root Extract: One of the reasons cancer is able to take hold is because the nutrients in the foods we consume aren't reaching the cells. Since stomach acid plays a key role in the digestion process it is wise to ensure that optimal conditions exist in the stomach. As people age the acid in their stomach that breaks down food for proper digestion becomes depleted. The addition of hydrochloric acid aids in the digestion and absorption of nutrients and assists the stomach in the breaking down process thereby reducing the energy required for digestion. Gentian, an ingredient in a wonderful bitter herbal, combined with Betaine HCL maintains a healthy pH in the stomach, supporting protein digestion, mineral absorption, small intestine pH and B12 absorption.

Essential Fatty Acids: Omega-3's are considered essential fatty acids. They are necessary for human health but the body can't make them — you must get them through food. Omega-3 fatty acids play a crucial role in brain function, as well as normal growth and development. They have also become popular because they may reduce the risk of heart disease. Research shows that omega-3 fatty acids reduce inflammation and may help lower risk of chronic diseases such as heart disease, cancer, and arthritis. Omega-3 fatty acids are highly concentrated in the brain and appear to be important for cognitive (brain memory and performance) and behavioral function.

Symptoms of omega-3 fatty acid deficiency include fatigue, poor memory, dry skin, heart problems, mood swings or depression, and poor circulation.

Other benefits of omega-3 fatty acids includes:
- Maintain overall cardiovascular and arterial health
- Support joint health, help to reduce inflammation and pain
- Support brain health, promoting concentration and long-term cognitive functions
- Promote mental well-being
- Support eye health

1 to 2 Tbsp of flax seed oil or 3 to 4 Tbsp of ground flax seed daily. If dealing with prostate issues, research suggests the use of ground flax seed rather than the oil is preferred. One teaspoon of Pharmax fish oil daily will meet the DHA needs of the body.

Vitamin B12, B6 and Folate: To maintain a healthy body, vitamin B12 is essential and according to the The American Journal of Clinical Nutrition, 39% of individuals tested had low-to-normal levels of B12 in their blood while 17% had levels low enough to cause symptoms of deficiency.

Health Benefits of Vitamin B12

- Maintains healthy nerve cells
- Maintains red blood cells
- Makes DNA, the genetic material in all cells
- Aids in proper digestion and the absorption of foods
- Helps with the synthesis of protein
- Helps metabolize carbohydrates and fats
- Plays an essential role in many other metabolic processes
- Aids in cell formation and cellular longevity

When B12 is combined with B6 and folate the benefits may include:

- Production of hydrochloric acid
- Absorption of fats and proteins
- Sodium and potassium balance
- Red blood cell formation
- Support for normal brain function
- Absorption of B12
- Support of the immune system
- Hormonal balance

It is important that B12 is in the Methylcobalamin form to ensure maximum absorption by the body.

Supplementation is not just what has been referred to as "expensive urine." It works with the body in the overall process of ensuring that nutrients that are needed to perform thousands of functions are readily available. Remember, if a cell is being created, the goal is to create the strongest, healthiest cell possible. This means there can be no nutrient deficiencies while this process is going on. And, it goes on every day.

Chapter Forty-Three: Can I Take Supplements While Using Conventional Approaches?

"Time and time again, throughout the history of medical practice, what was once considered as 'scientific' eventually becomes regarded as 'bad practice'."

—David Stewart

Can I be on the Recovery Diet while participating in conventional treatments such as chemotherapy and radiation? Organic vegetable juices will help combat the side effects of chemotherapy. There are over 2,000 papers cited worldwide on the benefits of antioxidants to patients during and after treatment. Antioxidants will protect against chemotherapy-induced side effects.

Some oncologists don't realize that antioxidants will actually protect against chemotherapy side effects and may even improve long-term survival in cancer patients. Through the years, several people have told us that when they made a significant dietary change as well as added nutritional supplementation, certain side effects of chemotherapy like, hair loss, nausea, need for blood transfusion, mouth sores, constipation, and several others seemed to have improved and were no longer challenges to contend with.

There are those who argue against nutritional supplementation during chemotherapy because they are concerned that antioxidants will protect cancer cells against free radical induced destruction. According to the research done by Dr. Russell Blaylock, the only way antioxidants have been shown to be harmful to cancer patients by increasing tumor growth or interfering with chemotherapy is when they have been administered as a sole or single entity.

He goes on to say that since 1932 the most common cause of death among cancer patients is starvation. It would seem that with the abundance of nutritional advancement, and the fact that even today, cancer patients are dying due to lack of nutrients for fear that those very same nutrients will feed the cancer cells, research should be on how to prevent people from starving to death while being treated for cancer. Even the Journal of the American Nutraceutical Association indicates considerable evidence that well-nourished cancer patients actually live longer than undernourished ones. The evidence is clear and readily available that there is no longer need to fear the nutrition, and that in fact, it needs to be consistently given to the person fighting cancer to strengthen the healthy cells to overcome the cancer cells.

There is little evidence that depicts any other negative implication on vitamin and mineral supplementation during conventional therapies.

Dr. Blaylock reviewed all of the available data on both sides of the issue and published an article in 2000 in the Journal of the American Nutraceutical Association where he concluded that the bulk of the evidence actually demonstrates great benefit to the cancer patient [1].

He cites Dr. Jerome Block, professor of medicine at the University of California at Los Angeles (UCLA) School of Medicine and former chief of medical oncology at the Harbor-UCLA Medical center as saying, "The hypotheses that antioxidants inhibition of free-radical activity may negate cytotoxic properties of some cancer therapies have been dependent on naive and inaccurate assumptions [2]."

He also references Dr. Charles Simone who has cited more than 350 studies, involving 2000 cancer patients that showed antioxidants extended the life span of cancer patients and improved quality of life. He included one of his own (Simone et al. 2000) involving 50 breast cancer patients who participated in either radiation or chemotherapy or both. All patients took large doses of various nutrients and antioxidants. He reported that 90% of them noted improvement in their physical symptoms, cognitive ability, sexual function and general well being. Not one person reported a worsening of symptoms.

Dr. Abraham Hoffer, MD, PhD. has treated more than 1100 cancer patients with high doses of vitamin C (most of whom were currently receiving chemotherapy). He concluded that their prolongation of life was heavily influenced by the use of various vitamins (Hoffer et al. 1993a; Hoffer et al. 1993b; Hoffer 1994; Hoffer 1996).

Antioxidants can enhance the efficacy of certain chemotherapy drugs. Dr. Blaylock sites several more studies to suggest to your oncologist that have demonstrated that antioxidant vitamins can actually enhance the efficacy of certain chemotherapy drugs on tumor cells which hopefully may convince them that antioxidants are an important addition to conventional treatment of cancers (Prasad et al. 1994; Prasad 1999; Prasad et al 2003).

Many doctors including Dr. Russell Blaylock have been treating cancer patients with nutritional supplementation either in supporting conventional methods or without them, and say they have found the patient to be stronger while battling the cancer and never have had a case where nutrition was detrimental to the patient. We just need to continue the process of educating those who have the most influence on our treatment options, that when a person maximizes certain nutrients and combinations of nutrients then the chances of him fighting off and recovering from disease is more likely to be quicker and require less recovery time and fewer invasive measures [3]

Science has become so intricate that now it has been proven that vitamins and minerals, phytonutrients, antioxidants, flavonoids, etc. can not only cause cancer cells to stop growing and subsequently die, but these very same nutrients will enable the healthy cells next to the cancer cells to maintain their strength and not allow any damage from chemotherapy or radiation. And what is more exciting is that these nutrients can actually enhance the effectiveness of the conventional therapies of chemotherapy and radiation while mitigating or preventing the most series side effects of these treatments.

Additional Studies:

From many studies over the past five decades, antioxidants are known to prevent cancer and other age-related diseases especially when taken long-term by healthy people [3].

In cancer patients or those at great risk of cancer, antioxidants in appropriate doses can also be of great benefit in treatment, taken in consultation with a nutrition-aware doctor [4].

Chapter Forty-Four: Daily Schedule of Supplements

Daily
- Fresh Air
- Prayer/Meditation
- Gentle Exercise
- Deep Breathing
- Forgiveness
- Plenty of Rest
- Humor

Upon Rising:
- Prayer/Meditation

7:00 am
- Iodine (nascent) supplement (on empty stomach); 1 to 2 drops
- BarleyMax® (1 tsp) mixed with 4 oz water (or taken dry)
- Digestive Enzyme capsule (1)
- B12-B6-Folate sublingual tablet (1)

8:00 am
- Juice (8 oz): carrot (70%) and vegetables (30%)
- Digestive Enzyme capsule (1)

8:30 am
- FiberCleanse (up to the first 90 days of The Hallelujah Recovery Diet; some people will require more cleansing than others) or B-Flax-D as directed

9:00 am
- BarleyMax® (1 tsp) mixed with 4 oz water (or taken dry)
- Digestive Enzyme capsule (1)

9:30 am
- Mid-Morning Snack – Cut veggies, or green smoothie with ¼ cup ground flax seed (minimal fruit)
- Digestive Enzyme capsule (1)
- Vitamin D3 capsule - 5,000 IU (1)
- Exercise, Sunshine, Rest, Deep Breathing

10:00 am
- Juice (8 oz): carrot (70%) and vegetables (30%)
- Digestive Enzyme capsule (1)

11:00 am
- Iodine (nascent) supplement (on empty stomach); 1 to 2 drops
- BarleyMax® (1 tsp) mixed with 4 oz water (or taken dry)
- Digestive Enzyme capsule (1)

12:00 noon – Lunch meal
- Digestive Enzyme capsules (2)
- Professional Strength Probiotics capsule (1)
- BioCurcumin capsule (1)
- Hydrochloric Acid (2)
- Salad – Whole or blended

1:00 pm
- Juice (8 oz): carrot (70%) and vegetables (30%)
- Digestive Enzyme capsule (1)

2:00 pm
- BarleyMax® (1 tsp) mixed with 4 oz water (or taken dry)
- Digestive Enzyme capsule (1)

2:30 pm
- Mid-Afternoon Snack (Cut veggies, or green smoothie)

- Digestive Enzyme capsule (1)
- Exercise, Sunshine, Rest, Deep Breathing

3:00 pm
- Juice (8 oz): carrot (70%) and vegetables (30%)
- Digestive Enzyme capsule (1)

4:00 pm
- Iodine (nascent) supplement (on empty stomach); 1 to 2 drops
- BarleyMax® (1 tsp) mixed with 4 oz water (or taken dry)
- Digestive Enzyme capsule (1)

5:00 pm – Supper meal
- Digestive Enzyme capsules (2)
- Professional Strength Probiotics capsule (1)
- B12-B6-Folate sublingual tablet (1)
- Prayer
- Salad – Whole or blended
- Hydrochloric Acid (2)
- Cooked food

6:00 pm
- Juice (8 oz): carrot (70%) and vegetables (30%)
- Digestive Enzyme capsule (1)

7:00 pm
* BarleyMax® (1 tsp) mixed with 4 oz water (or taken dry)
* Digestive Enzyme capsule (1)

8:00 pm
- Juice (8 oz): carrot (70%) and vegetables (30%)
- Digestive Enzyme capsule (1)

10:00 pm
- Sleep

This schedule can also be found in Appendix C. You can print a schedule from *www.UnravelTheMystery.com/downloads.*

Chapter Forty-Five: Highly Recommended Supplement

"Adam and Eve ate the first vitamins, including the package."
—E.R. Squibb

Melatonin

This supplement has been shown to protect against chemotherapy-induced weakened immune. In a randomized study by Lissoni et al. In 1999, people receiving chemotherapy also were given melatonin and it was found they had less hair loss, vomiting, nausea, stomach issues, red blood cell issues, blood platelet issues, lack of strength and fatigue. It would appear that adding melatonin to a chemotherapy regimen might prevent some toxic effects of the chemotherapy drugs.

Still other studies have also shown how melatonin has rescued bone marrow cells from death which is induced by chemotherapy compounds. (Maestroni et. Al 1994a; 1994b; 1998).

Depending on the type of cancer a person has, melatonin may be beneficial as an added supplement. It is not known how it will affect leukemia so those people may need to be cautious with its use. Prostate cancer men will need to get their blood tested for prolactin before they consider melatonin and ovarian cancer women have found better success in lower doses.

Selenium

Selenium is an essential trace mineral involved in a number of biological processes including kinase regulation, gene expression and immune function. Animal and epidemiological studies have suggested there may be an inverse relationship between selenium supplementation and cancer risk[1]. Low selenium levels have been linked to several different types of cancer. Selenium has anti-viral and anti-bacterial properties. Taken with vitamin E it can move heavy metals (especially mercury) from the body.

Zinc

Zinc, a trace mineral which, is vital for the functioning of numerous cellular processes, is critical for growth, and may play an important role in cancer outcome. The intracellular levels of this mineral are regulated through the coordinated expression of zinc transporters, which modulate both zinc influx as well as efflux. Zinc was first described in 1988 as an estrogen regulator with later work suggesting a role for this transporter in cancer growth and metastasis. Zinc is a requirement for all life on earth. Despite being the 27th most abundant element, the physiological importance of zinc is unparalleled. There are four general biological roles of zinc, which include its structural, signaling, catalytic, and regulatory functions. The ubiquity of zinc in biological processes lends itself to the idea that aberrations in zinc status may play a significant role in cellular dysfunction, including the development and/or progression of cancer. Evidence in support of this idea is extensive[2]. Zinc has long been used to help stimulate and support the immune system.

Ubiquinol

Ubiquinol is the antioxidant form of CoQ10 and is essential for mitochondrial synthesis of energy. It is the only known lipid-soluble antioxidant that is endogenously synthesized, protecting biological cell membranes against lipid peroxidation as well as regenerating other antioxidants such as vitamin C and vitamin E. Published clinical and experimental research shows that ubiquinol affects cardiovascular health, neuronal metabolism, renal health, and genes related to lipid/lipoprotein metabolism and inflammation.

Melanoma and breast cancer are two types of malignancies for which CoQ10 has demonstrated substantial clinical benefit.

A recent melanoma study compared the effects of administering alpha interferon with or without daily CoQ10 (400 mg). There was an astounding 10-fold lower risk of metastasizing in the CoQ10-supplemented group! This effect was even more pronounced for those with more advanced melanoma, where CoQ10-supplemented patients were 13 times less likely to develop metastasis. Alpha interferon is an immune boosting drug that can induce side effects so severe that patients have to discontinue it. In this study, only 22% of CoQ10-supplemented patients developed side effects while taking supplemental CoQ10 compared to 82% not taking supplemental CoQ10 [3][4].

Even the National Cancer Institute which has displayed bias against certain alternative therapies reports on the role that CoQ10 may play in cancer treatments.

Lycopene

Lycopene is a carotenoid, a natural pigment made by plants and various fruits and vegetables, including tomatoes, apricot, guava, and watermelon. Lycopene's absorption is improved with concurrent dietary fat intake. Lycopene inhibits androgen receptor expression in prostate cancer cells in vitro and, along with some of its metabolites, reduces prostate cancer cell proliferation and may modulate cell-cycle progression. Lycopene may also affect the insulin-like growth factor intracellular pathway in prostate cancer cells. Results from several in vitro and animal studies have indicated that lycopene may have chemopreventive effects for cancers of the prostate, skin, breast, lung, and liver; however, human trials have been inconsistent in their findings. Clinical trials utilizing lycopene in prostate cancer patients with various different clinical presentations (e.g., early stage, prostate-specific antigen (PSA) relapse, advanced disease) have yielded inconsistent results[5]. If I had prostate cancer, I would include the least sugar-ridden forms of lycopene rich foods realizing that the potential for food synergy is still a factor, and including these lycopene-rich, foods may attain results that may not have been indicated in clinical trials.

Section Six

❧

Alternative Treatment Options

> *"Each patient carries his own doctor inside him."*
> — Norman Cousins

According to the Life Extension book entitled *Disease Prevention and Treatment*, there are around 4 million people in America today who will survive cancer and live a full and productive life. The same book suggests that 1,500 people will die every day from cancer, which equates to a survival rate for cancer victims of 44%. These numbers would be difficult to validate since many of the people who die don't have cancer on their death certificate as the primary cause.

In our son's case, the wrong kind of cancer was placed on his death certificate and now it will not be counted in the appropriate statistics. The importance of this is that in recent history, there were two other students in his small high school that had the exact same kind of cancer that he did. But if anyone were to research this, his cancer would not show up in those stats.

One question that must be asked is how many of these deaths were the result of the treatment and how many were induced by disease?

The University of Texas MD Anderson Cancer Center (Houston) found that 99.3% of patients have heard of complementary medicine, and 68.7% of patients reported having used at least one unconventional therapy (Richardson et al. 2000). Since this research is 13 years old, it would seem likely that those numbers have both increased significantly.

Cancer isn't the same as it was 20 years ago. Charlotte Gerson has said in many interviews as well as in her book, *Healing the Gerson Way*, that the way she treats cancer isn't exactly the same way her father treated it years ago. She said it is stronger and more resistant than it was then.

We believe without any doubt that the Recovery Diet and selective supplementation of whole food minerals and antioxidants is the primary way to rebuild your body to fight against cancer. Yet, with the advent of some extraordinary measures we would be remiss if we didn't help you to identify them so you can make an informed decision on whether to add them to your artillery as you continue to battle this disease.

There are many alternative, complementary or stand-alone treatments that have been used successfully by practitioners both in the United States and across the world. These all can be used in conjunction with the Recovery Diet.

While cancer cells need to be killed (or reverted into normal cells), that is only one aspect of a natural cancer treatment. The treatment will likely need to build the immune system, shrink tumors, deal with microbes (which may be a cause of cancer and must be dealt with), deal with lactic acid in the bloodstream, deal with weakness (such as the cachexia cycle or a weak liver), and so on.

There are hundreds of alternative cancer treatments. There are many books written to describe the top ones. Unfortunately, for home use, there are likely less than two-dozen that can be considered strong enough to use in advanced cancer care. Some of these make sense from a logical perspective, don't cost a lot, and will not harm you in any case.

If we had cancer, we would consider adding some of these protocols in addition to the Recovery Diet, superfood supplementation and additional supplementation:

Home Based Supplemental Methods

Exercise – This is so important that a separate chapter has been designated in this book to convince you of the powerful changes your body will undertake when you add exercise into your cancer fighting regimen.

Hyperthermia – Far Infrared saunas provide a place where the body is exposed to high temperatures. High temperatures can kill cancer cells, usually without damage to normal tissues. In most countries of the world, hyperthermia is considered the 4th major modality of cancer therapy along with surgery, chemotherapy, and radiation. Only in the United States is it not at that status. In the United States it is used only as part of an alternative cancer treatment protocol.

Hyperthermia generates heat to create more blood supply to the area. Because cancers have such a high rate of metabolism, when they are warmed up with far infrared heat for example, they literally over-metabolize themselves to death. Some cancers are associated with viruses. You can make a body produce more heat shock proteins--one of the most common proteins in life, widely distributed all throughout nature. They allow healthy cells to persist in the face of adversity. Far Infrared saunas provide a form of whole-body hyperthermia that can improve your health by eliminating toxins from the body [1].

Some have found Hyperthermia to be very effective when used with a low dose of potentiated and targeted chemotherapy, also known as Insulin Potentiation Therapy (IPT).

Treating Candida – Many cancer patients have candida and without treating it simultaneously, the body must split its energy in fighting two battles. Many of these home-based methods will assist in fighting candida.

Protocel – A brown liquid formula that seems to have amazing effects on cancer. It is designed to specifically target cancer cells and weakens them and they finally die without disrupting any of the healthy cells in the body. The book entitled *Outsmart Your Cancer* by Tanya Harter Pierce devotes nearly 100 pages to this incredible product. It deserves great consideration and I would definitely place that in my top options to consider.

Ionic Foot Detox Machine – This machine does have controversy that surrounds it. However, it represents a significant advance in Energetic Medicine. It is a spa device, which appears to be associated with providing negative electron (Ionic) energy, enabling the body to accomplish detoxification, potential elimination of heavy metals, and balancing of inherent energy fields. As a therapeutic spa it seems to be an extremely useful adjunct to both Mainstream and Holistic medical therapies. Initial observations and anecdotal reports indicate this technology warrants further investigation. You can get these treatments from a health care provider or you can purchase a unit and take them at home.

Coffee Enemas – Coffee enemas are a way to remove circulating toxins and partial metabolites by dilating bile ducts and cleansing the liver. It is important that they be used in conjunction with juicing as the removal of toxins needs to be supported with extensive nutrition. The coffee administered by means of a cleansing enema stimulates an enzyme system in the liver known as glutathione S-transferase (GST) that removes a vast variety of free radicals (electrophiles) from the bloodstream. Under the influence of a coffee enema the GST enzyme system increases in activity to 650% above normal and removes electrophiles (free radicals) from the bloodstream. During the time coffee is being held in the intestines, all the blood in the body passes through the liver at least five times. The blood circulates through the liver every three minutes [2].

Vitamin B17 – Also known as nitrilosides or Laetrile. When the laetrile compound molecule comes across a cancer cell, it is broken down into 2 molecules of glucose: 1 molecule of hydrogen cyanide and 1 molecule of benzaldehyde. In the early days of laetrile research it was assumed that the hydrogen cyanide molecule was the major cancer cell killing molecule, but now it is known that it is the benzaldehyde molecule that is by far the major reason the cancer cell is killed.

The reason laetrile therapy takes so long to work, in spite of the marvelous design of the laetrile molecule, is because if the laetrile molecule happens to chemically react with the enzyme of a non-cancerous cell before it reacts with the enzyme of a cancerous cell the non-cancerous cell will break apart the laetrile molecule in such a way that it can no longer kill a cancer cell. Thus you have to take enough laetrile molecules, over a long enough time, that enough laetrile molecules coincidently (as far as we know) hits all of the cancer cells first. The second way that laetrile therapy works is in conjunction with the Recovery Diet. It is designed to build up the cancer fighting cells in the body, and let them work on the cancer cells. What they do is break down the enzymes surrounding the cancer cell so the white blood cells can identify and kill the cancer cell. One of the good side-effects of laetrile therapy is that more vitamin B12 is made in the body. With this in mind, make sure you supplement laetrile therapy with vitamin C. Vitamin C and vitamin B12 are, by themselves, an effective synergistic treatment for cancer.

If you want to know more about vitamin B17, watch the documentary "A World without Cancer" by G. Edward Griffin. This is quite an "old" documentary.

Vitamin B17 appears in abundance in untamed nature. Because B17 is bitter to the taste, in man's attempt to improve tastes and flavors for his own pleasure, he has eliminated bitter substances like B17 by selection and crossbreeding. It can be stated as a general rule that many of the foods that have been domesticated still contain the vitamin B17 in the part that is not eaten by modem man, such as the seeds in apricots. Listed in Appendix E is an evaluation of some of the more common foods that contain laetrile. Keep in mind that these are averages only and that specimens vary widely depending on variety, locale, soil, and climate.

Distilled Water – We strongly recommend Distilled water for the first 3 months on the Recovery Diet to assist in the detoxification process. It is best purchased in BPA free containers if possible or you can make your own from a fairly inexpensive machine.

Alkaline Water – After the 3 months of distilled water, we recommend Alkaline water. Ionized water increases alkalinity and uses its negative oxidation-reduction potential (ORP) to neutralize free radicals. Another important aspect that can be attributed to negatively charged, reduced water – low micro clustering of the water molecules. This process reduces the surface tension of the water and allows for solubility and cell permeability. Our studies found that the best machine to perform these functions is the Enagic SD501. You can find one on the internet.

Essiac Tea – Four simple ingredients of burdock root, sheep sorrel herb (powdered), slippery elm bark (powdered), Turkish rhubarb root (powdered). Lab tests show that sheep sorrel is the actual cancer killer and the other ingredients combine for a synergistic immune booster and blood purifier. The quality of the ingredients is the most important aspect of beneficial Essiac.

Pulsed Electromagnetic Field Therapy – several studies have found magnetic therapy has promising results in inhibiting tumor growth and deserves additional attention as an adjunctive therapy combined with other modalities to fight cancer. Magnetotherapy provides a non-invasive, safe, and easy method to directly treat the site of injury, the source of pain and inflammation, and other types of diseases and pathologies.

Proboost – This product is made from an animal that was raised in a country with strict standards on animal treatment and no known illnesses in these animals. Its purpose is to activate the white blood cells in an effort to boost the immune system. The thymus gland is responsible for maturing the T-cells with specific proteins so that these act as soldiers of the immune system. The T-cells are a key to regulating the immune system by maintaining the tempo of the B-cells which are antibody producers to a particular antigen. The T-cells also attack and destroy invading cells such as viruses and cancer cells. Initially when T-cells are created by the bone marrow, they are not able to perform their function until they are matured by the Thymic Protein A from the Thymus.

Moringa – The moringa tree has long been recognized by traditional healers as valuable in the treatment of tumors. Its cooked leaves have an estimated 17 times the calcium of milk, 10 times the vitamin A of carrots, 15 times the potassium of bananas, 25 times the iron of spinach and 4 times the protein of eggs. In addition to the leaves, the seed pods (drumstick) and other parts of the tree can be eaten as part of a tasty, nutritious dish. It seems however; the roots are where the medicine is [3][4].

Outside of Home Supplemental Methods

UVBI – Ultraviolet Blood Irradiation Therapy involves removing a very small volume of blood under sterile conditions, briefly exposing that blood to selected frequencies of Ultraviolet Light and re-infusing the blood back into the body. The blood is also treated with a very small amount of temporary acting anti-coagulant (heparin). UVBI is currently approved by the FDA for treating certain forms of lymph cancer and psoriasis. UVBI therapy is used clinically as both a specific (i.e. psoriasis, lymph cancer) and non-specific (chronic infections, chronic fatigue, auto-immune diseases, scleroderma, etc.) immune modulating therapy. Certain forms of cancer, auto-immune diseases, infections and tissue transplant rejection have all been published as benefiting from UVBI therapy. It is a process that several holistic doctors are using in an integrated plan to defeat cancer.

Hyperbaric Oxygen – Cancer exists in a low-oxygen environment and plentiful oxygen can kill it off. Hyperbaric oxygen therapy (HBOT) has also been shown to significantly reduce inflammation in the body, which is known to be a precursor to cancer. Thus it has the potential to be a simple alternative cancer treatment. HBOT involves increasing blood oxygen levels. 'Hyper' means increased and 'baric' relates to pressure. Oxygen is one of the gases in the air, and it's essential for life. Normally, oxygen makes up just over one fifth (21%) of air. In HBOT treatment, people breathe in pure (100%) oxygen. This is done by sitting in a chamber known as a hyperbaric oxygen chamber and using a mask or hood. Oxygen is carried around the body by the blood. Breathing in 100% (pure) oxygen under increased pressure allows extra oxygen to be taken up by the bloodstream and dissolved at a far greater rate. This extra oxygen can help where healing is slowed down by infection or where blood supply is limited by damage to the tissues. HBO treatment encourages new blood vessels to grow and carry additional blood, it increases the ability of the body's defense mechanisms to fight infection and kill bacteria, and helps reduce any swelling that may occur around the area.

A 2012 review by Moen suggests that this procedure will not stimulate tumor growth or enhance recurrence. Rather, the review suggests that the evidence supporting this method for tumor-inhibiting effects is strong and bears more recognition of this therapy [5].

Other significant points of HBOT:

1. Research shows it is already used to good effect when used with radiotherapy where it does seem to reduce tissue damage and side effects.
2. Some cancer centers use it to improve the assimilation of chemotherapy drugs.
3. On its own, in research with mice models, Hyperbaric Oxygen did not seem to offer any benefit in the fight against cancer. However, when used in combination with a Ketogenic Diet, albeit in mice models, the benefits were significant. Imagine what it would do when combined with the Hallelujah Recovery Diet!

Oral Health Care – One of the first things I would do if I was diagnosed with cancer, especially a breast tumor would be to go to a biological dentist and get mercury amalgams removed, root canals evaluated, cavitations repaired and any other dental work relating to gum and tissue health addressed. If you are not using an oral irrigation system daily, you should begin. I recommend the Hydrofloss oral irrigation system.

Root canals and other dental concerns are risk factors for various illnesses, including cancer. Pockets of bacterial infection can exist under the teeth and be undetectable using screening methods such as x-rays. This is especially true for teeth that have had root canals. These infections can persist for years without either the patients' or their doctors' and dentists' knowledge. Compounding this problem is the fact that bacteria and other toxins that can build up in root canals can be very difficult to eliminate. As a result, just as mercury vapors from amalgam fillings continually leech out to be absorbed by the body's tissues and organs, so too do harmful bacteria and related toxins leak out from root canals and the gums in general to depress immune function. Left untreated, these unhealthy microorganisms can severely weaken the immune system over time. It may be years before the cancer develops and no one thinks to connect it with the mouth. A Biological, or Holistic dentist is the only one you should see. They are specifically trained to remove both root canals and mercury fillings properly and completely. Do your research and be selective as not all biological dentists using this label are as knowledgeable as they need to be. Dentists and doctors indicating that upwards of 90% of breast cancer patients having a significant dental issue have written several articles. Others suffering from cancer may find great results after they get their oral pathology addressed as well.

To find a legitimate Biological dentist start searching here:
Huggins Applied Healing
5082 List Drive
Colorado Springs, CO 80919
Toll Free: (866) 948-4638
E-mail: info@drhuggins.com
www.hugginsappliedhealing.com
or
International Academy of Biological Dentistry and Medicine
(IABDM)
19122 Camellia Bend Circle
Spring, Texas 77379
Telephone: (281) 651-1745
www.iabdm.org

Ozone Therapy – Ozone is a blue colored form of oxygen (it's what makes the sky blue), and unlike regular oxygen, it is composed of three oxygen atoms instead of two. It is the addition of the third oxygen atom that makes ozone "supercharged" oxygen, and gives it all of its remarkable medical properties. Ozone is a potent regulator of the immune system. Ozone increases antioxidant protection more than any other therapy including vitamin C. Ozone is a powerful mitochondrial stimulant. Someone who has been fully trained should only administer it.

Enzyme Therapy – Enzyme therapy involves taking enzyme supplements as an alternative form of cancer treatment. Enzymes are natural proteins that stimulate and accelerate many biological reactions in the body. Digestive enzymes, many of which are made in the pancreas, break down food and help with the absorption of nutrients into the blood. Metabolic enzymes build new cells and repair damaged ones in the blood, tissues, and organs. Dr. Nicholas Gonzalez practices enzyme therapy in New York.

Radio Frequency Ablation (RFA) – High frequency electric current that is used to heat tumors from within. Inoperable tumors have been the target and this was initially done to provide relief only. We took our son to have this done. Unfortunately, by the time the doctor saw him, his tumor was too large for this procedure to be successful. This technique has become so valuable that in medical circles the word is, it may replace both surgery and radiation therapy. It is cost-effect, non-invasive, low-risk and the National Institutes of Health now consider RFA the most predictable, safest, and simplest method for thermal ablation in bone, liver, adrenal, kidney, prostate, breast and brain tumors. It has even been used in lung tumors.

Insulin Potentiation Therapy (IPT) – IPT is a true Stage IV alternative cancer treatment. It uses a combination of two orthodox drugs - insulin and a chemotherapy drug. Cancer cells have highly active insulin receptors. With IPT the insulin works on the cell membranes and allows chemotherapy to target cancer cells. Thus, it is the chemotherapy that kills the cancer cells, however, because of the insulin; the amount of chemotherapy needed is greatly reduced, meaning the side effects of the chemotherapy are greatly reduced. Thus, the chemotherapy is much more potent (hence the word: potentiation), much less chemotherapy is needed, and far less side effects are experienced.

Intravenous Vitamin C – An article published in the British Journal of Cancer Vol. 84, No.11, by Neil Riordan at the Riordan Clinic indicated that up to 46% of cancer patients have severe deficiencies in vitamin C. This procedure is excellent for infections, cellular recovery and when combined with Reishi mushrooms it enhances anti-tumor effects (Dr. Fukumi Morishiga). Interesting, how the synergy effect is seen again.

DMSO – Some alternative cancer centers use Dimethyl sulfoxide with some success. There is evidence that DMSO can cause cancerous cells to become benign. It may stop or slow the development of cancers, such as breast, ovarian, bladder and colorectal cancers. It is also promoted as an immune system booster.

DMSO Potentiation Therapy is used by some cancer centers to protect healthy cells from chemotherapy and to decrease side effects from the drugs. It seems to enhance the targeting action of drugs with cancer cells.

Several books have exceptional information about these various modalities.

The two I recommend are:

Outsmarting Cancer by Tanya Harter Pierce

Everything You Need To Know To Beat Cancer by Chris Woollams

Two other books that may be useful are:

Killing Cancer Not People by Robert G. Wright

Cancer-Free your Guide to Gentle, Non-toxic Healing by Bill Henderson

Section Seven

❧❧

Cancer Recovery Keys

Chapter Forty-Six: Healing Reactions

"I don't believe that there are any situations or any person on this planet who can not be helped, whose life can not be made better. And many of these situations can be cured. If your doctor does not know something, it does not mean that the knowledge does not exist elsewhere. No body is beyond hope. No body!"

—Natasha Campbell McBride

When your body begins to receive the vast amount of nutrients from the Hallelujah Recovery Diet day after day, it won't be long before it begins to make some big adjustments.

One of the first things we tell people is that when the body finally has enough energy, the first thing it will do is begin "housecleaning." This means that as good quality nutrition is added and stronger, healthier new cells are continuously being formed, the weak, sick, older cells will die off and will need to be removed.

If you have been on the Recovery Diet for a while and one day awaken and can't understand why you don't feel as well, you should congratulate yourself on the fact that you finally have accumulated enough nutrition and energy in your body to achieve a "healing crisis."

When toxic foods are eliminated, and we start eating living foods, especially fresh vegetable juices, the body is able to rebuild as well as cleanse. This internal cleansing results in toxins/poisons being emptied into the bloodstream, and is what many people refer to as detoxification. During this process, one may experience a range of both physical and mental discomfort that will subside over time, depending on the amount, degree, and length of time that a cleansing diet is sustained. Some may notice mild cleansing or detoxification signs, such as fatigue, mood swings and/or a headache, within a few days of making the change. A small percentage will experience severe detoxification indicators a few weeks later ,which may include diarrhea, depression, vomiting, or an unexplained rash. Each person is different, and each body reacts in different ways. What is important is that these symptoms are evidence that the body is in a cleansing mode. Eventually, as the "bad" gets eliminated and the "good" is put back in, symptoms start to abate, and the body starts functioning at a higher level of health.

Don't be discouraged or afraid. This process is vitally important to reach. One doctor tells his patients that when they start to vomit the entire staff erupts in applause encouraging the patient that they are removing the toxins and another layer of health will soon follow. He uses extreme detoxification methods in his practice that should only be done under a doctor's direction and care.

The Hallelujah Recovery Program promotes cleansing while the body rebuilds. This is different from the teachings of a lot of other programs. Many times people are encouraged to detoxify, or cleanse, the body first, and then work to rebuild the body. But the body is starved for nutrition so by feeding it high quality foods in the form of juices and BarleyMax® at the very start it will strengthen and rebuild while performing the function of cleansing. Therefore, it is essential to deal with both the toxicity and deficiency issues simultaneously.

Why does Detoxification occur?

The main function of the body is to create homeostasis- the state at which every part of the body is properly balanced and in a state of perfect health. Over the years, when that balance or homeostasis is upset due to lifestyle choices, the body starts to function in a constant mode of repair and restoration, working to keep you alive at all costs. To accomplish this, the body stores the toxic elements that have been forced upon it because it doesn't have the energy to do both tasks – repair and detoxify. The toxins may be stored deep within the tissues and cells. Unfortunately, it is when toxins are stored that real damage begins to occur in those areas, and signs of disease begin to manifest. As we begin making healthier nutrition and lifestyle choices, the body starts a cleansing process- eliminating the bad (toxins) and putting in the good (live nutrients) and the areas damaged by stored toxins begin to rebuild.

The cleansing process has several avenues of elimination:

1. Elimination through the bowels. One of the most important issues to address in detoxification is elimination. There are some indications that between 75-90% of Americans suffer from sluggish bowels. This can be a warning sign of greater health problems to come. If toxins from our body (dead cells, waste products, etc.) are not eliminated quickly, they can be re-absorbed into the body and result in a toxic buildup, which can ultimately contribute to the breakdown of the body and illness. Therefore, it is vital that bowel function be optimized in order to ensure rapid and efficient elimination of toxins.

2. Elimination through the skin. One way to help eliminate toxins is through dry skin brushing where the dead cells on the skin are brushed away. We lose over two pounds of toxins each day through our skin. Our skin is our largest organ and as such, when the bowels are not eliminating as they should, the toxins will try to get out any way that they can – the skin is one such avenue. This is why some people develop rashes or acne when their body goes through a cleansing process. Sores or rashes on the skin may be the last part of the body to heal as the body often heals from inside out.

3. Elimination through the lymph system. The lymph system is part of the immune system, and it assists the body in ridding itself of toxic elements; however, the lymph does not move through the body unless the body moves. Thus, exercise is a key component when it comes to dealing with signs of detoxification and rebuilding the immune system. An excellent way to move the lymph is through walking or rebounding for at least fifteen minutes every day.

4. Elimination through the mucous membranes. The mucous membranes trap toxins and help to move them out of the body; however, if the mucous is not kept at a thin consistency, the toxins may become trapped and sometimes infection will develop. Consuming an adequate amount of distilled or alkaline water (6-8 glasses per day) will help keep the mucous thin enough to flow out of the body rapidly.

What to do about the effects of Detoxification

When you go through detoxification you have several options to choose from:

Option 1: Do nothing and allow the body's detoxification to run its course. The body will only cleanse what it has the energy to deal with. Generally, these detoxification episodes last 3-7 days.

Option 2: Slow down the cleansing. Eat more cooked foods and cut back a little on the BarleyMax®. This generally results in an easing of the discomfort because the body is concentrating more of its energy on digesting and dealing with cooked foods than it is with cleansing and rebuilding. This is only recommended if the symptoms are too difficult to handle. The optimal method is to wait out the process and allow it to run its course without slowing it down.

Option 3: Speed it up! Help the body to cleanse more quickly. This entails eliminating solid foods; increasing water, juices and BarleyMax®; juice fasting and possibly even partaking in some water enemas or colonics. The symptoms won't disappear; in fact, they may even intensify for a short period of time. But when they are over, they usually don't reoccur in the same manner.

No matter which course you choose, getting rest is of the utmost importance. The body needs to reserve its strength for cleansing and rebuilding.

One of the reasons many people on The Hallelujah Recovery Diet do not experience severe cleansing is because of the 15% cooked food that is part of the program. It causes a slow-down in the release of toxins. They continue to be removed from the body, but at a much slower rate and over a longer period of time. That is why the cooked part is so important. Usually within the first two weeks, most people are over the symptoms of detoxification. However, there are instances where it may take over a year for the body to completely release all toxins, such as when a person has been exposed to environmental toxins, chemotherapy, radiation, excessive prescription drugs as well as the S.A.D.

Drinking plenty of water helps to dilute the toxins and move them out of the body more rapidly reducing some of the discomfort from detoxification.

The God-given intelligence of our cells is forever moving us toward full and complete homeostasis, or balance. While detoxification can be uncomfortable at times, it is nature's way of keeping us healthy.

So, if you believe you are going through or have gone through a detoxification episode – REJOICE!!! It means that your body and immune system are still recognizing when things are not as they should be and are busy putting it back in proper, working order.

Over time, as you stay on the diet and lifestyle, the detoxification episodes tend to get shorter and the length of time between them tends to get longer, as the body continues on its quest for health and well-being.

Chapter Forty-Seven: Exercise

"Sometimes the walk to the doctors is a better cure than the medicine you receive"
—Benny Bellamacina

There has been a growing movement that has shifted the way of thinking in the recovery of people. Years ago, people who were hospitalized were told to stay in their beds so they could recover. In the case of cancer, people stayed in their beds and hoped for the best. Today, the pendulum has begun to turn. Instead of staying sedentary through the cancer recovery process, people are being asked to get up and move.

Dr. Thierry Bouillet, MD, Medical Director of the Institute of Radiotherapy at the Avicenne Medical Center of the University of Paris, is also an expert in sports medicine who was intrigued with reading several recent studies that showed fewer cases of cancer among the most physically active patients as well as distinctly fewer relapses in those who remained active as compared to those who didn't.

He believes there are numerous ways that exercise will improve the body:

- When it reduces areas that store fat, it will reduce the areas that toxins are stored.
- It modifies and reduces our excess hormones that could stimulate growth of cancers.
- It reduces blood sugar levels and as a result, reduces the secretion of insulin and insulin growth factor (IGF) which can cause tissue inflammation and increase the growth and spread of tumors.

297

- It can even lower the level of inflammation in the blood.
- It has a protective effect on the immune system against stress from bad news.

He has also seen research that suggests that when a patient learns of bad news their NK (natural killer) cells count will reduce rapidly unless they have been exercising consistently and moderately. He has found great success in ensuring many of his cancer patients begin a moderate level of exercise when they begin their chemotherapy. The preferred method of exercise he uses is karate. He sees a lot of value between the movement of the exercise and the meaningful relationships that are formed. Dr. Bouillet is one of a growing number of doctors that see exercise as part of recovery.

Oncologists are slowly beginning to realize the idea that physical movement is one of the most proven methods to relieve fatigue that results from disease or from its treatment.

It must be noted that not all cancer patients can perform exercise from the beginning of their conventional treatment. Whether they have had surgery in places that require additional time for healing, or are extremely fatigued from nausea from chemotherapy, it is still important to work with a health care provider in all cases. But adding any form of light activity or movement is likely to benefit them.

Wendy Demark-Wahnefried, PhD, of Duke University wrote an editorial in the Journal of Clinical Oncology suggesting there is a reduction in cancer relapse rate of 50 to 60% with exercise. She actually compared exercise to one of the most revolutionary drug combinations of her time: Herceptin, combined with chemotherapy was considered "a major turning point in the eradication of suffering and death from cancer" [1]. But, physical exercise can provide benefits to people who have a broader variety of cancers than Herceptin could since it is typically used just for breast cancer.

Just remember, more is not always better when it comes to exercise. In fact, there is evidence that high intensity exercise, if done for a length of time, over time, can actually reduce the immune system and set the body up for disease. While battling cancer it is best not to push the body during exercise to the point that it needs to rebuild muscle or other body tissue. The body's energy needs to focus on healing from the cancer and not making repairs caused by exercise.

Examples of Exercise

Light yoga, karate, Pilates, gentle walking, light rebounding, light resistance training are all options that can assist the person with cancer in creating movement.

Exercise is an excellent way to increase metabolism, get fresh oxygen to the cells and hasten release of metabolic waste products. This also allows the body's natural production of life-enhancing endorphins to flood the bloodstream.

Several studies in the past few years have prompted such great results that overall, the message is clear: If you have cancer, you'll have a more successful fight against it and a better recovery afterward if you introduce light exercise. And, to avoid relapse, the combination of exercise and diet are likely to bring the greatest results over time.

Chapter Forty-Eight: Cancer Recovery Checklist

"Health is not valued until sickness comes."
—Thomas Fuller

Below is a checklist that you may find useful as you begin to weave through all of the well-meaning, well-intended mountains of guidance and information:

1. **Juicing** – As challenging as it can be to juice consistently, it is the best thing you can do for your body. Strive for 12 freshly extracted vegetable juices/ BarleyMax® each day. Solicit the help of those well meaning supporters who would likely bring over a casserole. Instead, give them a grocery list where they can bring you 5 pounds of carrots and some collard greens once or twice a week. Preferably they will be cleaned and ready to juice. The fresher the juice and the more you drink the more quickly the body will respond positively. Feed the army of Natural Killer Cells and starve the cancer cells! Use the juice and supplement log in Appendix A to help keep track of what to do and when. Remember, consuming juice allows 92% of the nutrients to reach cellular level as opposed to about 30% when the same food is chewed.

2. **Stay Hydrated** – Drink plenty of structured water, which comes from freshly extracted vegetable juices

and raw vegetables. Most people with cancer are de-hydrated. Water is needed to facilitate cell movement. It transports nutrients and carries away waste matter. While on the Recovery program you may not want to add much additional water. Adding more water after the juices may risk diluting the nutrients from the juices.

3. **Remove Toxic Foods** – Eliminate the foods that are causing the cancer: Meat, Dairy, White Flour, White Sugar and Salt and all processed "dead" foods while severely reducing those substances that feed cancer – natural sugars and healthy fats.

4. **Veggies, Veggies, Veggie**s – Consume large amounts of raw vegetables through smoothies, salads and blended salads and don't cheat! This isn't the time to eat less, it is the time to eat more!

5. **Minimize Toxin Exposure** – Replace or eliminate all avoidable toxins that are in your personal hygiene products: Hair dyes and shampoos, soaps, deodor-ant, cosmetics, lip balm, household cleaners, laundry soaps, dry cleaning, etc. that are commercially pur-chased all may have toxic substances. Place a water filter on the shower and consider a whole house wa-ter filtration system. Use a mask and gloves when handling any chemicals. Eliminate the use of plastic plates, plastic cups, plastic straws, plastic freezer bags, plastic storage containers, teflon non-stick, etc. Don't use the microwave and minimize microwave radia-tion exposure by applying biochips to all appliances and devices that emit radiation. Reduce time on the cell phone, sitting in front of computer screens, etc.

6. **Supplements/Detoxing** – Take whole-food supple-ments consistently; without forgetting. It can get monotonous consuming numerous pills every day throughout the day. Look at it this way, with the ex-ception of some detoxification symptoms, you won't lose your hair, you won't be terribly nauseous, you can still enjoy your family, you will still be able to work

and hundreds of other things that you would not be able to do if you chose an aggressive path. On the other hand, for those who still do choose the aggressive path, these supplements and the Recovery Diet may quite possibly prevent you from getting exceedingly sick with side effects as they have for many who have chosen to complement the different modalities.

7. **Hormones** – Get a hormone saliva test if battling a hormone-based cancer. Stop the introduction of outside hormones by drinking unchlorinated water that has never touched plastic, eliminating foods that have added estrogen-mimicking hormones. Consider herbs and other supplements that assist the body in "balancing hormones" which is helpful to reversing a hormone-based cancer. Supplements to consider include Ashwaganda, Maca, DIM etc. in conjunction with zero introduction of outside hormones. These can assist the body in regaining its hormonal balance.

8. **Begin Exercise Program** – All research points to a greater chance of successful recovery no matter what type or stage the cancer is if you add movement to your day. A slow walk, light weight lifting, rebounding, Pilates, all are great options. It is best for your body to keep the movement gentle. You don't need to be sore. You don't want to get to the point of exhaustion. This exercise is meant to assist your body in the detoxification process. You can rebuild your muscles later.

9. **Teeth** – Have your teeth and mouth evaluated by a biological dentist. Too much evidence proves unequivocally that the mouth has a direct link to the health of the entire body. Mercury amalgams, root canals and improper tooth extractions can cause cancer. Go to a dentist that has been specially trained to carefully remove these toxins in a way that will not compromise your health any further. Make him aware that you are battling this illness but don't de-

lay.

10. **Sleep** – Get adequate sleep every night. The body performs healing while you are asleep. There are cycles of detoxification that occur after midnight but well before the waking hours. Any hour that you sleep before midnight is a benefit to your recovery. Strive to be asleep before 10:00 pm and stay asleep as long as possible before sleep is interrupted. Keep the room dark. Eliminate as much EMF radiation from the room as possible. Melatonin taken before bed may assist with sleep difficulties. It has also recently been shown to have great anti-cancer benefits. Magnesium before bed is not only beneficial for sleep but also for bowel cleansing.

11. **Support** – Ensure you have a network of support. It has been proven that people with cancer will be more successful in overcoming the disease with increased survival rates when surrounded by loving, supportive, nurturing family and friends.

12. **Check Your Emotions** – Evidence suggests that unresolved anger, grief, guilt and negative thinking are powerful deterrents of cancer recovery and may in fact be instrumental in the cause of developing cancer. This means that body, mind and spirit all must be in harmony before the true physical recovery can take place.

13. **Evaluate Your Relationships** – Where is your mind regarding your present relationships; your past ones? Determine if you have unsettled emotions that you must come to terms with. "Bitterness is drinking a glass of poison and hoping the other person will die." When we brought our son to a toxicologist on his first visit, the doctor identified someone who our son had a strong negative emotional reaction to. The doctor told our son that he needed to forgive this person, whether or not they deserved it. He needed to forgive that person for his own sake. Remember, it is your own anger or hurt that is killing you and preventing

your recovery!

14. **Be Thankful** – Create a peaceful mind focused on gratitude. Keeping positive, peaceful thoughts are important to your recovery. Maintaining feelings of gratitude will keep you from concentrating on fear and hopelessness. This is the time to get outside of yourself and begin to look at others. The more time you spend thinking about others will help you see yourself as needed and important not as ill and in a hopeless situation.

15. **Pray** – Spend time each day in prayer and meditation. Having cancer requires mind over matter. It is important that you keep your mind in a state where you believe with every part of yourself that you will recover and that your body is a miraculous self-healing machine that will overcome this situation. Prayer can keep you in the frame of mind that maintains calm, peace, faith, hope and strength.

16. **Alternative Therapies** – Consider adding some of the alternative methods that have been discussed in the Alternative Treatments chapter. Your body is absolutely capable of repairing and restoring itself to better health. The alternative methods that are suggested may assist the body in its recovery process. It is not recommended to use all of these methods. However, many of them are natural, non-toxic approaches that will augment the Recovery Diet and give the body additional energy to beat the cancer. They would be great additions that should be considered.

"You only get one body; it is the temple of your soul. Even God is willing to dwell there. If you truly treat your body like a temple, it will serve you well for decades. If you abuse it you must be prepared for poor health and a lack of energy."
—Oli Hille

Chapter Forty-Nine: Living With(out) Cancer

"When you mature in your relationship with God you real-ize how suffering and patience are like eating your spiritual vegetables."

— Criss Jami

Living With(out) Cancer

The National Cancer Institute defines:
- Remission — A decrease in or disappearance of signs and symptoms of cancer.
- Partial Remission — Some, but not all, signs and symptoms of cancer have disappeared.
- Complete Remission — All signs and symptoms of cancer have disappeared, although cancer still may be in the body.

Many people who have chosen to change their diet and lifestyle have been able to see complete remission for many years and some for the remainder of their extended lives. The testimonies of just a few of those people can be found in the Real Life Stories chapter as well as thousands more can be found on *www.myHDiet.com*.

Others, for various reasons have been unable to obtain complete remission but have "lived with" controlled cancer in their bodies with reduced or no symptoms. One pastor friend of ours has been living with prostate cancer for over 17 years. He has been faithful on the

Hallelujah Diet, takes additional supplements and yet the stage 4 cancer that he was told would take him 17 years earlier, is now only a nuisance. It reminds him daily of the frailty of life, but he is an active, practicing head pastor of a large church and is nearing 80 years old.

The lesson we must learn here is that whether in complete or partial remission, you cannot allow cancer to infiltrate your minds to lead you to live in fear. The phrase "mind over matter" is aptly used here. People can overcome much if they don't allow their minds to succumb to their perceived reality of the situation. Perception is based on emotion. Reality is truth.

There are many worse things than "living with" cancer. Many people are working, living and loving each day knowing their cross in this life may be an illness that hasn't stopped them from experiencing abundant life. The key to "living with" cancer is the same as "living with" a spouse who is ill, or being a primary care provider for an elderly parent, or having a child with Down's Syndrome or another issue that requires your greater attention. The key is to have hope and faith that the One who allowed this situation is still in control and will continue to guide you each day sometimes moment by moment to not just "live with" the situation, but thrive in it. Look at Joni-Eareckson-Tada, a quadriplegic who for many years has never been capable of itching her nose, but who has broken free from that restraint and has painted beautiful pictures with her feet. She has started a ministry to provide wheel chairs in places to make other handicapped people able to access them.

Nick Fujicic has no limbs, yet he has a powerful ministry that is reaching the world with the message "You can still enjoy life and make a difference even if you aren't perfect!"

For anyone that has experienced remission by changing their diet and lifestyle, it must be noted that the body is only as strong as its next meal. In other words, to maintain this optimum level of health that reduced or removed the tumor, or other forms of cancer, the body is required to maintain a high level of nutrition intake. It may not require 12 juices each day once the cancer has been eliminated, but please note, if you choose to go back to the foods that you were eating when the disease first started, then you are setting yourself up to develop the cancer again.

Once your body has fully recovered, you can go from the Recovery Diet to the Hallelujah Diet, which will afford many more food opportunities. The Hallelujah Diet can provide more for your sweet tooth, possibly a little more healthy bread options, more living foods options that have been dehydrated so you can enjoy nuts, seeds, living potato chips and so much more. The Hallelujah Diet can be found on the website www.myHDiet.com.

We have seen people who have chosen to go back to the Standard American Diet and the unhealthy, toxic foods and within a year or two or longer, their cancer returned and it returned with a vengeance. Going back on the healthy diet and lifestyle may not be enough next time to kick the cancer again.

We strongly urge you to stay on course eating clean, whole, living foods so your diet will maintain the level of health that you were able to achieve.

Section Eight

❧❧

Preventing Cancer

> *"Health is the greatest possession. Contentment is the greatest treasure. Confidence is the greatest friend."*
> —Lao Tzu

Preventing Cancer

Although no one has the perfect cure, it is not hard to prevent cancer. Follow the guidelines below adding to them a positive attitude and you will likely find yourself healthier than you have ever been for many years to come.

1. Keep your weight under control. You want to avoid weight gain or increases in waist circumference after age 21.
2. Be physically active every day. Aim for 30 minutes of vigorous activity or 60 minutes of moderate activity every day on average.
3. Eat plant-based foods. They will maintain a strong immune system.
4. Eat your living foods on a dinner plate. Eat your cooked foods on a dessert plate.
5. Remove or severely limit all Toxic Foods. They promote and feed cancer.
6. Stay hydrated. Drink fresh vegetable juice and BarleyMax® everyday. 3 glasses of each through the day.
7. Limit consumption of refined salt.
8. Selective mineral and nutrient supplementation is key. No one can rely on just a "good diet" anymore.
9. Breastfeed infants (as appropriate) exclusively up to 6 months and continue as they start eating food.
10. Manage or change stress factors and your reactions toward them.
11. Eliminate as many toxins as possible that you drink, breathe, consume, wear, etc. Lifestyle changes are not hard and will pay great health dividends in the upcoming years.

12. Get periodic blood tests to ascertain your nutrient, vitamin and hormone levels. Once a year is a good amount.
13. Get 6-8 uninterrupted hours of sleep every night. Try not to change your sleeping habits on the weekends.
14. Consider going through a FiberCleanse detoxification at least once a year or after a period of unhealthy food consumption or stress.
15. Daily prayer and meditation are of paramount importance.
16. Remove all amalgams, infected root canals and repair cavitations. Take continuous care of your teeth and gums.

Section Nine

~~~

Real Life Stories

James S. – Prostate Cancer, Multiple Myeloma

Age at diagnosis: 68 – Recovery Diet only, no chemo or radiation
Type of cancer:
Prostate/multiple myeloma

Diagnosis date:
March, 2011

Scientific evidence of the diagnosis:
24 hour urine tests, prostate biopsy and blood tests

Diet:
100% Hallelujah Recovery Diet

Number of juices consumed each day?
6 carrot/vegetable juices

6 barley max juices

2 – 4oz wheat grass juices

Did you have any chemo, radiation or surgery BEFORE you started the Recovery diet?
No

How long were you on the Recovery Diet before you found your cancer was gone?
1 year

Scientific evidence to prove your cancer is gone:
Yes, blood tests and 24 hr urine tests

What can you say about the Hallelujah Diet Recovery Program?
It was extremely difficult trying to figure out what to eat in the beginning, but with the help of the website, my wife was able to figure out what to make for me without the oils, seeds, nuts or sugars. Olin Idol was always our 'go to' person in clarifying questions that we had. We wish we had a recovery diet recipe book to refer to, so thank you for writing it. After about 2 weeks, I began to feel really good and there were times that I forgot I was sick, as did my wife. After all the juicing, I really looked forward to eating the raw vegetable salads and especially that one cooked food.

Do you have any pictures or scans you would be willing to share with us?
The tests that found the cancer are the tests that eventually showed no cancer. No pictures or scans just reports.

Jordan R. – Medulloblastoma (Brain Cancer)

Age at diagnosis: 14 – Surgery to remove brain tumor plus Recovery Diet – No chemo or radiation

Type of cancer:
Medulloblastoma (Brain Cancer)

Diagnosis date:
December 9, 2012

Scientific evidence of the diagnosis:
CT Scan and MRI

Diet:
Recovery Diet

Number of juices consumed each day:
Started with 7-8 juices per day for 6 months then went to 5 per day for 4 months. Now still drinks 4 per day.

Any chemo, radiation or surgery BEFORE you started the Recovery diet:
Surgery only because the tumor was acting like a cork to drain fluid from his brain so in this case it was life threatening and needed immediate attention.

How did your oncologist react to you being on the diet while doing chemo, or being on the diet in general:
They turned us in for child abuse. A sheriff had to meet with us at our home. Then we had to appear at a meeting in front of Doctors, Child Services, Attorney General Reps, Sheriffs Rep, DCF Reps (Department of Children and Family).

How long were you on the Recovery Diet before you found your cancer was gone?
After the first MRI in April, 5 months after surgery, there was no evidence of recurrence. After another MRI in August, 9 months after surgery, there was no evidence of residual growth or anything.

Do you have scientific evidence to prove your cancer is gone?
MRI Results

What can you say about the Hallelujah Diet Recovery Program?
Basically it was a God-send for our family. We believe in it 100%.

Do you have any pictures or scans you would be willing to share with us?

We do have initial CT scan of the tumor and the MRI disk from April. Sadly the hospital did not want to give us anything else unless we 'purchased' it. (All the paperwork and medical files)

It's a long story, so many details. Sadly we have realized how corrupt and incompetent the medical industry is. We hurt for people that are sheep in their system.

Thank you for allowing us to share

Website created from his testimony- *www.harvestyourhealth.com*

Larry J. – Prostate Cancer, aggressive

Age at diagnosis: 72 – Recovery Diet only, no chemo or radiation – Diagnosed in 2005 – Has lived pain-free for 8 years

Type of cancer:
Aggressive prostate cancer.

Diagnosis date:
September 15, 2005

Scientific evidence of the diagnosis:
Biopsy

Diet:
Started Recovery Diet on October 15, 2005

Number of juices consumed each day:
Eight carrot juices per day

Any chemo, radiation or surgery BEFORE you started the Recovery diet?
No

How long were you on the Recovery Diet before you found your cancer was gone?
Never had test to determine if caner is gone. Quit having PSA tests. Body became very alkaline vs acidic.

Do you have scientific evidence to prove your cancer is gone?
No. Has been eight years. Why have tests if I would never submit to chemo, etc.?

What can you say about the Hallelujah Diet Recovery Program?
Very painless compared to chemo, etc.

Do you have any pictures or scans you would be willing to share with us?
Initial biopsy report is all that I have.

I will be 73 on January 31 and don't have any pain(s) whatsoever in my body. Our research indicates that cancer cannot survive in a high alkaline environment which I have. Donna was pronounced lupus free after adopting the vegan diet.

Michael V. – Stage 4 Lung Cancer, Spread to Bones and Spinal Cord

Age at diagnosis: 65 – Chemo plus Recovery Diet – Has 36 Pages of test results.

Type of cancer:
Stage 4 extended small cell lung cancer. The cancer had traveled to the bones in both hips and ball and sockets, and upper spinal cord.

Diagnosis date:
July 11, 2013 – Five days later full oxygen and a wheel chair.

Scientific evidence of the diagnosis:
Cat scans, Pet scans and Blood tests -- 36 pages

Diet:
The Recovery Diet

Number of juices you are drinking each day:
Still 12 juices a day. 6 Barley Max, 6 Carrot and green

Any chemo, radiation or surgery BEFORE you started the Recovery diet:
2 days of chemo. On day 3 of chemo, started only Barley Max 12 times a day until our juicer was delivered along with the supplements which was 6 days later.

Did you continue the Recovery diet while on chemo?
Yes, still on diet.

Did the Recovery diet relieve or reduce any of your symptoms from chemo or radiation?
Had NO pain through the chemo or radiation, doctors were surprised no bone pain and had bone cancer. Never took any medicines they prescribed.

Feel very strongly by the grace of God and juicing!!

How did your oncologist react to you being on the diet while doing chemo, or being on the diet in general?
Everyone at the hospital from the Oncologist to the Radiologist to the chemo nurses are very open to it. We even brought the juices to appointments and treatments! Radiologist noted juicing in her report dated 8-28-2013.

How long were you on the Recovery Diet before you found your cancer was gone?
July 23, 2013 to December 6, 2013

Scientific evidence to prove your cancer is gone:
Yes, scans blood test and reports

What can you say about the Hallelujah Diet Recovery Program?
I have already started 3 people I work with juicing. They have 4 a day. 2 Barley max and 2 carrot & green juices.

I tell everyone at work and anyone I'm talking to about the diet and Dot Scarpa the Health Minister that was kind enough to bring me into her home the week I had found out about my husband's cancer. She and her daughter had shown me all they had learned with the diet, from juicing to the correct foods to eat and where to shop for them. I have had someone come to my home to see how to juice as Dot had done for me. I truly believe that my husband would not be here today in the state of good health he is in, if it wasn't for the juicing, by the grace of God and chemo.

Nancy H. – Breast Cancer, Stage 1 Grade 3

Age at diagnosis: 62 – 4 rounds of Chemo+Bilateral Mastectomy plus Recovery Diet – Visited Lifestyle Center in Missouri
Type of cancer:
Breast Cancer, Stage 1 grade 3 – "Triple Negative"- Not related to hormones. Only 15% of women get this type

Diagnosis date:
April 2011

Scientific evidence of the diagnosis:
Yes – Mammogram, Biopsy

Diet:
Recovery Diet . Had been vegan for 2 years prior to cancer, added juices

and supplements

Number of juices consumed each day:
8 per day for the first 6 months

Any chemo, radiation or surgery BEFORE you started the Recovery diet?
1 round of chemo before going to lifestyle center in Missouri

3 more rounds of chemo

Bilateral mastectomy (then reconstructive surgery)- tumor was in right breast

Did you continue the Recovery diet while on chemo?
Yes

Did the Recovery diet relieve or reduce any of your symptoms from chemo or radiation?
Yes! Never got nauseous. Symptoms were minimal.

How long were you on the Recovery Diet before you found your cancer was gone?
6 months

Do you have scientific evidence to prove your cancer is gone?
Almost 3 years of clean scans and blood work:

PET scan- clean

CT scan and blood work every quarter- clean

What can you say about the Hallelujah Diet Recovery Program?
It's a great way to fight cancer or any type of disease.

Do you have any pictures or scans you would be willing to share with us?
Yes, diagnosis report and pictures

Had been vegan for 2 years after reading The China Study

Exercises regularly

Endured a lot of difficult times and stress at home. -- Believe stress contributed to the cancer

Pastor David B. –Prostate Cancer

Age at diagnosis: 78 – Recovery Diet only. No chemo or radiation

Type of cancer:
Prostate cancer

Diagnosis date:
January 10, 2013

Scientific evidence of the diagnosis:
Yes: Gleason reported 9 out of 10 for prostate, CAT scans, picture of where cancer spread to lymph nodes, and documents with PSA readings (went from 3 to 16.9 in 12 months – From Jan 2012 to Jan 2013)

Diet:
Recovery Diet Feb 2013

Number of juices consumed each day:
12 per day

Did you have any chemo, radiation or surgery BEFORE you started the Recovery diet?
Had a hormone shot in February 2013 and August 2013. No other treatments, lymph node biopsies were scheduled but not needed after second CAT scan showed no more cancer

Did you continue the Recovery diet while on chemo?
Never had chemo, still on Recover diet today

How long were you on the Recovery Diet before you found your cancer was gone?
4 months

Scientific evidence to prove your cancer is gone:
Second CAT scan in May 2013 reported cancer was gone and PSA went down to 0.5

What can you say about the Hallelujah Diet Recovery Program?
Absolutely wonderful! I would recommend it to others who are suffering.

Do you have any pictures or scans you would be willing to share for us?
Gleason report, picture of lymph nodes, and PSA reports

Had been taking medication for 8 years to reduce size of prostate so he could urinate – was told later by doctor that cancer is a potential side effect of this drug.

Additional benefits from diet change:

• *Lowered cholesterol*

• *Lowered blood pressure*

• *No more indigestion= no more medication needed for indigestion*

• *No more constipation*

• *No more dry itchy scalp*

Sandy R. – Breast Cancer

Age at diagnosis: 58 – Went to Lifestyle Center in Missouri

Surgical Biopsy – Recovery Diet plus Essential oils plus Infrared Sauna plus Alkaline Water plus Rebounder

No Chemo or radiation

Type of cancer:

Breast Cancer

Diagnosis date:

March 14, 2012

Scientific evidence of the diagnosis:

Surgical Biopsy (Lumpectomy) – Showed cancer cells, MRI-clean

Diet:

Started on 100% raw vegan diet 2 months before going to HA Lifestyle Center, then followed Recovery Diet

Ingested therapeutic grade Frankincense and Myrrh essential oils for 40 days

Number of juices consumed each day:

Alternated BarleyMax® and juice 6 times a day

Did you have any chemo, radiation or surgery BEFORE you started the Recovery diet?

Surgical biopsy

How did your oncologist react to you being on the diet while doing chemo, or being on the diet in general?

Integrative medical doctor-recommended and supported a raw vegan diet

How long were you on the Recovery Diet before you found your cancer was gone?

5 months

323

Do you have scientific evidence to prove your cancer is gone?
Thermal imaging scan in Sept 2012 -- clean, full body scan Dec 2012 and June 2013 – Completely cancer free

What can you say about the Hallelujah Diet Recovery Program?
It's a blessing. I loved it! It was the right place for me to be to learn how to eat what God's put here on the earth as our medicine.

Do you have any pictures or scans you would be willing to share with us?
Yes, reports.

Also used an infrared sauna, Alkaline water machine, whole-body vibration machine, rebounder, uses Young Living Essential Oils, and became a yoga instructor

Testimony was published at http://www.hahealthnews.com/halc/the-key-to-healing-breast-cancer/

Eleanor R. -- Breast Cancer

Age at diagnosis: 39
Type of cancer:
Early Stage 1 aggressive breast cancer

Diagnosis date:
2011

Scientific evidence of the diagnosis:
Mammograms

Diet:
As close to the recovery diet as possible-so a variation

Number of juices consumed each day?
2-3 juices a day plus green smoothies

Any chemo, radiation or surgery BEFORE you started the Recovery diet?
No, I immediately changed my diet then had surgery and radiation

Did the Recovery diet relieve or reduce any of your symptoms from chemo or radiation?
Relieved the symptoms of radiation. I was not tired and was able to work and keep up with my young children-ages 4 and 7 at the time.

How did your oncologist react to you being on the diet while doing

chemo, or being on the diet in general?
Told me that this was not the time to change my diet, but I did not listen and changed it anyway!!

How long were you on the Recovery Diet before you found your cancer was gone?
6 months

Do you have scientific evidence to prove your cancer is gone?
Mammograms for 2 years they have looked fantastic...boring in my doctor's words!!

What can you say about the Hallelujah Diet Recovery Program?
Awesome! Delicious! It works!!

Do you have any pictures or scans you would be willing to share with us?
I am willing to sign something so that my doctors office can release this info to you.

Lifestyle Centers

If you believe you need further assistance in adopting this lifestyle, there are three Hallelujah Lifestyle Centers that are waiting for your visit. Although they are not a medical facility their specialty is in teaching people how to incorporate all of the components that you learned in this book. You and 6 or so other guests will spend a week in a lovely home perfectly designed to help you learn how to juice in the spacious kitchen, ensure that you exercise each day and spend time out in the sun. You will get further education on the miraculous self-healing body and receive a number of great tips on how to create a living foods kitchen and pantry. They will send you home with many recipes to try and enjoy.

The best way to learn anything is to actually do it. These centers are here to teach you the practical tips and how to apply the Recovery Diet into your daily life. There is one in North Carolina, West Virginia and Florida. Take a look at the website *www.halifestylecenters.com* and give them a call. Their nurturing, loving approach will feed your soul as well as your body. It is a great time to immerse yourself into this life-giving program.

FAQ

What if I go back to SAD foods?

Your body is only as strong as the cells that it most recently created. If a person reverts back to the Standard American Diet, there is a chance the body will weaken from the lack of strong nutrients in the food and in time usually within three years, the body can succumb to the weakened immune system and the potential for cancer recurrence is quite high. Through the last 22 years we have observed that some people who have chosen to bring the SAD foods into their diets after overcoming cancer through nutrition, have re-developed it and the Hallelujah Recovery Diet was not strong enough to overcome it a second time. Cancer cells mutate and become extraordinarily strong. The SAD food introduction is taking a great risk.

How long do I need to do this?

This diet must be followed in its entirety for at least 12 months. Remember, cancer can take 10-20 years to develop into what you are experiencing right now. It will take time to rebuild your immune system to create a strong army to fight it and once the cancer is gone, the diet will still be needed to repair the immune system from the fight it just went through. Lots of nutrients are needed to ensure that all organs, tissues and cells have time to rebuild and create an alkaline environment. This all will take time. It may take 15-18 months.

Once you have reached complete recovery, you can return to eating a little more fat, maybe in the form of nuts, seeds, avocados, Veganaise. You can slowly introduce more honey, maple syrup, and other natural sweeteners. But you can never return to the Standard American Diet. Those killer foods can never again be a part of your diet.

Why do I remove the pulp from juice before I drink it?

This program recommends that to obtain the optimal amount of nutrition, fiber should be extracted from the juice before it is consumed. All vegetable juices should be consumed without the pulp in them. Fiber is extremely important. It assists in the elimination of toxins and removal of them through the bowels. The optimal way to get the fiber is through eating the fresh, raw vegetables and leafy greens twice a day in the large salads. Blended salads and smoothies can provide additional fiber as well. The juices will do their job best when the fiber has been removed. Remember, drinking the juice from a carrot allows over 90% of the nutrients to reach cellular level as opposed to 30% when the same carrot is chewed.

Why must I stay on the Hallelujah Diet Recovery program for at least 12 months?

Most cancers that affect adults can take from 10-20 years to develop. Therefore, to assist your body in the process of recovery, it may take up to 12 months and sometimes up to 18 months on this high nutrient program before the cancer has been eradicated and the immune system as well as other vital organs to sufficiently recover and regain control in the body. It seems amazing though, that it can take 10 years to develop it, but within less than 2 years, it can be not only controlled but often turned into remission.

This diet may seem restrictive at first glance, but unlike chemotherapy, radiation or even surgery where your entire life must be placed on hold during these treatments and the residual effects of them can be life changing, but likely in negative way, the Hallelujah Diet recovery program merely assists you in giving your body all the nutrients daily for it to successfully eliminate the toxins, rebuild its immune system and subsequently develop a strong, living body that will sustain health for a long time.

Will antioxidants interfere with the effectiveness of chemotherapy?

There are no studies that even remotely suggest this is true. In fact, there are numerous studies that prove that a patient participating in chemotherapy will be more successful when taking supplements that include antioxidants, vitamins, minerals and enzymes and probiotics. See the special section in this book to assist you.

The lack of awareness of these studies may prompt oncologists to be wary of the combination but you, the patient, can bring this to their attention and demand that the two must be used together.

What if you can only get in 6-8 juices on certain days, will the program still work?

We suggest the optimal program because there are very sick people who need every drop of nutrient that the juice will provide. We have had testimonies of those who were unable to maintain 12 juices daily yet, removed the negative foods, thoughts, etc. And were able to make a complete recovery with a few less juices each day but still high amounts of raw vegetables were included.

I hate exercise. Can I just do the program and still get good results?

Although, we have no way of knowing how you personally will react, we can only say that when the body is removing toxins daily through exercise and other measures, there is a greater likelihood that the nutrients will be delivered to the cells to enhance their effectiveness thereby improving the likelihood that they will breakdown the cancer cells and subsequently create the conditions for the body to recover.

Do I have to drink water while drinking all of the juices?

There is no great need to continue to drink water throughout the day. In fact, it is best to avoid water after you have consumed juice since you don't want to dilute the nutrients. If you can get all 12 of the juices into your body each day, you may still find yourself thirsty. If that is the case, the best water to drink is distilled water. You would be best served if you could make your own distilled water since nearly all distilled water comes in plastic, BPA containers that will likely leach the chemical into the pure distilled water. If you cannot make your own distilled water, then purchase only in plastic containers that have not been exposed to fluorescent light that can break down the plastic quickly or those containers that have not been exposed to heat.

It is recommended that you stay on the distilled water for at least 3 months and longer if needed. This water has a strong detoxification effect and will work in conjunction with the other supplements to detoxify the body. After the 90 days, consider adding HydroBoost, which will make the distilled water less aggressive while replenishing the body with minerals in a form that can be easily assimilated within the body.

What if I miss my supplements? Can I double up?

Supplements are not like prescription drugs. They work best when taken consistently either with or without food as indicated. The purpose of supplements is to act as as an accompaniment to the nutritious food to enhance the effectiveness of the food and to build the cells and strengthen the immune system. Do not double up, but try to maintain a consistency in taking them.

What about organic ingredients?

If you live in an area where organic produce is readily available, those are the optimal foods to eat. You may find them in health food stores or even in some higher end grocery stores. However, if they look as if they have traveled a long distance, and are wilted, dry or wrinkly, then, the next best option is to find a local grower who may have fresh produce that may have minimal pesticides and herbicides on it. Finally, if you cannot find either, then purchase the produce you find in your local supermarket, wash it well and peel the outside where the pesticides would likely congregate most.

Can I have a massage with cancer?

People with cancer should avoid very deep massage. Gentler types may be safer. Some people worry that having a massage when you have cancer may make the cancer cells travel to other parts of the body due to lymphatic circulation. No research has proved this to be true.

If you are having radiation you should avoid massaging the treated area to avoid risk of cancer spreading. And don't have massage to any area of your body where the skin is broken, bleeding or bruised.

Several small studies have been done to see if massage would assist cancer patients in pain, fatigue, nausea, anxiety, and depression. The integrity of the studies has been in question so there really isn't any strong documentation to support these.

What if my doctor does not support this?

We can't tell you what to do. We can only provide you with studies, research, clinical evidence and anecdotal evidence so you may be ready to share any or all of it with your doctor. Remember, this is your body and you will be responsible for the consequences. Second opinion anyone?

Can children follow this program if they have cancer?

A modified version of the diet can be useful for children; however, they are still growing and will need additional nutritional support in the form of cooked vegetables. They will also require a different amount of supplementation since the recommended amounts are for adult bodies.

If I have to eat smaller salads during the hours I drink my juice, how long must I wait after I consume my juice before I begin to eat the smaller salads?

It is best to delay adding the solids for 20-30 minutes to allow the juices time to reach the cells and do their work.

What if I lose too much weight on this program?

Significant weight loss can occur on the recovery program. Major detoxification is taking place.

Many toxins are stored in fat cells therefore the less fat cells on the body, the more likely toxins will be eliminated. When people say that you are too thin, remember that they are seeing you from a perspective of what the average American looks like. Most people who lose weight may see their ribs and hip bones. That is actually not too thin.

What is more important is your energy level. You can expect days where your body is working so hard that you have the feeling that you are fatigued. However, this is to be expected as well. The body is undergoing a major transformation and it needs all the energy it can get.

If you feel that you need to stop losing the weight, you can increase the amount of cooked vegetables and beans into your diet. These additional calories will assist you in this goal of maintaining a little more weight. This food may also give you more energy. Remember though, the cooked food cannot replace any of the other juices or raw foods.

Conclusion

After years of reviewing studies, analyzing data, researching nutrition, and learning about toxins and environmental effects there are several conclusions that we can draw from these efforts:

The environment and the way our society has set itself up for the benefit of convenience and technological advancement, has wreaked havoc with our hormones. From the food additives to the fluorescent lighting to the diesel exhaust, and the chlorine plus hundreds of other factors, our endocrine system and our delicate hormone balance is constantly becoming imbalanced. So many xenoestrogens are plaguing us daily that over time, this will weaken our thyroid, adrenals and ultimately our hormone balance causing us to succumb to numerous cancers that were not so prevalent even 10 years ago.

We use the word synergy often in this book relating to what happens when two or more components combine. Sometimes it creates positive results like when vitamins A and D combine. The result is greater than the two individual vitamins alone. There are some powerful, positive synergistic effects from food! However, after all of the reviewing of the various toxins, we have come to the conclusion, that there are very few studies being done on the synergistic effects of two or more toxins that combine. We know what happens when we consume fluoride, and we know what happens when we consume chlorine, but what happens when we consume them together? It would seem, with what little research is available, that the two carcinogens together may be more dangerous to the body than when exposed individually. Ironically, in this particular example, it is highly likely that your body will be exposed to them simultaneously. The challenge is not knowing all of the damage they are causing. Just because the damage may be occurring slowly, doesn't mean that you won't live long enough to experience the full effect.

It is wise not to wait for the government or any administrative body to test the combinations of these carcinogens and finally inform us of their dangers and what we should do to avoid them. There are too many to test and the combinations would outnumber the actual toxins themselves. It is best to recognize that the world we live in is filled with many seen and unseen toxins that we are exposed to every hour of every day. We need to evaluate what we can live with and what we must live without. It is best to do this before a cancer diagnosis is made but that will definitely put everything into perspective. Sometimes, it takes that type of diagnosis for us to realize that what we thought was so important really means nothing at all.

Ask yourself these questions:

Is that newest smart phone really going to make you look smart after 10 years of radiation exposure? Do you have to have wireless internet when you don't know what it can do to your body long term? Is the extra time it takes to warm up a bowl of soup on the stove top too much effort? Is switching from plastic to glass really an issue? Can you find another "favorite" skin care product? Can your neighbors live with your dandelions?

A clean, efficient and strengthened immune system that isn't weighed down with attacking allergens, toxins or inflammation is free to wage war on things like infection, inflammation, and cell mutations.

Your immune system requires proper cell food to function at its best. Eating high-quality, nutrient-rich foods is the primary way to give your body strength it needs to overcome and prevent disease.

We can't forget detoxification. Avoiding exposure to toxins in our industrialized world is nearly impossible, unless you live in a giant bubble. Therefore, it's important to eat foods that flush toxins from the body, so toxins don't accumulate. Yes, the body detoxifies itself naturally, but given the ever-increasing amount of toxins in our everyday environments, it's important to make sure this function is efficient.

Some antioxidants like glutathione help clean the liver and neutralize the effects of harmful medications for people dealing with chronic disease like cancer, making it an important part of cancer nutrition. Detoxification is key when fighting infections, because dead bacteria (such as Candida) can release harmful neurotoxins. If you're trying to recover, it makes no sense to make it more difficult. Detoxification is also key when losing weight because toxins can remain stored in fat tissue. As that weight is shed, years of accumulated toxins are released into the bloodstream.

Eat the foods that promote healthy urination, bowel movements and support liver function, as these are the primary elimination points within the body. The more vegetables, fresh water and juices you give to your body, the more it can rejuvenate and repair the areas that need attention. Don't give up and don't give in.

Don't forget the companion to this book, *Unravel the Mystery: Simple, Effective, Nutritious Recipes to Fight Cancer*. It is available through *myHDiet.com*.

As Dr. Blaylock says, "Almost all recurrence of cancer can be avoided by consuming a strong diet and supplementation for the rest of the life of the person."

Once you have eliminated the disease and have also given ample time for the vital organs to recover and regain their strength, which can take from 12 to 15 to sometimes even 18 months, you will need to continue to support them with nutrition for them to stay in peak performance and not allow them to weaken from inferior nutrition.

Then, we suggest you move to the Hallelujah Diet at that time. While it is less restrictive it is still a nutrient dense program that helps to keep the body working smoothly. There are many avenues of support to teach you the additional foods and recipes that you will be able to enjoy. Our website www.myHDiet.com has hundreds of recipes at your fingertips and they are free.

Another great opportunity for learning is 60 Days To Reclaim Your Health video program. My husband, Paul and I developed this to help people put into practice the principles needed to combat disease. Each day you will receive an email that will teach you even more about this incredible way of eating for your health. You will watch us in our kitchen, creating great recipes and discussing and teaching practical, time and money saving tips to continue this lifestyle. Check it out at *www.juiceupyourlife.com*. Click on the Reclaim your Health program and start learning more.

As you find yourself gaining more energy and restoring your health, you will likely be more encouraged to research this incredible connection between nutrition and health. An excellent place to start is on our website at this location: *www.myHDiet.com*

After living this lifestyle for nearly twenty years, I have learned much about the incredible human machine, how it thrives when given quality air, pure water, many nutrients and calming peace. This message has been shared with hundreds of thousands of people in the last 25 years. Many people who were told to go home and prepare to die, are alive today celebrating birthdays, anniversaries and creating memories they never thought would be possible.

When God designed man he made an incredible creation. 6,000 years later the body is as marvelous now as it was then. Unlike the automobile there has never been any recalls and there has never been any need for revisions or reconfiguration. The body has the capacity to repair, restore, replace and recover. That gift was given to you when you were born and it is still available for you today. Even the natural aging process that everyone goes through won't turn off the healing mechanism.

Compared to Creation and Biblical times, the environment where the human body exists today has changed. Today, the human body must balance the poor air quality, the poor water quality and the constant barrage of radiation that surrounds it day and night. It must do the best it can to extract whatever nourishment is available from the processed, dead but convenient sources of fuel that it is being fed. The human body today, is so over stimulated by cell phones, email, hundreds of TV stations, radio, and appointments that silence and stillness are nowhere to be found.

In spite of the different environment, the human body is still amazing. Unleash the power from within. Take the important step of faith. Make the changes that were outlined in this book. As you do, continue to remember that you were designed by the most intelligent creator whose IQ is far beyond the reach of any mortal. Your body has the capacity and the capability to change its own destiny. Give it the fuel it needs and then… get out of the way!

Appendix A

Daily Routine Chart

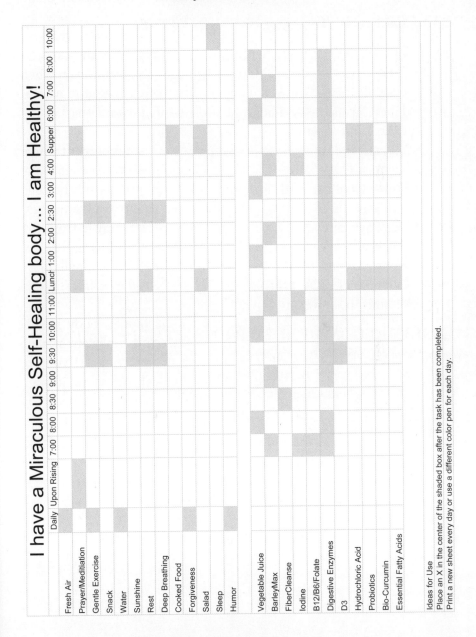

Download and print a copy from *www.UnravelTheMystery.com.*

Appendix B

CANCER FIGHTING SUPPLEMENT LIST

ESSENTIAL SUPPLEMENTS:

- BarleyMax® – Available in Regular, Berry, Mint or Capsules
- FiberCleanse – Available in unflavored, green apple, lemon and capsules
- Nascent Iodine
- Vitamin D3 – 5,000 IU
- Professional Strength Probiotics
- Bio-Curcumin
- Digestive Enzymes
- Betaine Hydrochloric Acid (HCL) Pepsin & Gentian Root Extract
- Flora Flax Oil W/DHA
- Vitamin B12, B6 and Folate

HIGHLY RECOMMENDED PRODUCT/SUPPLEMENTS:

- *Unravel the Mystery: Simple, Effective, Nutritious Recipes to Fight Cancer* by Ann Malkmus
- Pharmax Fish Oil – One teaspoon daily
- Ubiquinol
- Melatonin

RECOMMENDED PRODUCTS & SUPPLEMENTS:

- The Hallelujah Diet book by Rev. George Malkmus
- 60 Days to Reclaim Your Health – On-line video program
- Getting Started On The Hallelujah Diet DVD Set

Appendix C

Daily Routine

Nutritional Supplementation/Daily Schedule Of Supplements

Daily
- Fresh Air
- Prayer/Meditation
- Gentle Exercise
- Deep Breathing
- Forgiveness
- Plenty of Rest
- Humor

Upon Rising:
- Prayer/Meditation

7:00 am
- Iodine (nascent) supplement (on empty stomach); 1 to 2 drops
- BarleyMax® (1 tsp) mixed with 4 oz water (or taken dry)
- Digestive Enzyme capsule (1)
- B12-B6-Folate sublingual tablet (1)

8:00 am
- Juice (8 oz): carrot (70%) and vegetables (30%)
- Digestive Enzyme capsule (1)

8:30 am
- FiberCleanse (up to the first 90 days of The Hallelujah Recovery Diet; some people will require more cleansing than others) or B-Flax-D as directed

9:00 am
- BarleyMax® (1 tsp) mixed with 4 oz water (or taken dry)
- Digestive Enzyme capsule (1)

9:30 am
- Mid-Morning Snack – Cut veggies, or green smoothie with ¼ cup ground flax seed (minimal fruit)
- Digestive Enzyme capsule (1)
- Vitamin D3 capsule - 5,000 IU (1)
- Exercise, Sunshine, Rest, Deep Breathing

10:00 am
- Juice (8 oz): carrot (70%) and vegetables (30%)
- Digestive Enzyme capsule (1)

11:00 am
- Iodine (nascent) supplement (on empty stomach); 1 to 2 drops
- BarleyMax® (1 tsp) mixed with 4 oz water (or taken dry)
- Digestive Enzyme capsule (1)

12:00 noon – Lunch meal
- Digestive Enzyme capsules (2)
- Professional Strength Probiotics capsule (1)
- BioCurcumin capsule (1)
- Hydrochloric Acid (2)
- Salad – Whole or blended

1:00 pm
- Juice (8 oz): carrot (70%) and vegetables (30%)
- Digestive Enzyme capsule (1)

2:00 pm
- BarleyMax® (1 tsp) mixed with 4 oz water (or taken dry)
- Digestive Enzyme capsule (1)

2:30 pm
- Mid-Afternoon Snack (Cut veggies, or green smoothie)
- Digestive Enzyme capsule (1)
- Exercise, Sunshine, Rest, Deep Breathing

3:00 pm
- Juice (8 oz): carrot (70%) and vegetables (30%)
- Digestive Enzyme capsule (1)

4:00 pm
- Iodine (nascent) supplement (on empty stomach); 1 to 2 drops
- BarleyMax® (1 tsp) mixed with 4 oz water (or taken dry)
- Digestive Enzyme capsule (1)

5:00 pm – Supper meal
- Digestive Enzyme capsules (2)
- Professional Strength Probiotics capsule (1)
- B12-B6-Folate sublingual tablet (1)
- Prayer
- Salad – Whole or blended
- Hydrochloric Acid (2)
- Cooked food

6:00 pm
- Juice (8 oz): carrot (70%) and vegetables (30%)
- Digestive Enzyme capsule (1)

7:00 pm
- BarleyMax® (1 tsp) mixed with 4 oz water (or taken dry)
- Digestive Enzyme capsule (1)

8:00 pm
- Juice (8 oz): carrot (70%) and vegetables (30%)
- Digestive Enzyme capsule (1)

10:00 pm
- Sleep

Appendix D

MSG, Truth in Labeling

Table 2: Names of common ingredients that contain processed free glutamic acid (MSG)[1]
or
create MSG during processing

Names of ingredients that **always** contain processed free glutamic acid:	Names of ingredients that **often** contain or produce processed free glutamic acid during processing:	The following are ingredients suspected of containing or creating sufficient processed free glutamic acid to serve as MSG-reaction triggers in **HIGHLY SENSITIVE** people:
Glutamic acid (E 620)[2]		
Glutamate (E 620)		
Monosodium glutamate (E 621)	Carrageenan (E 407)	Corn starch
Monopotassium glutamate (E 622)	Bouillon and broth	Corn syrup
Calcium glutamate (E 623)	Stock	Modified food starch
Monoammonium glutamate (E 624)	Any "flavors" or "flavoring"	Lipolyzed butter fat
Magnesium glutamate (E 625)	Maltodextrin	Dextrose
Natrium glutamate	Citric acid, Citrate (E 330)	Rice syrup
Anything "hydrolyzed"	Anything "ultra-pasteurized"	Brown rice syrup
Any "hydrolyzed protein"	Barley malt	Milk powder
Calcium caseinate, Sodium caseinate	Pectin (E 440)	Reduced fat milk (skim; 1%; 2%)
Yeast extract	Malt extract	most things "low fat" or "no fat"
Yeast food, Yeast nutrient	Seasonings	anything "enriched"
Autolyzed yeast		anything "vitamin enriched"
Gelatin		anything "pasteurized"
Textured protein		Annatto
Whey protein		Vinegar
Whey protein concentrate		Balsamic vinegar
Whey protein isolate		
Soy protein		Amino acid chelate
Soy protein concentrate		
Soy protein isolate		Citrate, aspartate, and
Anything "protein"		glutamate used as chelating
Anything "protein fortified"		agents with mineral
Soy sauce		supplements.
Soy sauce extract		
Protease		
Anything "enzyme modified"		
Anything containing "enzymes"		
Anything "fermented"		
Vetsin		
Ajinomoto		
Umami		

(1) Glutamic acid found **in unadulterated protein** does not cause adverse reactions. To cause adverse reactions, the glutamic acid must have been processed/manufactured or come from protein that has been fermented.

(2) E numbers are use in Europe in place of food additive names.

Appendix E

Foods Containing B17 (Nitrilosides)

Fruits	Range*
Blackberry, domestic	low
Blackberry, wild	high
Boysenberry	med.
Choke cherry	high
Wild crabapple	high
Market cranberry	low
Swedish cranberry	high
Currant	med.
Elderberry	med.
Gooseberry	med.
Huckleberry	med.
Loganberry	med.
Mulberry	med.
Quince	med.
Raspberry	med.

Nuts (all raw)	Range*
Bitter almond	high
Cashew	low
Macadamia	med. to high

Seeds	Range*
Apple seeds	high
Apricot seed	high
Buckwheat	med.
Cherry seed	high
Flax	med.
Millet	med.
Nectarine seed	high
Peach seed	high
Pear seeds	high
Plum seed	high
Prune seed	high
Squash seeds	med.

Sprouts	Range*
Bamboo	high
Fava	med.
Garbanzo	med.
Mung	med.

Tubers	Range*
Cassava	high
Sweet Potato	low
Yams	low

Beans	Range*
Black	low
Black-eyed peas	low
Fava	high
Garbanzo	low to med.
Green pea	low
kidney	low to med.
Lentils	med.
Lima, U.S.	low
Lima, Burma	med.
Mung	med. to high
Shell	low

Leaves	Range*
Alfalfa	high
Beet tops	low
Eucalyptus	high
Spinach	low
Water cress	low

Range*
High -- above 500 mgs. nitrilosides per 100 grams food
Medium -- above 100 mgs. per 100 grams food
Low -- below 100 mgs. per 100 grams food

Endnotes

References

Chapter 1
1. 1992 study, The American Heart Association's Council on Cardiopulmonary and Critical Care, and a 2002 study, International Agency for Research on Cancer—an affiliate of the World Health Organization.

Chapter 2
1. Anand P, Kunnumakkara AB, Kunnumakara AB, et al. (September 2008). "Cancer is a preventable disease that requires major lifestyle changes". Pharm. Res. 25 (9): 2097–116.
2. Pagano JS, Blaser M, Buendia MA, et al. (December 2004). "Infectious agents and cancer: criteria for a causal relation."Semin. Cancer Biol. 14 (6): 453–71.
3. Samaras, Vassilis; Rafailidis, Petros I.; Mourtzoukou, Eleni G.; Peppas, George; Falagas, Matthew E. (May 2010). "Chronic bacterial and parasitic infections and cancer: a review". The Journal of Infection in Developing Countries 4 (5): 267–281.

Chapter 3
1. King WD, Marrett LD. Case-control study of bladder cancer and chlorination by-products in treated water Cancer Causes Control. Department of Community Health and Epidemiology, Queen's University, Kingston, Ontario, Canada.1996 Nov;7(6):596-604.
2. McDonald TA, Komulainen H. Carcinogenicity of the chlorination disinfection by-product MX. J Environ Sci Health C Environ Carcinog Ecotoxicol Rev. 2005;23(2):163-214.
3. http://hosted.ap.org/specials/interactives/pharmawater_site/day1_01.html
4. http://www.who.int/water_sanitation_health/emerging/info_sheet   pharmaceuticals/en/index.html
5. http://www.epa.gov/eerd/research/pharmaceuticals.html
6. Science News, Vol. 130 no. 12, pgs. 177-192.

Chapter 4
1. Taylor A, Taylor NC. Effect of Fluoride on tumor growth. Proc Soc Exper Biol Med 65:252-255, 1965.
2. Yiamouyannis J. Fluoride: The Aging Factor. Delaware, Ohio: Health Action Press, 1993, pp.73-90.
3. Lasne C, et. Al Transforming activities of sodium fluoride in cultured Syrian hamster embryo and BALB/3T3 cells. Cell Biol Toxicol: 311-324, 1988.
4. Izuora 2011; Whyte 2006; USDA 2005.

Chapter 5

1. Fourth National Report on Human Exposure to Environmental Chemicals (Fourth Report), CDC's National Health and Nutrition Examination Survey (NHANES) 2003–2004.

2. Jenny L. Carwile, Xiaoyun Ye, Xiaoliu Zhou, Anotonia M. Calafat, Karin B. Michels "Canned Soup Consumption and Urinary Bishphenol A: A Randomized Crossover Trial,", JAMA, online Nov. 22, 2011; in Nov. 23/30 print issue.

3. Bisphenol-A and human oocyte maturation in vitro. Hum. Reprod. first published online July 30, 2013.

4. D. Li, Z. Zhou, D. Qing, Y. He, T. Wu, M. Miao, J. Wang, X. Weng, J.R. Ferber, L.J. Herrinton, Q. Zhu, E. Gao, H. Checkoway, and W. Yuan."Occupational exposure to bisphenol-A (BPA) and the risk of Self-Reported Male Sexual Dysfunction." Hum. Reprod. Advance Access published on November 10, 2009.

5. De-Kun Li mail, Maohua Miao, ZhiJun Zhou, Chunhua Wu, Huijing Shi, Xiaoqin Liu, Siqi Wang, Wei Yuan. Urine Bisphenol-A Level in Relation to Obesity and Overweight in School-Age Children. June 12, 2013.

6. Kathleen M. Donohue, Rachel L. Miller, Matthew S. Perzanowski, Allan C. Just, LoriA.Hoepner, SrikeshArunajadai, Stephen Canfield, David Resnick, Antonia M. Calafat, Frederica P. Perera, Robin M. Whyatt. Prenatal and postnatal bisphenol A exposure and asthma development among inner-city children. Journal of Allergy and Clinical Immunology, 2013; 131 (3): 736.

7. http://www.medicalnewstoday.com/articles/250454.php

8. http://www.medicalnewstoday.com/articles/247741.php

9. http://www.medicalnewstoday.com/articles/236477.php

10. http://www.medicalnewstoday.com/articles/234786.php

11. http://www.medicalnewstoday.com/articles/220724.php

12. http://www.medicalnewstoday.com/articles/210765.php

13. http://www.medicalnewstoday.com/articles/206102.php

14. http://www.medicalnewstoday.com/articles/200239.php

15. http://www.medicalnewstoday.com/articles/196811.php

16. http://www.medicalnewstoday.com/articles/189576.php

17. http://www.medicalnewstoday.com/articles/173973.php

18. Keri RA, Ho SM, Hunt PA, Knudsen KE, Soto AM, Prins GS. An evaluation of evidence for the carcinogenic activity of bisphenol A. Reprod Toxicol. 2007 Aug-Sep;24(2):240-52.

19. Welshons WV, Nagel SC, vom Saal FS. Endocrine mechanisms mediating effects of bisphenol A at levels of human exposure. Large effects from small exposures. III. Department of Biomedical Sciences, E102 Veterinary Medicine, University of Missouri-Columbia, Columbia, Missouri 65211-5120, USA.

Chapter 6

1. Environmental Working Group's PFCs: A family of chemicals that contaminate the world.

Chapter 7

1. Pathophysiology. 2013 Apr;20(2):123-9.
2. Davis DL, Kesari S, Soskolne CL, Miller AB, Stein Y.
   Environmental Health Trust, P.O. Box 58, Teton Village, WY 83025, USA.
3. Dr. Lita Lee ,Health Effects of Microwave Radiation - Microwave Ovens, and in the March and September 1991 issues of Earthletter.
4. Hardell 2008. Malignant brain tumour (glioma) study - reported at RRT International Conference on EMF and Health - a global issue, September 2008. Found a 5-fold increase in glioma risk for those starting mobile phone use under 20 years of age indicating the age group at first use is highly significant.
5. Alvaro A. de Salles, Giovani Bulla, Claudio E. Fernaacutendez Rodriguez, Electromagnetic Absorption in the Head of Adults and Children Due to Mobile Phone Operation Close to the Head. Electrical Engineering Department, Federal University of Rio Grande do Sul (UFRGS), Porto Alegre, Brasil.
6. Santini R, Seigne M, Bonhomme-Faivre L., Studies on symptoms in vicinity of a mobile phone base station. (2002), Pathol Biol (Paris), 2002 Jul; 50(6):369-73
7. Wolf R M.D., Wolf D M.D. (2004), Increase incidence of cancer near a cell-phone transmitter station, International Journal of Cancer Prevention, vol. 1, nr. 2, April 2004.
8. Eger H, Hagen K U, Lucas B, Vogel P, Voit H (2004), Einfluss der räumlichen Nähe von Mobilfunksendeanlagen auf die Krebsinzidenz, Umwelt-Medizin-Gesellschaft, 17. Jahrgang, Ausgabe 4/2004, S. 273-356.
9. H. Chiang, G.D. Yao, Q.S. Fang, K.Q. Wang, D.Z. Lu, Y.K. Zhou. Health Effects of Environmental Electromagnetic Fields. Journal Electromagnetic Biology and Medicine, Volume 8, Issue 1 1989, pages 127-131.
10. Brenner, David, J. and Eric J. Hall, Risk of cancer from diagnostic X-rays, The Lancet, Volume 363, Issue 9427, Page 2192, 26 June 2004.
11. Qishen P, Guo BJ, Kolman A. Radioprotective effect of extract from Spirulina platensis in mouse bone marrow cells studied by using the micronucleus test. Toxicol Lett. 1989 Aug;48(2):165-9.
12. Yong LC, Petersen MR, Sigurdson AJ, Sampson LA, Ward EM. High dietary antioxidant intakes are associated with decreased chromosome translocation frequency in airline pilots. Am J Clin Nutr. 2009 Nov;90(5):1402-10.
13. Chen B, Zhou XC. Protective effect of natural dietary antioxidants on space radiation-induced damages. Space Med Med Eng (Beijing). 2003;16 Suppl:514-8.
14. Badr FM, El Habit OH, Harraz MM. Radioprotective effect of melatonin assessed by measuring chromosomal damage in mitotic and meiotic cells. Mutat Res. 1999 Aug 18;444(2):367-72.
15. Koc M, Buyukokuroglu ME, Taysi S. The effect of melatonin on peripheral blood cells during total body irradiation in rats. Biol Pharm Bull. 2002 May;25(5):656-7.
16. Shetty TK, Satav JG, Nair CK. Protection of DNA and microsomal membranes in vitro by Glycyrrhiza glabra L. against gamma irradiation. Phytother Res. 2002 Sep;16(6):576-8.

17. Singh I, Sharma A, Nunia V, Goyal PK. Radioprotection of Swiss albino mice by Emblica officinalis. Phytother Res. 2005 May;19(5):444-6.

Chapter 8
1. Erik Dohlman USDA.gov, Trade and Food Safety, Chapter 6, Mycotoxin Hazards and Regulations.
2. Elisa V Bandera, Urmila Chandran, Brian Buckley, Yong Lin, Sastry Isukapalli, Ian Marshall, Melony King, Helmut Zarbl. Urinary mycoestrogens, body size and breast development in New Jersey girls. Full Free Text. Sci Total Environ. 2011 Oct 3.
3. Hans P van Egmond, Ronald C Schothorst, Marco A Jonker. Regulations relating to mycotoxins in food: perspectives in a global and European context. Anal Bioanal Chem. 2007 Sep ;389(1):147-57.

Chapter 9
1. Mercury exposure and risks from dental amalgam in the US population, post-2000. Sci Total Environ. 2011 Sep 15 ;409(20):4257-68.
2. http://www.burtongoldberg.com/page78.html
3. Increased levels of transition metals in breast cancer tissue. Neuro Endocrinol Lett. 2006 Dec. 27 Suppl 1:36-9.
4. Mary Beth Martin, et al. Estrogen-like activity of metals in MCF-7 breast cancer cells. Endocrinology. 2003 Jun ;144(6):2425-36.
5. http://www.burtongoldberg.com/page78.html
6. Järup L, Hazards of heavy metal contamination. Br Med Bull. 2003;68:167-82.
7. Cancer Research March 15, 2012: 72:1457.
8. Los Angeles Times March 15, 2012.
9. Breast Cancer and the Environment: A Life Course Approach, The Institute of Medicine (IOM), December 7, 2011
10. Silva N, Peiris-John R, Wickremasinghe R, Senanayake H, Sathiakumar N. J Appl Toxicol. Cadmium a metalloestrogen: are we convinced? 2012 May;32(5):318-32.

Chapter 10
1. F. Mannello, D. Ligi, M. Canale Aluminium, carbonyls and cytokines in human nipple aspirate fluids: Possible relationship between inflammation, oxidative stress and breast cancer microenvironment Original Research Article. Journal of Inorganic Biochemistry, Volume 128, November 2013, Pages 250-256.
2. Philippa D. Darbre, Ayse Bakir, Elzira Iskakova. Effect of aluminum on migratory and invasive properties of MCF-7 human breast cancer cells in culture. Original Research Article. Journal of Inorganic Biochemistry, Volume 128, November 2013, Pages 245-249.
3. Philippa D. Darbre, Ferdinando Mannello, Christopher Exley, Aluminium and breast cancer: Sources of exposure, tissue measurements and mechanisms of toxicological actions onbreast biology Original Research Article. Journal of Inorganic Biochemistry, Volume 128, November 2013, Pages 257-261.

4. Sappino, A.-P., Buser, R., Lesne, L., Gimelli, S., Béna, F., Belin, D. and Mandriota, S. J. Aluminium chloride promotes anchorage-independent growth in human mammary epithelial cells. Journal of Applied Toxicology. 2012.
5. McGrath KG (December 2003). An earlier age of breast cancer diagnosis related to more frequent use of antiperspirants/deodorants and underarm shaving (PDF). European Journal of Cancer Prevention 12 (6): 479–85.
6. http://www.drpepi.com/aluminum-poisoning.php

Chapter 11
1. Measurement of paraben concentrations in human breast tissue at serial locations across the breast from axilla to sternum. J Appl Toxicol. 2012 Mar; 32(3):219-32.
2. Parabens detection in different zones of the human breast: consideration of source and implications of findings. J Appl Toxicol. 2012 May; 32(5):305-9.

Chapter 12
1. https://www.hugginsappliedhealing.com/mercury-toxicity.php
2. http://oneradionetwork.com/health/hal-huggins-dds-ms-slaying-the-dental-dragons-dentistry-controls-immunity-july-16-2013.

Chapter 13
1. Sood AK, et al Adrenergic modulation of focal adhesion kinase protects human ovarian cancer cells from anoikis. J Clin Invest. 2010 May;120(5):1515-23.
2. Thaker PH et al. Chronic stress promotes tumor growth and angiogenesis in a mouse model of ovarian carcinoma. Nat Med 12:939-44, 8/2006.
3. Archana S. Nagaraja, Guillermo N. Armaiz-Pena, Susan K. Lutgendorf and Anil K. Sood Why stress is bad for cancer patience. The journal of Clinical Investigation Vol. 123, Issue 2 (February 1, 2013) J Clin Invest. 2013;123(2):558–560.
4. J.K. Kiecolt-Glaser and R. Glaser, Psychoneuroimmunology and Cancer: Fact or Fiction? European Journal of Cancer, Vol. 35, No. 11, pp. 1603±1607, 1999
5. Goodkin et. Al. 1986; Darmon 1993.

Chapter 14
1. Dr Ute Nothlings, of the Cancer Research Center at the University of Hawaii, Honolulu, Hawaii, 2005.
2. Herner, A., et. al., In J Cancer 2011; 129: 2349-59.▨
3. Speyer, C.L., et. al., Breast Cancer Res Treat 2012; 132: 565-73.
4. Kobylewski, S. and Jacobson, M.F., In J Occup Environ Health 2012; 18: 220-46.
5. Axon, A., et. al., Toxicology 2012; 298: 40-51.
6. ibid
7. Blaylock, Russell, Dangerous Food Additives That Damage Your Health, The Blaylock Wellness Report July, 2013.
8. Chunyang Liao, Fang Liu, Kurunthachalam Kannan, Occurrence of and dietary exposure to parabens in foodstuffs from the United States. Environ Sci Technol.

2013 Apr 16 ;47(8):3918-25.

Chapter 15
1. Michael C. R. Alavanja et. al Use of Agricultural Pesticides and Prostate Cancer Risk in the Agricultural Health Study Cohort Am. J. Epidemiol. (2003) 157 (9): 800-814.
2. Helen H. McDuffie, et al. Non-Hodgkin's Lymphoma and Specific Pesticide Exposures in Men Cross-Canada Study of Pesticides and Health Cancer Epidemiol Biomarkers Prev November 2001 10; 1155.
3. Lawrence S. Engel, et al. Pesticide Use and Breast Cancer Risk among Farmers' Wives in the Agricultural Health Study Am. J. Epidemiol. (2005) 161 (2):121-135.
4. Koutros S, Beane Freeman LE, Lubin JH, Heltshe SL, Andreotti G, Barry KH, DellaValle CT, Hoppin JA, Sandler DP, Lynch CF, Blair A, Alavanja MC. Risk of total and aggressive prostate cancer and pesticide use in the Agricultural Health Study. Am J Epidemiol. 2013 Jan 1;177(1):59-74.

Chapter 16
1. http://www.ewg.org/foodnews/summary.php
2. http://www.responsibletechnology.org
3. Mark Townsend, Why soya is a hidden destroyer, Daily Express, March 12, 1999.
4. A. Pusztai and S. Bardocz, GMO in animal nutrition: potential benefits and risks, Chapter 17, Biology of Nutrition in Growing Animals, R. Mosenthin, J. Zentek and T. Zebrowska (Eds.) Elsevier, October 2005.
5. Hye-Yung Yum, Soo-Young Lee, Kyung-Eun Lee, Myung-Hyun Sohn, Kyu-Earn Kim, Genetically Modified and Wild Soybeans: An immunologic comparison, Allergy and Asthma Proceedings 26, no. 3 (May–June 2005): 210-216(7).
6. Manuela Malatesta, et al, Ultrastructural Analysis of Pancreatic Acinar Cells from Mice Fed on Genetically modified Soybean, Journal of Anatomy 201, no. 5 (November 2002): 409.
7. M. Malatesta, M. Biggiogera, E. Manuali, M. B. L. Rocchi, B. Baldelli, G. Gazzanelli, Fine Structural Analyses of Pancreatic Acinar Cell Nuclei from Mice Fed on GM Soybean, Eur J Histochem 47 (2003): 385–388.
8. Scott H. Sicherer et al., Prevalence of peanut and tree nut allergy in the United States determined by means of a random digit.
dial telephone survey: A 5-year follow-up study, Journal of Allergy and Clinical Immunology, March 2003, vol. 112, n 6, 1203-1207.
9. J. R. Latham, et al., The Mutational Consequences of Plant Transformation, The Journal of Biomedicine and Biotechnology 2006.
10. Allison Wilson, et. al., Transformation-induced mutations in transgenic plants: Analysis and biosafety implications, Biotechnology and Genetic Engineering Reviews – Vol. 23, December 2006.
11. J. R. Latham, et al., The Mutational Consequences of Plant Transformation, The Journal of Biomedicine and Biotechnology 2006.

12. Allison Wilson, et. al., Transformation-induced mutations in transgenic plants: Analysis and biosafety implications, Biotechnology and Genetic Engineering Reviews – Vol. 23, December 2006.

14. Arpad Pusztai, Can science give us the tools for recognizing possible health risks of GM food, Nutrition and Health, 2002, Vol 16 Pp 73-84.

15. John M. Burns, 13-Week Dietary Subchronic Comparison Study with MON 863 Corn in Rats Preceded by a 1-Week Baseline Food Consumption Determination with PMI Certified Rodent Diet #5002, December 17, 2002.

16. R. Tudisco, P. Lombardi, F. Bovera, D. d'Angelo, M. I. Cutrignelli, V. Mastellone, V. Terzi, L. Avallone, F. Infascelli, Genetically Modified Soya Bean in Rabbit Feeding: Detection of DNA Fragments and Evaluation of Metabolic Effects by Enzymatic Analysis, Animal Science 82 (2006): 193–199.

17 Oliveri et al., Temporary Depression of Transcription in Mouse Pre-implantation Embryos from Mice Fed on Genetically Modified Soybean, 48th Symposium of the Society for Histochemistry, Lake Maggiore (Italy), September 7–10, 2006.

18. Irina Ermakova, Experimental Evidence of GMO Hazards, Presentation at Scientists for a GM Free Europe, EU Parliament, Brussels, June 12, 2007.

Chapter 17

1. David E. Nelson, MD, MPH, Dwayne W. Jarman, DVM, MPH, Jürgen Rehm, PhD, Thomas K. Greenfield, PhD, Grégoire Rey, PhD, William C. Kerr, PhD, Paige Miller, PhD, MPH, Kevin D. Shield, MHSc, Yu Ye, MA, and Timothy S. Naimi, MD, MPH Alcohol-Attributable Cancer Deaths and Years of Potential Life Lost in the United States. American Journal of Public Health | April 2013, Vol 103.

Chapter 18

1. Public Health Nutr. 2011 Apr;14(4):568-74. doi: 10.1017.

2. Norat T, Bingham S, Ferrari P, et al, Meat, fish, and colorectal cancer risk: the European Prospective Investigation into cancer and nutrition.

3. Nöthlings U, Wilkens LR, Murphy SP, Hankin JH, Henderson BE, Kolonel LN. Meat and fat intake as risk factors for pancreatic cancer: the multiethnic cohort study. J Natl Cancer Inst. 2005 Oct 5;97(19):1458-65; 2005 Jun 15;97(12):906-16.

Chapter 19

1. Newmark, Harold L., Heaney, Robert P; Nutrition and cancer Department of Chemical Biology, Rutgers, The State University of New Jersey, 2010.

1. Chan JM, Stampfer MJ, Ma J, Gann PH, Gaziano JM, Giovannucci E. Dairy products, calcium, and prostate cancer risk in the Physicians' Health Study. Am J Clin Nutr. 2001;74:549-554.

2. Ferrer, JF, Kenyon SJ, Gupta P. Milk of dairy cows frequently contains a leukemogenic virus. Science 213: 1014-1016, 1981.

3. Larsson SC, Orsini N, Wolk A. Milk, milk products and lactose intake and ovarian cancer risk: a meta-analysis of epidemiological studies. Int J Cancer.

2006;118(2):431-441.

Chapter 20
1. Nicholas A Graham, Martik Tahmasian, Bitika Kohli, Evangelia Komisopoulou, Maggie Zhu, Igor Vivanco, Michael A Teitell, Hong Wu, Antoni Ribas, Roger S Lo, Ingo K Mellinghoff, Paul S Mischel, Thomas G Graeber. Glucose deprivation activates a metabolic and signaling amplification loop leading to cell death. Molecular Systems Biology, 2012.
2. Rainer J Klement and Ulrike Kämmerer; Is there a role for carbohydrate restriction in the treatment and prevention of cancer? Nutr Metab (Lond). 2011; 8: 75; Published online 2011 October 26.
3. Mantovani A, Allavena P, Sica A, Balkwill F.; Cancer-related inflammation; Nature. 2008 Jul 24;454.
4. http://www.watercure.com/dehydrationandcancerlecturedvd.aspx
5. http://www.cancer.ucla.edu/index.aspx?recordid=385&page=644
6. http://cancerres.aacrjournals.org/content/71/13/4484.full

Chapter 21
1. Dunn et al "JGF 1 Alters Drug Sensitivity of HBL 100 Human Breast Cancer Cells by Inhibition of Apoptosis Induce by Diverse Anticancer drugs" Cancer Research no. 15 (1997): 2687-93.

Chapter 22
1. Vos MB, Kimmons JE, Gillespie C, et al. Dietary fructose consumption among US children and adults: the third national health and nutrition examination survey. J Med. 2008;10(7):160.
2. Montonen J, Jarvinen R, Heliovaara M, et al. Food consumption and the incidence of type II diabetes mellitus. Eur J Clin Nutr. 2005;59:441-448.
3. Stanhope KL, Schwarz JM, Keim NL, et al. Consuming fructose-sweetened, not glucose-sweetened, beverages increases visceral adiposity and lipids and decreases insulin sensitivity in overweight/obese humans. J Clin Invest. 2009;119:1322-1334.
4. Perez-Pozo SE, Schold J, Nakagawa T, et al. Excessive fructose intake induces the features of metabolic syndrome in healthy adult men: role of uric acid in the hypertensive response. Int J Obes (Lond). 2010;34:454-461.
5. Meyer KA, Kushi LH, Jacobs DR, et al. Carbohydrates, dietary fiber, and incident type 2 diabetes in older women. Am J Clin Nutr. 2000;71:921-930.
6. Port AM, Ruth AR, Istfan NW. Fructose consumption and cancer: is there a connection? Curr Opin Endocrinol Diabetes Obes. 2012;19(5):367-374.
7. Mueller NT, Odegaared A, Anderson K, et al. Soft drink and juice consumption and risk of pancreatic cancer: the Singapore Chinese health study. Cancer Epidemiol Biomarkers Prev. 2010;19(2):447-455.
8. Larsson SC, Bergkvist L, Wolk A. Consumption of sugar and sugar sweetened foods and the risk of pancreatic cancer in a prospective study. Am J Clin Nutr.

2006;84(5):1171-1176.14.

9. Jansen RJ, Robinson DP, Stolzenberg-Solomon RZ, et al. Fruit and vegetable consumption is inversely associated with having pancreatic cancer. Cancer Causes Control. 2011;22(12):1613-1625.
10. United States Department of Agriculture. http://www.usda.gov/factbook/chapter2.pdf.
11. Liu H, Huang D, McArthur DL, et al. Fructose induces transketolase flux to promote pancreatic cancer growth. Cancer Res. 2010;70:6368-6376.

Chapter 23

1. Schernhammer ES, Bertrand KA, Birmann BM, Sampson L, Willett WW, Feskanich D. Consumption of artificial sweetener– and sugar-containing soda and risk of lymphoma and leukemia in men and women. Am J Clin Nutr. 2012.

Chapter 24

1. Xiao-Qin Wang, Paul D Terry, and Hong Yan Xiao-Qin Wang, Hong Yan, Department of Epidemiology, School of Medicine, Xi'an Jiaotong University, Xi'an 710061, Shaanxi Province, China.
2. The Benefits of Himalayan Salt; Global Healing Center, Published on May 15, 2009, Last Updated on September 10, 2013.

Chapter 25

1. Tannenbaum and Silverstone, 1953; Tannenbaum, 1959.
2. Carroll, 1975; Carroll and Khor, 1975.
3. U.S. Department of Health and Human Services, 1988; National Research Council, 1982, 1989.
4. National Research Council, 1982, 1989; Welsch, 1992.
5. Carroll 1994; Rose and Connolly, 1991.

Chapter 26

1. Quoted from a letter by Donald Miller, M.D. Professor of Surgery, University of Washington.
2. Paraphrased from the affidavit to congress on August 13, 2002 Dr. Boyd Haley Professor and Chair, Department of Chemistry University of Kentucky.
3. Paraphrased from the NIOSH Mixed Exposures Research Agenda.
4. Effects of Mercury from Mother's Dental Amalgam and other sources on the fetus and infants, B. Windham (Ed), 2007.

Section 2

1. Ames BN, Wakimoto P. Are vitamin and mineral deficiencies a major cancer risk? Nat Rev Cancer. 2002 Sep;2(9):694-704.

Chapter 29

1. http://www.hacres.com/pdf/documents/research-BarleyMax®-Protects-DNA.pdf

2. Collins B, Horska A, Hotten P, Riddoch C, Collins A. Kiwifruit protects against oxidative DNA damage in human cells and in vitro. Nutr Cancer. 2001;39(1):148-53.
3. Gill CIR, Haldar S, Porter S, et al. The effect of cruciferous and leguminous sprouts on genotoxicity, in vitro and in vivo. Cancer Epidemiol Biomarkers Prev. 2004;13(7):1199-205.
4. Porrini M, Riso P, Oriani G. Spinach and tomato consumption increases lymphocyte DNA resistance to oxidative stress but this is not related to cell carotenoid concentrations. Eur J Nutr. 2002;41(3):95-100.
5. Guarnieri S, Riso P, Porrini M. Orange juice vs vitamin C: effect on hydrogen peroxide-induced DNA damage in mononuclear blood cells. Br. J. Nutr. 2007;97(4):639-643.
6. Rieger MA, Parlesak A, Pool-Zobel BL, Rechkemmer G, Bode C. A diet high in fat and meat but low in dietary fibre increases the genotoxic potential of 'faecal water'. Carcinogenesis. 1999;20(12):2311-6.

Chapter 30
1. Environmental Working Group (EWG) http://www.ewg.org/foodnews/list. php

Chapter 34
1. http://abcnews.go.com/sections/2020/2020/2020_010330_sleep.html

Chapter 35
1. M. Nathaniel Mead, Benefits of Sunlight: A Bright Spot for Human Health, Environ Health Perspect. 2008 April; 116(4): A160–A167.

Chapter 38
1. Collins B, Horska A, Hotten P, Riddoch C, Collins A. Kiwifruit protects against oxidative DNA damage in human cells and in vitro. Nutr Cancer. 2001;39(1):148-53.
2. Gill CIR, Haldar S, Porter S, et al. The effect of cruciferous and leguminous sprouts on genotoxicity, in vitro and in vivo. Cancer Epidemiol Biomarkers Prev. 2004;13(7):1199-205.
3. Porrini M, Riso P, Oriani G. Spinach and tomato consumption increases lymphocyte DNA resistance to oxidative stress but this is not related to cell carotenoid concentrations. Eur J Nutr. 2002;41(3):95-100.
4. Guarnieri S, Riso P, Porrini M. Orange juice vs vitamin C: effect on hydrogen peroxide-induced DNA damage in mononuclear blood cells. Br. J. Nutr. 2007;97(4):639-643.
5. Rieger MA, Parlesak A, Pool-Zobel BL, Rechkemmer G, Bode C. A diet high in fat and meat but low in dietary fibre increases the genotoxic potential of 'faecal water'. Carcinogenesis. 1999;20(12):2311-6.
6. Donaldson, MS. Nutrition and cancer: A review of the evidence for an anti-cancer diet. Nutrition Journal 2004 3:19 Review.
7. Krajmalnik-Brown R, Ilhan ZE, Kang DW, DiBaise JK. Nutr Clin Pract. 2012

Apr;27(2):201-14. Effects of gut microbes on nutrient absorption and energy regulation. Epub 2012 Feb 24.

8. Donaldson, MS. A Carotenoid Health Index Based on Plasma Carotenoids and Health Outcomes. Nutrients. 2011;3(12):1003–1022.
9. Asparagus For Cancer published in Cancer News Journal, Dec 1979, United Kingdom.
10. Peter Rose, Kathy Faulkner, Gary Williamson, and Richard Mithen, 7-Methylsulfinylheptyl and 8-methylsulfinyloctyl isothiocyanates from watercress are potent inducers of phase II enzymes, Carcinogenesis, August 15, 2000.

Chapter 43
1. Blaylock RL. A review of conventional cancer prevention and treatment and the adjunctive use of nutraceutical supplements and antioxidant: is there a danger or a significant benefit? J Am Nutri Assoc 3:17-35, 2000.
2. Block, JB, Evans MS. A review of recent results addressing the potential interactions of antioxidants with cancer drug therapy. J Amer Nutr Assoc 4:11-20, 2001.
3. Hickey S, Saul, AW (2008) Vitamin C: The Real Story. Basic Health Publications.
4. Gonzalez MJ, Miranda-Massari JR, Saul AW (2009) I Have Cancer: What Should I Do? Your Orthomolecular Guide for Cancer Management. Basic Health Publications.

Chapter 45
1. National Cancer Institute at the National institutes of Health. Prostate Cancer, Nutrition and Dietary Supplements (PDQ)/Selenium.
2. Grattan Bruce J., Freake Hedley C. Zinc and Cancer: Implications for LIV-1 in Breast Cancer. Nutrients. 2012 July; 4(7): 648–675.
3. Melanoma Res. 2007 Jun 17(3):177-83.
4. National Cancer Institute at the National institutes of Health. Prostate Cancer, Nutrition and Dietary Supplements (PDQ)/Lycopene.
5   Moen I, Stuhr LE., Hyperbaric oxygen therapy and cancer – a review. Target Oncol 2012 Dec;7(4):233-42.

Section 6
1. Van der Zee J. Heating the patient: A promising approach? Annals of Oncology 2002; 13:1173-1184.
2. Gerson, Charlotte. Healing The Gerson Way, 2013
4. Bharali R, J Tabassum, MRH Azad (2003) Chemomodulatory effect of Moringa oleifera, Lam, on hepatic carcinogen metabolizing enzymes, antioxidant parameters and skin papillomagenesis in mice. Asian Pacific Journal of Cancer Prevention 4: 131-139.
5. Murakami A, Y Kitazono, S Jiwajinda, K Koshimizu, and H Ohigashi (1998) Niaziminin, a thiocarbamate from the leaves of Moringa oleifera, holds a strict structural requirement for inhibition of tumor-promoter- induced Epstein-Barr virus activation. Planta Medica 64: 319-323.

Chapter 47
1. This quote is from Andrew C. von Eschenbach, MD, director of the National Cancer Institute National Cancer Institute, "Herceptin Combined with Chemotherapy Improves Disease-Free Survival for Patients with Early-Stage Breast Cancer," 2005.

Index

Index

I

J

K

O

P

Pancreas, 15, 20, 105, 116, 124, 141, 260, 286
Pancreatic, 93, 111, 121, 127-128, 220, 238, 349-352
Panoramic, 85
Papaya, 101, 106, 191
Paraben, 79-80, 97-98, 348
Parabens, 3, 79-82, 91, 97-98, 348
Parasites, 29-30
Parasitic infections, 30, 344
Parsley, 72, 174, 249
Parsnips, 240
Pasta, 97, 158
Pastas, 125, 157
Pasteurized, 116, 176, 342
Pathogenic, 84-85, 213
Pathogens, 33
Pathology, 70, 83, 85-86, 285
Peanut, 104, 140, 349
Peanuts, 67-68, 104
Peas, 190, 343
Pectin, 342
Peeled, 173, 249
Peeling, 173
Peppers, 97, 190, 201
Pepsin, 261, 338
Perchlorate, 63, 72-73
Perfluorinated, 49
Perfluoro, 51
Perfluorocarbons, 22
Periodontal, 39, 84
Periods, 193
Peroxidation, 65, 274
Peroxide, 184, 186, 353
Pesticide, 100, 106, 173, 190-191, 349
Pesticides, 3, 20, 22, 24, 77, 99-101, 109, 143, 146, 152, 187, 189-190, 258, 330, 349
Pharmax, 157, 262, 338
Pharynx, 238
Phenols, 244
Phlegm, 198
Phosphatase, 116, 180
Phosphate, 116, 137
Phosphorus, 76
Photolytic, 50

Photosynthesis, 218
Phthalides, 203
Physiological, 72, 87, 98, 144, 208, 274
Physiology, 187
Phytochemicals, 163, 178, 225, 237, 241, 244-246
Phytoestrogens, 239
Phytonutrients, 187, 193-194, 241, 246, 267
Phytosterols, 241
Pigment, 245, 275
Pilates, 299, 303
Pineal, 223
Pineapples, 190
Plastic bottles, 44, 229
Plastics, 20, 22, 43, 229
Platelet, 246, 273
Pneumonia, 20
Pneumonitis, 68
Pollutants, 24, 26, 36, 49, 69, 228
Polluted, 32, 212, 228
Pollution, 25, 50, 144, 212
Polycarbonate, 43-44
Polychlorinated, 22
Polyphenols, 222, 245
Polysaccharides, 242
Polyunsaturated, 140
Pork, 109, 111, 158
Positive stress, 199
Postmenopausal, 221
Postnatal, 345
Potassium, 63, 96, 178, 202, 263, 283
Potatoes, 71, 97, 105, 157, 190-191
Potentiation, 286-287
Pots, 76
Poultry, 110-112, 177
Prayer, 232-233, 269, 271, 305, 313, 339, 341
Pregnancy, 25
Premalignant, 241
Premature, 67-68, 217
Premenstrual, 223
Prenatal, 45, 345
Preservative, 92-93, 97, 124, 135, 237
Preservatives, 3, 80-82, 91, 124
Preventing cancer, 4, 238, 311-313
Prevention, 26, 44, 64, 76, 80, 88, 150, 238, 278, 346, 348, 351, 354
Primary routes, 195, 198
Probiotics, 240, 260-261, 329

X

Y

Z